THE COVID SPECTRUM

THEORETICAL AND EXPERIENTIAL REFLECTIONS FROM INDIA AND BEYOND

Edited by

Kanchana Mahadevan
Satishchandra Kumar
Meher Bhoot
Rajesh Kharat

Foreword by Slavoj Žižek

SPEAKING TIGER

in association with

University of Mumbai

SPEAKING TIGER BOOKS LLP
125A, Ground Floor, Shahpur Jat, near Asiad Village,
New Delhi 110049

First published by Speaking Tiger Books 2021

ISBN: 978-93-5447-145-2
eISBN: 978-93-5447-150-6

10 9 8 7 6 5 4 3 2 1

Typeset in Sabon Roman by SÜRYA, New Delhi
Printed at Chaman Enterprises, New Delhi

Meher Bhoot is Associate Professor and Head at the Department of German, University of Mumbai since 2013. Her areas of specialization are German Literature with a focus on Literature of the German Minorities, Postcolonial Studies, and Culture Studies, and her areas of interest are European Cultural History and European History of Art. She is an active member of the German Institute's partnership with the Universities of Göttingen and Freiburg in Germany. Under the aegis of this partnership, she was a Guest Professor at the Department of Intercultural German Studies, University of Göttingen, Germany in 2017. She is a DAAD Fellow since 2004 and has also been a recipient of the Rotary Cultural and Ambassadorial Scholarship (1997–98). Apart from her published articles, some of the co-edited volumes include *Revisiting Günter Grass: Voices from India and Germany*, *Interkulturelle Momente*, and *Einfach menschlich*. She has also coedited textbooks for short courses on teaching Marathi to non-native speakers, including *Communicative Marathi for Nurses* and *Communicative Marathi for Rickshaw and Taxi Drivers*, *Communicative Marathi for Government Officials* and *Communicative Marathi for Bank Employees*. She is the co-editor of *Sambhāṣaṇ*, an interdisciplinary humanities online journal of the University of Mumbai.

Rajesh Kharat is Dean, Humanities, University of Mumbai (on Deputation), Professor and former Chairperson, Centre for South Asian Studies, Jawarharlal Nehru University, New Delhi. He has an MA in Political Science from University of Pune and has completed his MPhil and PhD from CSAS, JNU, New Delhi. He has been actively teaching since 1991. He has published several books and over 30 research papers. He has authored three books, namely, *Bhutan in SAARC: Role of a Small State in Regional Alliance* (1999/2000), *Foreign Policy of Bhutan* (2005), and *Tibetan Refugees in India* (2003). He has edited two books, *Bhutan: Political Transition and Democratisation* (2016) and *Bhutan: Contemporary Issues and Perspectives* (2015). He has completed five major research projects in India and abroad on themes related to contemporary South Asia. He recently established the School of International Relations and Strategic Studies at the University of Mumbai. He is also the honorary editor of *Sambhāṣaṇ* an interdisciplinary humanities online journal of the University of Mumbai. He is also Visitor's Representative at the Executive Council of Mahatma Gandhi Central University, Bihar.

Satishchandra Kumar is Professor and Head at the Department of Applied Psychology & Counselling Centre, University of Mumbai. He is also the former Co-ordinator of the Mahatma Gandhi Peace Centre. He is the recipient of the Summer Fellowship from Albert Ellis Institute New York. He also had a scholarship for supervised training under the Enneagram Professional Training Programme created by Helen Palmer, San Francisco, USA. He was awarded the Research Fellowship by the Indian Council of Social Science Research (ICSSR), New Delhi. He has published in international peer-reviewed journals like *Journal of Personality and Social Psychology*, *Psychological Science*, *British Journal of Guidance and Counselling*, and has contributed to a Sage volume of *Eminent Indian Psychologists: 100 Years of Psychology in India*. He has published more than 40 research papers in national and internationally renowned journals. Apart from research publications, some of the edited books include *Beyond the Ordinary: Stories that Inspire and Challenge* and *Some Outstanding Women of India*. His area of research interest is Industrial/Organizational Psychology, which includes positive psychology, engagement at the workplace, and stress and coping at the workplace. He is a reviewer on various international journals and book boards. He is also the co-editor of *Sambhāṣaṇ*, an interdisciplinary humanities online journal of the University of Mumbai.

Kanchana Mahadevan is Professor and Head at the Department of Philosophy, University of Mumbai. She was a visiting professor (2016) and a visiting research scholar (2019) at LUISS University, Rome. She has been a senior fellow at the Justitia Amplificata, Goethe University Frankfurt and Bad Homburg (2018) and at the Moore Institute, National University of Ireland, Galway (2019). She teaches and researches in feminist philosophy, continental thought, critical theory, and political philosophy. She also works in the interdisciplinary areas of aesthetics and film. Her book *Between Femininity and Feminism: Colonial and Postcolonial Perspectives on Care* (2014) examines the relevance of Western feminist philosophy in the Indian context, while bringing Western feminism into dialogue with its Indian counterpart. Her publications on Ambedkar explore his rearticulation of democracy from the Indian perspective. In her recently published research papers on care ethics, she has explored its critical potential in relation to health work and the cosmopolitan character of care. She is the editor of *Sambhāṣaṇ*, an interdisciplinary humanities online journal of the University of Mumbai.

To caregivers...

CONTENTS

PART II: EXPERIENTIAL REFLECTIONS, NARRATIVES AND STRATEGIES

Reflections on Health and Wellness

Learning Narratives

FOREWORD

LIGHT AT THE END OF THE TUNNEL? YES, BUT...

Slavoj Žižek

Our media has been telling us over and over again that we are at the 'beginning of the end' of the pandemic. This, in spite of the consistently rising numbers of infections and deaths. However, millions are already vaccinated so there is now at least the proverbial light at the end of the tunnel. Despite worries about how we will survive the next few months, or even longer, there are sighs of relief. This relief is much deserved as what was so depressing about the pandemic was precisely that there was no clear exit in sight—the feeling of the end of the world dragged on without end. Now, as it begins to look like the nightmare will be over soon, we will try to obliterate it from our memory and return to normalcy as soon as possible. Some intellectuals who are keen on finding a deeper meaning in every catastrophe, even evoke the famous verses from Friedrich Hölderlin's hymn to Patmos—'Wo aber Gefahr ist, wächst das Rettende auch' (But where the danger is, that which saves is also growing)—as relevant to our predicament (Volk 2020). In what does this relevance reside precisely? Is it simply the science that saved us by inventing vaccines in record time? Is it that the pandemic reminded us of our mortality and vulnerability and thus cured us of our arrogance: we are part of nature, not its masters?

It would be much more appropriate to turn Hölderlin's verses around: 'But where that which saves us is growing, there are dangers also.' These dangers are multiple; let's begin with World Health Organization (WHO) experts' warning that 'even though the coronavirus pandemic has been very severe, it is "not necessarily the big one"', and that 'the world will have to learn to live with COVID-19' (Davey 2020). Not only is the

COVID pandemic far from over, but new pandemics are also on the horizon as global warming, fires, and droughts continue to ruin our environment; the economic effects of the pandemic will strike later, giving a new boost to social protests; our lives will continue to be under digital control; mental health problems will explode. We will have to learn to live not just with COVID-19 but with all this medley of interconnected phenomena. This is why we are now going through the most dangerous moment of the entire pandemic. To relax now would be like falling asleep behind the wheel of a car speeding down a winding road. We have to make numerous decisions that cannot all be grounded in science. It is now the time to make radical political choices.

True, science may save us. Greta Thunberg was right about trusting science, but in true scientific spirit, we should also admit two things noted by Jürgen Habermas (Schwering 2020): 1) We didn't just learn new things, we also got to know how many things we don't know; and 2) we were forced to act in such an impenetrable situation not knowing what effects our acts would have. This not-knowing does not concern only the pandemic—we at least have experts there—but even more its economic, social, and psychic consequences. It is not simply that we don't know what's going on, we *know* that we *don't know*, and this not-knowing is itself a social fact; it is inscribed into how our institutions act.

Taking another step further—it is not just that we know more and more what and how much we don't know, it sometimes appears as if reality itself acts as if it has forgotten its own laws. We know the joke about 'knowledge in the real'—a stone knows the law it must obey when it is falling down, etc. But the basic lesson of quantum physics is that nature itself doesn't know all its laws, and this is why Albert Einstein reacted with such anxiety to quantum physics and its basic premise of the indeterminacy of nature. For Einstein, this simply meant that quantum physics is an incomplete theory that ignores certain unknown variables. There is a supreme irony in the fact that, although both Einstein and Niels Bohr were atheists, their most famous exchange is about God: Einstein remarked, 'God does not play dice,' and Bohr snapped back, 'Stop telling God what to do.' Their disagreement was not about God but about the nature of our universe. Einstein couldn't accept that nature itself is in some sense 'incomplete'. The pandemic seems to have proven Bohr right.

This indeterminacy that reaches all the way down to the subatomic level opens up the space for our intervention, but only if we fully assume it. That is, only if we reject determinism in both its main versions—naturalism and divine providence. A Slovene theologian who advocated keeping churches open in spite of the quarantine regulations answered the reproach that many lives will be lost by simply stating, 'The mission of the church is not health but salvation.' The death and suffering of thousands doesn't matter when it comes to salvation in eternity through God.

This is what Mother Teresa was doing in Kolkata: her mission was to take care of 'the hungry, the naked, the homeless, the crippled, the blind, the lepers, all those people who feel unwanted, unloved, uncared for throughout society, people that have become a burden to the society and are shunned by everyone' ('Missionaries', 2021). But, as critics have demonstrated, more than their health, she took care of their salvation and deathbed conversion to Catholicism. So we can easily imagine what she would have been doing now when the pandemic is ravaging the world: no vaccination, not even respirators, just the spiritual solace in a grey environment for the last hours of their lives. And we can also imagine what will happen in the near future if the pandemic explodes even more (through new mutations of the virus) and render vaccines inefficient—people will be dying at rates even more alarming than from the Spanish flu and, lacking any vision of how to contain the pandemic, our authorities will resign themselves to just providing care for the dying, including pills for painless death, while the Church will offer mass conversions to diminish the depression with the promise of salvation for the faithful.

Our ultimate choice is between carrying on with the present

despair or annihilation. The correct choice is the decision to assume despair and utter hopelessness of our predicament—only if we pass through this zero-point will we be able to construct a new society. The wrong step may lead us to a new divided society with the privileged living in isolated bubbles and the majority vegetating in barbaric conditions. Today more than ever, egalitarianism is not just a vague ideal but an urgent necessity—vaccines for all, universal healthcare, global struggle against the global warming. Here is a small unexpected sign in this direction: Uğur Şahin, BioNTech's CEO, a Turk living in Germany who played a key role in inventing the best vaccine, said in an interview at the end of 2020, 'At the moment, it doesn't look good—a hole is appearing because there's a lack of other approved vaccines and we have to fill the gap with our own vaccine' ('Coronavirus live', 2021). This was a wonderful moment when the CEO of a company wanted his competitors to get stronger because he knows that only together can we win the struggle against the pandemic.

So maybe the proper way to conclude is to repeat the well-known warning that is sometimes added to the idea of the light at the end of the tunnel: let's make sure that this light is not the light of another train rushing towards us from the other side of the tunnel.

INTRODUCTION

UNCERTAIN CONSOCIATES, UNSETTLING CONDITIONS: THE PREDICAMENT OF COVID-19

Kanchana Mahadevan, Satishchandra Kumar, Meher Bhoot, Rajesh Kharat

This book brings together a gamut of responses from research papers and commentaries to poetry, from across continents, to the unabating pandemic that discern COVID-19 as driving accepted ways of life into an 'unprecedented' (Lal 2020, 1) tailspin. They explore some of the neo-normals that have come to stay (at least for over fifteen months), such as lockdown, quarantine, virtual worlds, surveillance, inequalities, and fragile public health systems. These phenomena have overturned set distinctions between life and non-life, the individual and the collective, or, for that matter, the public and the private. They have, thereby, transfigured the process of living in primordial ways. The essays in the anthology examine the possibilities of reconfiguring boundaries imposed by symptoms such as the 'infodemic' and forced separation. Some of them explore the expanding role of digital technology in engaging with the emancipatory consequences of the present extraordinary conditions to open up possibilities for generating dialogues by imagining, critiquing, and coping. However, such potential is also limited because of the persistence of digital divides that make the very act of dialogue impossible. This volume also focuses on the extent to which the COVID-19 pandemic is exceptional, given that current responses have often referred to the history of pandemics. Questions of inequality, authoritarianism, welfare, trauma, and sustainability have arisen as we combat a pandemic a century after the Spanish flu. The theoretical and experiential reflections in this volume are situated within and across diverse disciplines of the humanities and social sciences; indeed, they also reveal an interdisciplinary spirit in engaging with the pandemic in ways that transcend medicalization and scientism. In this context, the anthology engages with the difficulties of arriving at any easy conclusions from theoretical and experiential perspectives—beginning with Slavoj Žižek's foreword: 'Light at the End of the Tunnel? Yes, But…'.

The theoretical writings in the first part of this book describe the ontology of vulnerability aggravated by the pandemic while turning to possibilities of living together in egalitarian, enabling, and empowering ways. Vulnerability or 'precariousness' (Butler 2009, 2) reveals that life itself is not evenly available but is experienced and aspired through loss, such as death or disease. The latter do not merely indicate the limits of finitude (ibid., 14), but rather reveal the interrelatedness of diverse forms of life and non-life as an existential situation of vulnerability, into which all living beings are thrown, underscoring the absence of stable meanings or a common universal purpose. However, the situation is not simply one where human beings affirm their hubris through projects, whether singular or collective, outside the determinisms of the situation. The distinctiveness of the human being has been called into question in the course of struggling and sharing existence with non-human others, such as viruses. Thus, the contingent processes of life together with heterogeneous beings make it impossible to affirm any hierarchy of living beings culminating in the human being, in the league of philosophers such as Aristotle, Descartes, Kant, or the existentialists. Intermingled but fading lines between plants, animals, human beings, and untold other forces reveal the extent to which lives and non-lives in their diverse forms are exposed to each other. To inhabit the world with others who are different is to reside with the inimical as well.

The term virus comes from the Latin *vīrus* or 'venom, poisonous fluid, acrid element in a substance, a secretion with medical or magical properties'.[1] Such dwelling also blurs the

1. *Merriam-Webster.com Dictionary*, s.v. 'virus'.

divide between self and other, often through their ingestion. The mandatory self-isolation during the present pandemic fractures the idea of a seamless human collectivity combating the virus on a war path. Self-isolation underscores the need for human beings to cope with what is most unlike them, viruses, and to reside with them (for which there are no guarantees). It makes us envisage contact in ways that go beyond the human touch, as Brunella Antomarini argues in her paper for 'contact in absentia'. Since human beings learn to live with the pandemic by physically distancing themselves, the virtual space has become a relevant representation of communication. As the very idea of vaccination shows, to become immune, one has to take a minor dose of the very virus that one is struggling against so that it can be reproduced in the human body to create an immune-response.[2] Being catapulted into a common predicament of disease is hardly a consolation, since one has to get beyond the human mode of life to live with entities that inhabit domains between life and non-life in ways that are ecological.

Being fragile exposes the human being to other living beings and conversely beings who differ from human beings are also exposed to human thought and praxis (Butler 2009, 2). Such interdependence of self and other(s) assumes different modes of relationships. Of being handed over to the foreign, which can host human beings (as ecologies do), or making room for foreign entities that inflict themselves on human hosts (as viruses do). The vulnerability in a world ridden with corona, thus, does not merely pose a challenge of living with human diversity of race, nation, or gender following Judith Butler, but it has also explicitly posed the challenge of occupying the world with entities hostile to human life. Further, living together in heterogeneous contexts of biology and geography (as well as those of society, politics, and so forth, which Butler has narrated)

2. It is the lack of such determinate boundaries that propels Habermas, a critic of Nietzchean thought, to profess his resistance to social Darwinist interpretations of Nietzsche, on account of his exposure to Nietzsche during his adolescent period (Schwering 2020).

has moments of conciliation, consonance, and conflict. One can neither disavow nor overcome conflicts by affirming human projects, nor can one seek refuge in the tenuous conciliatory and consonant moments that are impermanent. Both kinds of moments, those of harmony and struggle, are inexplicable from the scientific or metaphysical points of view. The search for firm explanations has only bred conspiracy theories, as the essay by Andrew Edgar maintains. The unpredictability of living with strangers, including viruses, counters all forms of determinism. One cannot fully cognize or recognize situations of vulnerability, and hence, one has to suspend the desire to cognize and replace it with the ability to apprehend (ibid., 2–5). As Žižek notes, reflecting in his paper on 'The Great Reset', one cannot read a deeper meaning into the pandemic as retribution nor profess to fathom it thoroughly. In experiencing the pandemic, one has to contend with 'existential uncertainties' (Schwering 2020), given the failure of systems such as health and welfare. Thus, for better or for worse, there are no experts to give the human race a thorough knowledge, or delineate the consequences or prospects of the virus (ibid.).

In spite of its all-pervasiveness, vulnerability itself is not equally experienced by all, as Joan Tronto has deliberated in her essay 'The Limits of Responsible Caring in the COVID-19 Pandemic'. Social hierarchies of race, caste, class, disability, and gender frame the extent to which hierarchies are experienced. Tronto observes how disparities in conjunction with the pandemic have led to the breakdown of relationships of care in public contexts. Thus, institutions have to step in to alleviate the immediate human misery in the larger ontology. Hence, philosophically responding to the pandemic, Sebastiano Maffettone advocates thinking with sensitivity for inclusive public policies in his 'Pandemic: Philosophy and Public Policy'. Such visions of kinder institutions and policies are critical, given the problematic responses that we have witnessed at the institutional level.

The pandemic continues to rage on in waves, underlining the inevitability and anguish of being alone and away from family, friends, and communities. Isolation introduces order within the disorder of an ever-expanding contagion. The latter demands the act of sequestering oneself as a commitment to being a responsible individual who values human life. Since every single human being can potentially spread the disease, being alone appears to be the only way to contain it. Coping strategies abound with Foucauldian self-disciplinary practices of self-isolation. Additionally, institutional measures are also introduced to effectively circumscribe the ongoing disease by separating human beings from each other. Camus in *The Plague* narrates the predicament of locking the gates to the town, when unprepared parents, children, and spouses are 'without the least warning, hopelessly cut off, prevented from seeing one another again…' (1948, 133). Thus, lockdowns, quarantines, and contactless ration supplies become normalization techniques of seclusion (Foucault 1979, 195–200). Such manoeuvres that collapse the divide between volition and coercion have often undertaken the latter form for the sick. They are coerced into seclusion in quarantine centres and isolation wards of hospitals as well as their homes. They are kept on watch during their seclusion to record and contain the disease. Foucault defines surveillance as a crucial aspect of epidemic management, premised upon segregating the sick (ibid.). But disease outbreaks do not necessarily isolate only through orderly physical seclusion; the Indian context, for instance, reveals that disorder also performs a disciplining role for the State and institutions, as the qualitatively different modes of isolation, despite their 'strict spatial partitioning' (ibid., 195) disclose. Thus, overcrowded hospitals segregate masses of people who are in physical contact with each other, reinforcing their vulnerability to disease, but also isolating them psychologically. Pandita Ramabai's 1897 observations on the dangerous exploitative consequences of epidemics, especially for women, kept in detention in overflowing plague hospitals in India (Kosambi 2016, 231–33), have assumed renewed significance in light of what we know about how hospitals treat COVID-19 patients. The long walks home by migrants to their villages from cities during the national lockdown of the summer of 2020 exposed them not only to hunger and life-threatening dehydration but also to disease, as they trekked for several days on highways crowded with thousands of others like them (Lal 2020, 68–78; Misra 2021; Sharma 2021). In the cities, the lockdown forced millions to stay confined in poorly ventilated single-room dwellings they shared with four, six, even a dozen others. Reports on the current pandemic reveal that the terrain of 'spatial partitioning' is not static as Foucault implied (1979, 195). Rather, there are diverse movements and privileges within them. Being alone is a protective shield only for those with privileges of voluntary self-isolation. Such privileges are signs of social capital in which class, caste, and gender intersect. For those without access to such capital, being alone further reinforces the vulnerability to disease. Pandemics have shown that modes of being alone are mediated by the social.

The competitive struggles for sustenance or the inherent conflict of being with others are not the only possibilities unfastened by a pandemic. Alternate notions of relationships hinge on claims made by others, given the inevitability of interdependence. Sanjay Reddy's piece on the 'Return of the Normative' during COVID-19 critiques the current crisis as rooted in the persistent lack of economic policy during 'normal' times where 'market' economics is assumed to be absolute. He argues for commitment to normative inclusiveness as well as case specificity in addressing the problems of the pandemic from the economic point of view (which is also rooted in the social, political, philosophical, and ecological dimensions). Reddy's essay reveals that 'the obligations "we" have are precisely those that disrupt any established notion of the "we"' (Butler 2009, 14). The stratified societies we inhabit do not allow for invoking ready-made solidarities and imposing top-down rules for resolving crises. Solidarities would rather have to be created by engaging with conflicts of interests at the grassroots level, taking the public social domain into consideration. Such responsibility cannot merely be rooted in rules of following protocols of hygiene or medicine. It requires nourishment and sustenance of life against all the odds and losses that drive it (ibid.). Sustaining life requires the ability to empathize with the suffering of others in an attempt to mitigate it. The ethical obligations raised in the context of the pandemic are foregrounded by Ernest Hess-Lüttich in his essay 'Discourse, Crisis and Corona'.

The ecological and institutional contexts of the present pandemic have revealed the obligation of being compassionate as a normative necessity. Despite human beings being physically cut off from each other, compassion forges bonds in the public domain that help mitigate mounting losses and suffering. Compassion's Latin roots in *pati*, or to suffer, and *com*, or being with the sufferer, suggest the notion of *compati*, implying suffering *with* the other. It connotes a common existential condition of lives that simultaneously undergo suffering and empathize with one another. The pandemic demands that we should be, even nudges us towards being, responsible to and for others in the interdependent circle of vulnerability in compassionate ways. It has most explicitly highlighted the impossibility of thinking about the self without at the same time thinking about others. In this context, Maurice Hamington's essay flags the problem of privilege and social unrest in times of the 'great pause' of the pandemic. He argues for a caring world not simply limited to social institutions but as an existential fabric. Given the tenuous and overlapping relation between self and other, compassion for others is also related to the self. As Kristen Neff notes, self-compassion involves the same empathy to one's own self as one would have towards the suffering of others (2012).

Rather than the cognitive 'know thyself', the affective 'care for thyself' is, as Foucault notes, an 'art of existence' going back to ancient Greek thinkers (Foucault 1988, 43–44). Foucault enlists the many forms it takes, such as adopting the attitude of making the self an object of care (*cura sui*), giving attention to civic and domestic tasks and removing pathos or purification (on a medicalized note) through exercises, meditative practices, and activities. All of this leads to a 'conversion to self' (ibid.,

64–65). However, one has to think about self-care by going beyond Foucault, in ways that are linked to larger ecologies in light of Tronto's and Hamington's caution against those with privilege retreating into their oases. Like compassion, self-compassion requires one to engage with and feel for one's suffering along with the suffering of others. Moreover, one has to adopt a non-judgemental, existentialist perspective to the failures and limitations of one's own self. The interdependence of compassion and self-compassion can be addressed through acts of consolation, kindness, and storytelling.

Compassion is not pity, nor is self-compassion narcissism; they are rather integral to healing therapeutic practices. Gordon Flett (2018) observed that self-compassion and the capacity to soothe oneself results in the constructive process of dialogue with oneself. Instead of indulging in self-blame, one begins to matter to oneself, which expands to others mattering as well. Thus, self-compassion teaches us to be less harsh on others and on ourselves. Harshness towards oneself may extend to others as acts of violence. Yet, non-violent and peaceful relations with both self and others do not simply happen spontaneously. Their compassionate and self-compassionate foundations have to be built through intervention, often therapeutic, as Neff has argued. In this process, the therapist or counsellor has to accept the complex relationship with the patient without being invasive or autocratic. This requires the therapist to adopt a perspective of self-acceptance so that it is transmitted to support and care for patients (Henry et al. 1990).

~

The experiential second part of the book reveals that 'precarious' lives are not simply human but encompass a whole ecology of lived experiences. In the spirit of Mary Shelley's 1826 dystopian work *The Last Man* (1998), they narrate the labyrinthine containments of disease, strife, anxieties, and miseries through the sweeping waves of a pandemic. However, rather than induce hopelessness, the experiential essays become acts of hope, desires to connect, and strategies for coping, and aspirations for the community. All of these are signs of being alive and wanting to live.

Reading Shelley in non-European contexts, such as India, raises an uncomfortable question: Does she construe the plague as a disease originating in the East and transmitting to the West? In her novel, the plague begins in Constantinople before it starts spreading globally. Her protagonist, Lionel Verney, both visits Constantinople and has a chance contact with an African suffering from the plague in his own home in London. Such a reading has parallels with contemporary racist and discriminatory interpretations of COVID-19. Indeed, the very idea of a 'last man' who is immune to the onslaught of engulfing illness is problematic, as noted by Peter Melville (2007). But is the 'last man' Verney an observer who is outside the spread of epidemics around him? Verney's susceptibility to disease is ample evidence of his frangibility. His encounter with the dying African man's 'convulsive grasp' (Shelley 1998, 265), from which Verney severed himself 'with mixed horror and impatience' (ibid.), has been interpreted in diverse ways, as a phenomenon of inoculation fortifying 'the last man', or as Verney's racist abhorrence and even as a ray of hope towards human bonds across race.[3] The encounter has to be read in the context of Shelley's critique of the contagion view of plague as transmitting through bodily contact; as Anne McWhir (1998, 2002) noted, Shelley was apprehensive about the contagion view of the plague. Shelley discerned disease to be in the air, a boundless mysterious force without origins, beyond human control, that can randomly affect anyone. Hence, it's the air that brings the dying African together with the 'last man', hinting at a possible camaraderie between total strangers who are powerless. The inevitability of illness spreading forecloses all borders closing, since it afflicts everyone regardless of continents and race. Verney's brush with an unnamed African in the grip of a plague could be read, following Melville, as indicating the priority of his family ties and perhaps nationalism. Verney

3. See Melville (2007) for an account of these diverse readings.

refused to get distracted by a stranger 'with mixed horror and impatience' (Shelley 1998, 265). His horror could have been directed to the plague and his impatience to his ardent desire to be with his own son Alfred who was ill with plague and who eventually died (Melville 2007, 834–37). His compassion was confined to his own family, race, and nation. But then, this is precisely why it becomes so difficult to endure the plague.

Other passages in Shelley's text depict Verney's tirade against xenophobia against Asians as based on falsely regarding the plague as contagious (ibid., 832); for 'she had trod every nook of our spacious globe' (Shelley 1998, 332). This is particularly relevant in recent times when the virus has been a pretext for inflicting violence, stigma, and trauma (Ruiz et al. 2020; Bhattacharya et al. 2020). The encounter scene continues to remain significant in the contemporary context of failing to acknowledge the interdependence of the self and others, as well as failing to be compassionate. Following Melville, Shelley's narration can hardly be understood in an absolute manner as its incompleteness does not foreclose determinate meaning (1998, 842). The encounter scene indicates Verney's short-sightedness in really understanding the need to forge bonds even with those who are foreign, as this alone would open up the possibility of countering air-borne incursions of the plague, 'devastatingly democratic in its destruction' (Melville 2007, 834), with clean air that translates itself to ecological sensitivity. This would parallel interpretations of Shelley's 'last man' as a critique of controlling quarantine measures premised upon contagiousness of disease (McWhir 2002, 28–29) and an absence of compassion for strangers. One might add to McWhir and Melville that it enables a postcolonial critical reading of Shelley, of the impossibility of naming the East, or any other part of the world, as the starting point of disease, which has no origin.

The essays in this anthology do not become condemned to quarantine; they explode from confinement, reflecting human frailty in the continuing search for meaning and desire to communicate. They vocalize the significance of consolation, care, and reconciliation given the inevitability of vulnerability that has been foregrounded by the pandemic as an inescapable aspect of being. The pandemic has unfurled innumerable vistas of being responsible and supportive to susceptibilities of interdependent lives, making both healing and health tangible possibilities, rather than pipe dreams. In this context, this book engages with the question of the extent to which a contagious disease compels and inspires human beings to engage with existentialist questions of renewing life with creativity and imagination, while being haunted by their own mortality.

The reflections on health by İclal Eskioğlu Aydın, Ada Kot, and Yvonne Sandoval reveal the centrality of collectivity and care in the pursuit of wellness. Vinay Lal narrates the possibility of pursuing such goals in institutional contexts by discussing healthcare in Cuba. The narratives by Sara Dang, Aarti Ramaswami, Peggy Sax, Arundhati Sharma, Elena Baskina, and Masha Tiunova showcase how an emphasis on interaction can strengthen learning despite the inevitable distancing measures that now prevail. Ruxandra Anghel, Basantsingh Deerpaul, Raji Manjari Pokhrel, and Prathama Raghavan invoke compassionate and self-compassionate strategies of coping with the changes of the new normal. Jude Clark, Lata Dyaram, Kirtika Kain, Dave Sookhoo, Alison Scott-Baumann and Hina Shahid reflect on the stark traces of social dichotomies and discrimination that persist in digital contexts, and which have been reinforced during the pandemic. Some of them focus on the cognitive potential emanating from the suffering of the pandemic. These reflections also identify memory as a difficult and therapeutic partner in moments of isolation. They also gesture towards modes of healing that address social disparities. Christopher Norris's poem, which serves as the epilogue to the book, revisits the pandemic twenty years later to reveal that one cannot simplistically claim to have overcome it; the original event of the pandemic has splintered in unexpected directions because of our 'precarious' and ecological lives.

All the essays are contextualized in their specific social/historical locations, enabling comparative perspectives across continents and cultures to examine affinities and differences.

New modes of consanguinity, emerging from isolation, resonate in their reflections. Their deliberations on the complex character of COVID-19, as both disabling and enabling, emerge from arts, humanities, and social sciences to open new possibilities for learning and living. They unfold empathetic and democratic modes of engaging with obligations to those who are familiar and those who are distant 'others' during a period of distress. And they enunciate the extent to which a contagious disease compels human beings, who are haunted by their own mortality without ready-made solidarities, to embark on questions of renewing life by relating to non-human life with creativity and imagination.

PART I

THEORIZING THE PANDEMIC

PAUSE, PRIVILEGE, SACRIFICE, AND A MORE CARING SOCIETY

Maurice Hamington

> An advantage of quarantine is that it can be used to think afresh. Clearing the mind of clutter and thinking how to live in an altered world is the task at hand.
>
> —John Gray (2020)

The current COVID-19 pandemic has an unusual side-effect compared to other existential threats that human beings face—it has afforded some people the opportunity to stop and reflect on their place and purpose in the world. Because of the stay-at-home and social distancing directives, many individuals have more time alone, away from the rush of work and commutes, for added moments of contemplation. The constant push for productivity under the dominant international neoliberal capitalist market paradigm makes for an unrelenting pace of life and work. This daily rapid velocity does not allow most people to take stock of personal and social contexts nor to think about where humanity is headed. A number of commentators have referred to the present condition under the pandemic as the 'Great Pause' (Blanchard 2020).

However, this moniker smacks of privilege. For frontline workers, essential workers, and those who struggle to subsist there is no pause but merely more burden in doing their jobs and surviving. As Australian professor of community development Peter Westoby describes in speaking to South African archivist for the Nelson Mandela Foundation, Verne Harris, 'For the privileged the pandemic has been a giant pause, a kind of resting moment for contemplation, more yoga, perhaps alcohol detox and goodness knows what else. For the poor it has been catastrophic—and we now talk of the hunger pandemic unfolding in your [African] continent' (2020, 6). Much of the international pandemic has placed a microscope to personal and social privilege as those who have the resources are much more likely to both avoid the disease and weather the resultant economic downturn. This brief commentary explores the moral potential of the current Great Pause for rethinking privilege and perhaps considering what it might take, including embracing sacrifice, to enact a more caring society.

CARE THEORY

In the 1980s, a new name was applied to the fundamental and life-sustaining work of caring for one another—care ethics. Although care is essential to human existence, moral theorists generally overlooked care in favour of systems of adjudicating right and wrong such as rules, rights, and consequences as the heart of ethics. Feminist thinkers, dissatisfied with traditional approaches to moral philosophy proposed a relational-based morality that valued experience, context, and emotion in a more holistic moral framework (Gilligan 1982; Noddings 1984). Since its original formulation almost forty years ago, care ethics has burgeoned across disciplines including the development of critical political analyses (Tronto 1993; Engster 2007). Beyond morality, the entanglements of care include epistemological (Dalmiya 2016; Puig de la Bellacasa 2017) and ontological (Shiu-Ching 2016) dimensions, which is why a more accurate term to describe this field of study might be the broader notion of 'care theory'.

At a very basic level, care, as it is described by the scholars who study it, entails *inquiry*, *connection*, and *action*. Inquiry is necessary because all good care entails knowledge of the particular needs of the one cared for as well as the general knowledge of proficiency in care delivery. For example, physicians will provide the best care if they combine their professional skills with what they learn from the circumstances of their particular patients (Hamington 2018). Connection describes the compelling motivational aspect of care, including emotions which often manifest as empathy (Slote 2007). The one who cares feels with the other in some way, which makes the caring abiding and deeper than superficial hospitality. Finally, care entails action. Care is a practice (Held 2006, 36–38) and not simply a disposition towards others. The one cared for is the ultimate arbiter of care's effectiveness and must experience care activity on his or her behalf.

Care theory is an appropriate lens of analysis for addressing the current pandemic, as several authors have demonstrated (Branicki 2020, 5–6; Wirth et al. 2020). During the international COVID-19 crisis, we care for ourselves, care for others in need, and consider the best methods for caring for our community and society. Such efforts require inquiry—learning about the disease and its transmission as well as the circumstances of those vulnerable to the disease; connection—in terms of understanding the fear and pain of community members; and, action—tangible practices needed to protect ourselves and others, that mitigate suffering. Care has a temporal dimension to it: one can act in ways that meet immediate needs but a robust care also extends to caring for the long term. For example, feeding the poor is an important act in the moment, but figuring out systems to sustain everyone over a longer horizon is also a valuable act of care. As we contemplate caring for one another during the great pause, we have an opportunity to reflect on what would it mean to put systems of lasting care in place that could help people endure through life's challenges. In the present world context, where there is so much wealth and resources juxtaposed against precarious squalor, a question of collective sacrifice arises: What are we willing to give up to care for others in our society?

SACRIFICE

One of the under-theorized aspects of care is the role of sacrifice. Care connotes many positive feelings, as we like to be cared for and we can derive a great deal of joy from caring for others (Noddings 1984, 132–47). However, as anyone who has cared for others knows, caring also entails attentiveness, time, patience, resources, and effort: a sacrifice. A vexing aspect of the COVID-19 pandemic is that it is an entangled social challenge that is not easily addressed by the dominant international paradigm of neoliberalism. Generally, neoliberalism seeks individualistic and competitive market-based solutions to problems. As George Monbiot describes, 'Neoliberalism sees competition as the defining characteristic of human relations. It redefines citizens as consumers, whose democratic choices are best exercised by buying and selling, a process that rewards merit and punishes inefficiency. It maintains that "the market" delivers benefits that could never be achieved by planning' (2016). However, the pandemic necessitated a collaborative, non-market based, worldwide effort that included making individual sacrifices for the greater good. In other words, caring, and more specifically, caring sacrifice is required to address disparate social privilege. Even before the pandemic, neoliberalism was failing to meet the challenges of contemporary social issues. John Gray claims, 'With all its talk of freedom and choice, liberalism was in practice the experiment of dissolving traditional sources of social cohesion and political legitimacy and replacing them with the promise of rising material living standards. This experiment has now run its course' (2020).

Some countries and communities are better suited than others to make the caring sacrifices needed in this moment. Anti-mask, anti-social distancing, anti-vaccine protests, as well as efforts to open economies too early exemplify flawed commitment to the caring sacrifice needed to confront the epidemic.

Inge van Nistelrooij is a Dutch care scholar who offered the first major examination of care ethics and sacrifice. She finds the subject of sacrifice crucial in establishing one's moral agency and moral identity. Nistelrooij contends that coming to terms with self-sacrifice is essential in defining one's commitment to care:

> Self-sacrifice in caring is a practice that is directed at an other, others, the self, the world, aiming at a 'higher good' in which the self simultaneously realizes the self's identity. Self-sacrifice

> stands in the tension between fragility and autonomy, and it is inevitably ambiguous and uncertain. Self-sacrifice in caring for another is understandable only when intersubjectivity is seen, not as a balance between the self and the other, but as a relation of intertwined identities. Self-sacrifice in caring on a political level requires an understanding of the community as found on a desire to live together. Self-sacrifice in caring requires as well that caring be understood against the horizon of meanings that are embraced in caring. Finally, self-sacrifice in caring entails inevitable conflicts and struggle on all levels—identity, intersubjectivity, community, and horizons of meaning. (2015, 290)

Nistelrooij applies a social and political lens of care to sacrifice and delineates the complexity of self-sacrifice's entanglements. In this understanding, care is both means and ends: care is the higher good with its 'horizon of meanings' which society seeks as well as a method to achieve that good. The COVID-19 pandemic, then, can be considered a test of moral values and commitments. What do we care about? Can we sacrifice sporting events, family get-togethers, concerts, and travel to better care for others? Are those individuals with privileges willing to sacrifice for the long-run reconstruction of society for the benefit of its most vulnerable members? During the Great Pause, these questions prompted by the pandemic experience about our collective values can be a source of moral reflection on society beyond the present crisis.

PRIVILEGE AND REFLECTION

The global pandemic has highlighted the role of power and privilege in mitigating precarity. Differences are less pronounced in some countries than others, but market capitalism has provided some with the resources to reduce the chances of catching COVID-19 through social distancing and access to better healthcare. Although ostensibly, everyone is susceptible to the virus, the wealthy are less likely to contract the disease and more likely to receive better treatment. Although the advantage of privilege in this crisis is worldwide, it is particularly stark in large heterogeneous nations such as India and the United States. So the opportunity to pause and reflect on the bigger-picture questions of social and political surrounding is a privilege of those who have the health and wherewithal to make the time and space for such contemplation. Furthermore, the skill and ability to engage in reflection is also a privilege granted by education and training to think about social issues in an informed and critical manner. My point is that there is no escaping the fact that privilege is tied to what I am asking for in this commentary—that we rethink our social values and practices to use this moment as a springboard toward a more caring society. The fact of my privilege in writing this commentary and the fact of your privilege in reading it is not a value judgement because the real moral test of privilege is how we use our advantages to make the world a better place.

The dominant modern paradigm of neoliberalism places value on productivity and the free market which accelerate the scale of privilege. It creates resource 'winners' and 'losers' and has little use for empathy and connection. For example, neoliberal philosophy is generally opposed to progressive income tax that can build caring infrastructure and the welfare state. Neoliberalism also accelerates the pace of life in service of monetized work and devalues ethical reflection (or any aspect of the humanities that cannot compete in the marketplace). Furthermore, the neoliberal emphasis on individual freedom overlooks solutions, particularly sacrificial ones, in service of the greater good. Political theorist Isabell Lorey describes those in power as actively or at least complicitly contributing to an intentional precarity through the philosophy and values of neoliberalism. She describes neoliberalism as engaging in the 'demolition and restructuring of collective security systems' (2015, 5). Neoliberalism has thus contributed to vulnerabilities that exacerbated the impact of the present pandemic as well as making the world more susceptible to future crises. Although forms of care can be bought and sold, deep responsive care is antithetical to neoliberalism. Positive change requires a commitment to care and move away from unfettered neoliberal values.

A CARING MOVEMENT BORN OF TRAGEDY

> A crisis arises because a prevailing governance paradigm is ill-suited to new circumstances, and the crisis itself eventually generates modifications to the prevailing paradigm.
>
> —Alasdair Roberts (2020, 1140–41)

The Great Pause is a tremendous opportunity for the world to imagine better, more caring social structures thus using the present crisis to motivate moral progress. Joan Tronto describes how making care a central value in democratic life will 'require a rethinking of many existing social institutions, political institutions, and practices' (2013, 178). However, the movement towards a more caring world will consist of more than calculated policy changes. It will require a determination that appeals to the world's intellect as well as its emotion to create a comprehensive commitment to care. Recalling my earlier assertion that care consists of inquiry, connection, and action, a caring society must draw upon expanding our knowledge of one another (particularly those who are unfamiliar to us) and our contexts in a manner that binds with empathy to foment real change in the world. The Movement for Black Lives is one example of structural social change beginning to happen.

The Movement for Black Lives began as a response to the acquittal of George Zimmerman who murdered Trayvon Martin in 2013. In that year, three Black organizers—Patrisse Cullors, Alicia Garza, and Opal Tometi—founded an intersectional and inclusive movement under the banner of #BlackLivesMatter (Black Lives Matter). On 25 May 2020, in the midst of the pandemic, George Floyd died on a street in Minneapolis, Minnesota, after having been pinned to the pavement as a white police officer, Derek Chauvin, knelt on Floyd's neck for nearly eight minutes. Although this violent form of police racism is particularly endemic to the United States, the world has witnessed a rise in xenophobic narratives and violence (United Nations 2016). Racism is a very old human scourge but the will to engage with this problem now seems in part to be tied to the pandemic crisis. Surveys indicated that the pandemic not only gave people more time to participate in protests and think about changing society but they may have also found compassion because of their own pandemic-related hardships (Arora 2020). Institutions of care differ in effectiveness from country to country and although as a developed nation the United States has a particularly weak system of social welfare support, the pandemic has revealed structural challenges around the globe (Mohammed 2020). The cry 'Black Lives Matter' is a demand for care—not just platitudes or superficial rules of equality but sacrificial acts of care. The caring action might entail reparations, increased social services, guaranteed income, law enforcement reform, jurisprudence reform, and/or education reform, most of which will involve change and sacrifice as taxing those with the requisite resources is an important means for funding these changes. However, the Movement for Black Lives addresses the experience of one particular oppressed and vulnerable community. There are many others. A caring society will have mechanisms for listening to and responding to its various at-risk communities.

The Great Pause can be a time to rethink social values and practices in order to expand and deepen the circle of care. Stanford psychologist Jamil Zaki notes that 'people who endure great suffering often become *more* empathic as a result' (2019, 25). He refers to this as 'altruism born of suffering' (ibid., 26). We are in a moment of collective suffering. The number of people who have died or become ill because of COVID-19 is staggering. Even those who have been privileged enough to avoid illness have had the disease touch a family member, or acquaintance, or at the very least witnessed the suffering of others through the media. As John Gray claims, 'A sense of fragility is everywhere. It is not only society that feels shaky. So does the human position in the world' (2020). We can leverage this moment of shared suffering to empathize and fuel a movement to make our respective societies more caring, transcending the narratives of neoliberalism and xenophobia. What is ultimately hopeful in Zaki's analysis of empathy is that there is an element of moral agency to it. We can make changes in our lives to turn up our empathy (2019, 38). He even cites social research that indicates we can overcome tribal differences through empathetic tuning (ibid., 44). That is what we need in this moment.

If we turn up our empathy we can allow our collective suffering to drive our imagination and foment the political will to co-create a more caring society.

CONSPIRACY THEORIES, FAKE NEWS, AND COVID-19

Andrew Edgar

INTRODUCTION

The COVID-19 pandemic has been accompanied by constant misinformation (including conspiracy theories and fake news) about whether it really exists or not, and if it does exist, its origins, severity, and possible remedies. This misinformation has led to ineffectual policies being implemented for combating the virus—especially when the misinformation is believed and propagated by the leaders of national governments—and inadvisable and risky behaviour being adopted by potential victims of the virus. We might even say that misinformation corrupts our ability to hold a well-informed and reasonable conversation about how we are to engage with the pandemic.

Those who believe and act upon the misinformation find it more convincing and satisfying than scientific and medical explanations, and this poses a profound challenge to healthcare professionals. But we must acknowledge that stories grounded in misinformation answer to a deep-seated need to give meaning and coherence to a profoundly confusing and disorientating situation. Misinformation cannot simply be dismissed. There must be an engagement, a conversation, between medical science and those who believe in and propagate misinformation, so that we begin to understand the reasons why so many people find conspiracy theories compelling. Only then might the medical experts find ways to communicate the medical facts that answer to those insecurities and give people a sense of purpose and coherence despite the apparent chaos of the pandemic.

Healthcare professionals need to understand misinformation and its appeal in order to be able to re-establish a conversation with the people they are striving to help and protect.

NARRATIVE MEDICINE

A narrative approach presupposes that human beings are, to use Mary Paumier Jones's phrase, 'storytelling animals' (1996). That is not merely to remark that story-telling is a universal feature of human culture, but rather to recognize the complex and subtle roles played by story-telling within different cultures. Paul Ricoeur argued that it is through stories or narratives that a person's sense of identity is constructed (Ricoeur 1991). The answer to the question 'Who am I?' is grounded in a story, or a series of stories. If asked who I am, I respond by evoking stories about my personal life and that of my family, perhaps also about my country or community, the religion I espouse, or even the profession to which I belong. Personal identity, then, lies not in some permanent and unchanging substance, such as Descartes's 'thinking thing' (Descartes 1996, 54), but rather in the capacity of human agents to bring the relevant details of their lives together into more or less coherent narratives.

Such narratives are not fixed but will be changed and developed as the person's experiences change. Nor are such narratives mere neutral chronicles of remembered events and actions. Rather, they will be imbued with normative judgements and passions, as I proudly perceive the good that I (and my community) have done and shamefully condemn the bad. Further, I have a sense of myself as a continuing being in so far as I can tell a story of my past and project that story into the future. These stories will, therefore, ground my actions precisely because I will strive to enact a future self that is coherent with what has transpired before (building on my past successes, and correcting or atoning for past failures and weaknesses).

Such stories are not just personal affairs. Humans are cultural and social beings, necessarily developing within communities that have rich cultures and histories. Our personal narratives thus draw upon the stories that are circulated in our culture, be these fairy tales and legends, religious narratives and histories, or the tales conveyed by popular and high culture in novels, movies and, perhaps, even video games. Such stories give us templates to construct our own narratives as well as exemplars of both admirable and contemptible behaviour. As social beings, our sense of personal identity will depend on our sense of belonging to certain groups, and thus upon the stories that are told by and about those groups. Stories are thus a crucial part of my conversation with others. I typically justify my actions to others by telling stories, and I listen to the stories that others tell of me and my community, and in so far as those stories judge me, for good or ill, I may modify my own story and the actions that follow from it.

The importance of story-telling in medicine is increasingly recognized and indeed has spawned the sub-discipline of narrative medicine (Charon 2006). What is of crucial significance here is the way in which illness can disrupt our stories. The unexpected nature of an illness, and the manner in which it inhibits our actions, can make the way in which we project our story into the (near) future feel nonsensical. The patient can feel overwhelmed by the immediacy of events, so that there is no time in which to impose or discover a sense of coherence or progression.

Arthur Frank classified the attempt to tell stories about such experiences as 'chaos narratives'—'its plot imagines life never getting better. Stories are chaotic in their absence of narrative order. Events are told as the storyteller experiences life: without sequence or discernible causality' (Frank 1995, 97). The chaos narrative is, in many respects, an anti-narrative, or a mark of the failure to tell a story. It is a painful, incoherent expression of suffering and confusion. It gives the patient no grounds upon which to act, for it undermines their very sense of themselves as a person, with a past continuing coherently into the future.

Ideally, as sense is made of the condition, by both the patient and their physicians and carers, what Frank calls a 'restitution narrative' can be told. Such a narrative emerges from Talcott Parson's concept of the sick-role (Frank 1995, 5–6). Here, it is presupposed that illness is acute. One falls ill and thereby enters the sick-role. This offers certain privileges (such as remission from performing work or household duties) but also certain obligations, including complying with medical instructions and following the prescribed therapeutic regime. Such obligations restore a sense of agency, and indeed one's sense of self. One strives to recover so that one can return to one's everyday life and pick up the stories one told about oneself before one fell ill. You become once more the person you were and who you intend to be. The story of one's illness can then be told as a more or less brief hiatus in the ongoing story of one's life. The illness may be an important experience, helping to modify and enrich one's sense of self, and of how one projects oneself into the future (for example, in recognizing one's vulnerability one takes better care of oneself, or determines to use one's time more productively). Yet the illness may be a mere aside, having little impact upon the story of one's life as a whole. In either case, the illness is in the past, a memory, rather than a living part of one's story.

Frank argued that this dominant and pervasive story is problematic as it does not respond to the prevalence of chronic illness in modern society. Chronic illness is not a hiatus but rather entails a fundamental change in the identity, and thus the story, of the patient. The identity of the chronically ill person becomes entwined with the illness—the illness is not a memory but something ever-present—and this can potentially undermine a good deal of the sense and coherence of the old story the person told of themselves, and especially the way in which that story is projected into the future. (Consider this example. A woman puts off having children in order to focus on her career. She aims to provide a secure home for her children by being professionally successful. Her story is clear and coherent. Yet, unexpectedly, this woman has to undergo a hysterectomy before she decides to have a child. Her life story is fundamentally changed. A past, which was once prudent planning for the future, has become time wasted; the future, which promised successful motherhood, has become empty.) The chronically ill person is thus thrown into what Frank calls a 'quest' (Frank 1995, 115ff) to find a new story and new identity, acknowledging how their sense of self must change but also allowing them to 'bear witness' (ibid., 165), and thereby communicate their new needs, frustrations—and perhaps opportunities—to others.

Frank's model of three narratives (restitution, chaos, and quest) has ramifications for how the COVID-19 pandemic is understood. COVID-19 has, in effect, engendered a chaos narrative writ large. Scientific attempts to explain and understand the disease seem tentative or ineffectual. Especially in the early stages of the onset of the infection, the official narratives about the virus tended to focus, unavoidably, on a lack of medical knowledge, and thus upon the degree of uncertainty of the outcomes and effectiveness of the medical interventions and public health policies that were being implemented. There was uncertainty about the origins of the virus and its initial transition from animal to human populations; how contagious and deadly it was; who was most at risk; whether having contracted the virus one acquired immunity; and so on. Scientific and medical honesty and openness thus reinforced the impression that COVID-19 was an incomprehensible event, and an example of what the French existentialist Albert Camus might call the absurd—a confrontation between the human need for meaning and coherence and the 'unreasonable silence of the world' (Camus 1975, 32).

This scientific honesty is deeply problematic. In itself, it undermines a profoundly important narrative of the Enlightenment, such that, as modern rational science has developed, it has given human beings the tools to understand and control nature. This narrative, in turn, renders older forms of story-telling irrational and superstitious. Thus COVID-19 cannot officially be declared an act of divine retribution, such as plagues in the European Middle Ages might have been understood. Such religious interpretations, while wrong and ineffective from the perspective of modern science, gave rise to meaningful narratives (in opposition to the scientific chaos narrative). Perhaps the only things that modern medicine could offer that provided a sense of coherence and progress were the infection and mortality statistics gathered by various countries.

One could watch these numbers increase, rather like watching a cricketer's total of runs accumulate during a long innings. But even these numbers were undermined by stories about the way in which data are collected, and thus the figures' unreliability.

COVID-19, it may then be suggested, engendered a chaos narrative precisely because it resisted the sort of Enlightenment narratives that accompanied previous global crises and emergencies. Pandemics and medical emergencies, such as SARS, MARS, and Ebola outbreaks, were contained within relatively discrete geographical locations. Public health policies and medical interventions appeared to work. Science understood and controlled the threat posed by nature. Even with Ebola, with its very high mortality rates and huge toll on human suffering, the medical interventions controlled and eventually suppressed the disease. Similarly, other natural emergencies, such as the 2010 Haiti earthquake, Hurricane Katrina in 2005, or innumerable flooding incidents across the world, lent themselves to similar stories, all akin to Frank's restitution narrative. A localized region is afflicted. International and government aid is administered, following sound scientific advice. The region gradually recovers.

CONSPIRACY THEORY AND FAKE NEWS

Butter and Knight offered the following characterization of conspiracy theories: They assumed that everything has been planned and nothing happens by coincidence; they divided the world strictly into the evil conspirators and the innocent victims of their plot; and they claimed that the conspiracy works in secret and does not reveal itself even after it has reached (Butter and Knight 2020b, 1).

Fenster noted that the conspiracists see themselves as defenders of a moral order (that is placed in danger by the conspiracy). As such, conspiracy narratives do not merely make sense of a seemingly chaotic and threatening world, but also do much to give the believer a sense of identity, not merely as an individual, but as a member of an (enlightened) group (Fenster 1999, 119). As such, conspiracy theories may be understood as a resource in the constitution of a narrative sense of self-identity. Not least, the conspiracy theory articulates a distinction between self and other, or us and them.

Fenster highlighted conspiracy theories' rejection of accident or coincidence and insistence upon everything being planned. This serves to reinforce the place that fake news might have within them. The conspiracy theory strives to bring together into a coherent whole disparate material. Chaos is rendered meaningful, Camus' 'silence' made to speak, and complexity reduced (albeit that conspiracy theories can be extremely intricate). Thus, at the root of many conspiracy theories concerning COVID-19 lies the assertion that the virus was manufactured, rather than one occurring naturally (despite there being strong scientific evidence against this assertion). The virus does not then accidentally transfer from animals to humans. It is intentionally introduced into the human population by someone, seeing it as threatening the moral order. In a classic version of a conspiracy theory, this threatening agent is identified as Bill Gates.[1] The Gates Foundation is argued to have manufactured the virus as a pretext for embarking upon a mass vaccination programme, through which, in some versions of the story, a sinister nano-technology will be introduced into the global population, allowing Gates to control that population or inculcate it into a new form of global economy. That the Gates Foundation sponsored a conference on pandemics in late 2019 is crucial evidence. Nothing is accidental, not least the timing of a conference in relation to the outbreak of a pandemic. Other threats to the moral order, in other conspiracy theories, include China (with China's Nation Biosafety Laboratory being

1. It may be noted that the conspiracy theories concerning COVID-19 frequently draw upon or link into existing conspiracy theories. So, the Gates Foundation is seen as a threat in many theories. More worryingly, theories may draw upon and exacerbate existing social divides, prejudices, and instances of xenophobia, not least in marking out the distinction between 'us', the believers in the conspiracy, and 'them', the perpetrators of the conspiracy.

situated a mere thirty-two kilometres from Wuhan, where the first outbreak was identified), and from a Russian perspective the USA, although reputedly Russian theorist Aleksandr Dugin presents it as a punishment for globalization. Other versions suggest that COVID-19 is a bio-weapon created in Canada and stolen by the Chinese, or created in the US and spread, unwittingly, by a US contestant at the 2019 World Military Games that took place in Wuhan.[2]

Such theories are not necessarily a threat to public health, and might just be treated as amusing asides. If the conspiracist believes that the virus is real, and indeed if the danger posed by the virus is compounded by the threat of being vaccinated by the Gates Foundation, then the conspiracist might be expected to do all that is possible to help suppress the virus (and thus thwart Gates, thereby protecting the moral order). Conspiracy theories become problematic, it may be suggested, when they propagate misinformation concerning the threat and very existence of the virus.

Conspiracy theories are not identical to fake news though (Butter and Knight 2020b, 2). Fake news can be composed of discrete claims and need not be grounded in the broader narrative of a conspiracy. Further, while conspiracists may generally be assumed to be sincere in their beliefs, fake news is frequently manufactured maliciously. The narrative sense of self of the propagator of fake news is thus potentially very different to that of the conspiracist. Nonetheless, if sincerely believed, fake news does imply that official news channels are deceptive (and hence potentially a threat and part of a conspiracy against the moral order). Further, they offer a firm ground upon which to act, and it is precisely in this that fake news poses a danger during the COVID-19 pandemic.

The greatest threat lies in the denial of the existence of COVID-19. In one rather engaging conspiracy theory, COVID-19

2. These versions of COVID-19 conspiracy theories, and many more, have been sourced from issues of the magazine *Fortean Times*, between April and August 2020.

is thought up in order to perpetrate a global lockdown. This is because the Earth is threatened with destruction by an asteroid, and lockdown ensures that all of us will spend our last days with our family and loved ones. Other, more sinister versions propose that the virus is an excuse for lockdown, and that lockdown in turn is a form of social control, preventing social protests or other threats against those who threaten the moral order. More subtly, many spurious remedies for COVID-19 have been proposed, including alcohol, heat, vitamin C, salt water, garlic, and chlorine dioxide, as well as hydroxychloroquine. Such remedies may be a threat in themselves (one woman apparently died from eating an excessive amount of raw garlic) as well as offering the user no protection (or at best minimal protection) against the virus.

This prevalence of fake news and conspiracy theory may be explained by returning to the claim above that COVID-19 has predominantly yielded chaos narratives. Frank's chaos narrative entails that the individual agent's grounds for acting—for making coherent and meaningful decisions as to their future—are undermined. They are left passive and the victims of forces that are beyond their control. So too, the very science that strives to understand COVID-19 appears to leave us, as individuals and communities, passive. We exist in a world of utter contingency, of mere facts and data that have no deeper meaning. Not only is our health threatened, but our economic security, too, as the global economy contracts. Even those at work have to face radically different, and potentially risky, working practices, and may be confronted with uncomfortable choices between protecting their health and their livelihood. Hard-won skills and competences may be rendered useless. It becomes increasingly difficult to project any sense of one's self into a post-COVID-19 future, or even make sense of one's past and what one attempted to achieve with one's life during that time.

In the face of chaos, conspiracies and fake news offer meaningful and coherent stories. They fill the gap vacated by the banishment of the pre-modern appeal to divine judgement.

(Indeed, some religious leaders have interpreted COVID-19 in this manner, as well as assuming that one could not contract the virus within a holy place such as a church or temple.) Conspiracy theory and fake news replace the ambiguity and uncertainty of medical science by clear and simple remedies, and crucially, beliefs upon which one can act with apparent confidence. While the official chaos narrative disempowers, the conspiracy theory transforms COVID-19 into the basis for greater empowerment (be this by simply dosing oneself with vitamin C, or by exercising one's duty as a conspiracist to defend the threatened moral order). In addition, one's sense of identity is strengthened (as part of the group that has seen through the hoax, and who has a clear opponent.)

CONCLUDING REMARKS

Conspiracy theories and fake news fill a gap left by the Enlightenment narrative of medical science. This gap might be termed a 'hermeneutic' gap as it refers to a loss of any sense of meaning during the pandemic. As storytelling animals, humans rely upon coherent narratives to make sense of themselves, and the physical and social environments in which they live. It is through such stories that they are able to evaluate and decide their future actions. COVID-19 so radically and abruptly changed our environment that it rendered our old stories and ways of making sense of our actions largely redundant. Medical science in its pursuit of the truth of COVID-19, and thus of effective vaccinations and public health policies through which the virus could be suppressed, could not offer compelling stories, but only a chaos narrative.

This leaves us the question as to whether there are equivalents to Frank's restitution narrative and quest narratives in the case of COVID-19. A restitution narrative presupposes that the pandemic is an acute event (similar to many other natural disasters). Citizens would thus have an obligation, not unlike that of the patient within the sick-role, to submit themselves to the advice of the medical authorities. Yet this narrative appears to have failed because of the uncertainty of the medical science. It may then be suggested that what is required are quest narratives as an attractive alternative to conspiracies and fake news. That is to say that COVID-19 is not understood as an acute event but as something that has become a fundamental part of who we are, akin to a chronic illness. Both as individuals and as communities we are 'COVID-sufferers'.

Such narratives would be important precisely because they would meet the need that conspiracy theories and fake news fulfil, but to positive rather than negative effect. It may tentatively be suggested that such narratives lie in speculations about there being a better and more just world post COVID. Narratives are beginning to be formed that argue for COVID-19 as an opportunity to reassess humanity's environmental impact and to move towards more just and equitable societies (not least through the revitalization of the Black Lives Matter movement in the midst of the pandemic). A careful consideration of conspiracy theory plays a role in such speculation, precisely in so far as conspiracy theories may be understood as being symptomatic of deep social concerns and insecurities. Conspiracy theorists and those who believe fake news cannot simply be excluded from any conversation merely on the grounds that their views do not align with those of the scientific and political establishment. Rather, speculative conversations about the future must articulate a world in which the insecurities of conspiracy theorists, be they fears of economic and social redundancy, thanks to globalization and technological advance, or the threat of state apparatuses that are neither transparent nor democratically accountable, are addressed, albeit almost certainly not in the way that the conspiracist expects.

COVID-19 will not be revealed to be part of a conspiracy, by Bill Gates or anyone else, to undermine our freedoms, but it might be understood as an accident that made us newly aware of our social, political, and indeed scientific problems and vulnerabilities, and how we might address them. Quest narratives of who we want to be, individually and collectively, post COVID, are thus beginning to be written.

CONTACT IN ABSENTIA: TOWARDS A CYBERTOUCH

Brunella Antomarini

> There is nothing in the universe that does not touch us.
>
> —Leibniz, *Discourse on Metaphysics*

The recent circumstances of the COVID-19 pandemic, while requiring humans to make the great effort of keeping mutual distance, have also been an opportunity to test the plasticity of their sensory systems. Particularly when communicating via screen, we have undergone the so-called 'Zoom fatigue'. But why is talking via video streaming or even video recording so tiresome? Why do we have mixed feelings—from rejection to caution, to pleasure and uncertainty, to trust and distrust—about communicating online? What makes it different—if in physical presence, too, we simply sit, speak, listen, and do keep a distance, while the rest of our static bodies do not seem to have a share in the ongoing communication? What does it mean to 'communicate', if voice and meaning are not, apparently, the whole story?

That we move in a doubled space is nothing new. Since the telephone, we have learnt to decouple space from place. Or going further back in time, theatre would give the audience the impression of being where it is not, and in Renaissance painting, the technique of geometric perspective introduced the sense of participating in a space that was elsewhere (Lister et al. 2009, 115 and ff.). For at least one century, we have had to learn to watch a movie and to cope with the filmic space—from Bergson to Benjamin, McLuhan, and Deleuze, we know how that technological cyberspace needed to be *learnt* and has been naturalized in our cognitive systems. But now, on the occasion of the lockdown, what marks another change and causes the fatigue is the fact that, in that artificial space, we are required to *act* in a 3D/2D space. And while film actors still move in a common environment which, however edited and manipulated, is physically shared with other people, we, the online speakers, share and do not share the same space, undergoing a disturbing interference between the space where the screen is placed, the place where we are (doubled on screen), and the space where the interlocutors are, looming from behind them. This space within a space confuses our bodies—which space is our body occupying? Which air is our voice crossing to reach which destination? We move our hands and head and we utter sounds in a way that is not totally instinctive. It's as if we struggle to reach what is actually out of reach. We look for ways to pierce that impenetrable depth that in real presence we can potentially reach. We sense a loss of the target. The continuity of the presence fades quickly through the possible on and off of video or audio. Not that the intermittence of attention has been caused by digital presence—the attention span has a natural limit and we naturally tend to defend ourselves by switching from one focus to another one.

Walter Benjamin noticed it at the dawn of the cinema—anticipating and preparing Lyotard's notion of the inhuman, or Virilio's dromology. According to Benjamin, the cinema has modified perception in a way that allows for an intermittence of attention and distraction, a continuous on/off state in which the sense of presence is weakened. Concentration in distraction (Benjamin 2000, 18) reveals the illusory condition of stable attention, which simply does not exist: either it is an imposition, or a commonplace. There is a physiological need to protect our organisms from mediatic manipulation by keeping a critical distance, like keeping an open eye in sleep. So while we need to enjoy a pleasant sensorial elicitation, we also need to beware of its possible manipulation.

A SCREEN IS NOT A CANVAS

While communicating through a screen, we are aware of being divided but our body is not, or at least is not prepared for the self-division. If the digital culture has decreased distances and we live in a global village, the need to use online communication lets a new kind of distance emerge: through the digital state, we are able to observe and experience *ourselves* as what is not at hand. We act at a distance from ourselves, being looked at from the others' points of view; it is not the faraway environment that gets closer, but it is we who are closer to distant people and more distant from ourselves. If these technologies have destroyed distance, as McLuhan stated, being on screen introduces an indefinite distance: in fact, the space where we experience ourselves (this McLuhan could not envisage) is unknown. We are a perspectival point of view and a vanishing point at the same time. The phenomenological description of seeing while being seen (in the sense meant by Husserl, Merleau-Ponty, and Lacan, among others) is now reversed—we *see* that point of space where we are not. The fatigue consists then in pretending to keep our identity while being aware that it is mostly deprived of control—we are not just in the constant mutual adjustment with the others, through their feedback, but we linger in a space with poor feedback—which is reduced to the explicit meaning and inflection of the voice but cannot be activated by the implicit micro-means of communication. On screen, it is difficult to focus on anything particularly relevant. The image of the interlocutor appears flat and opaque. And we know that the same happens to us. But we hardly accept that indifference as our brain/mind looks for ways to make the conversation meaningful, or poignant, or persuasive, similar to how we can count on many details in real presence, from the motion of bodies and hands to eye expressions, to the atmosphere given by smell and sound. And this dynamic being reciprocal, the whole communication risks failure to building *real* conversations (where 'real' means a mutual retroaction to those micro-means of communication). A screen is not a canvas where an illusory perspective is carefully rendered, in which we can virtually move and touch distant objects.

Should we conclude that a perceptual catastrophe is the inescapable consequence of the new and increasingly frequent phenomenon of remote communication?

Or are there hints of a paradigm shift that could result in a deeper perceptual self-consciousness and empowerment comparable to the one that occurred after the emergence of telephone or the cinema?

ENACTIVE VISION

Our brains are put under pressure, and we strive more and more quickly to find ways to cross the space between us and our interlocutors. As Alva Noe's innovative theory of visual perception points out, seeing has less to do with images than with tentative ways to *touch* the environment, which is necessarily mobile and partially grasped. Looking at something means to perceive one part of the actual entity and to be able to physically interact with it and figure out the unperceived parts of it, whereas *focusing* on something means to choose the relevance of a virtual action that would turn the part into a whole perception. But surely our attempts remain unstable, circumstantial, or emotional. A picture is a living presence we inevitably endow with a meaning:

> Indeed, I would venture to say that it is just this fact of the presence-as-absence structure of pictures that explains their remarkable, somehow fundamental power, what has been called their *Lebendigkeit*. (Noe 2012, 85)

Noe's perspective of 'making up' for the absent part in a picture is now reinforced by our instability when on screen we perceive ourselves perceive—we test the various possibilities of dealing with an absent object in a way similar to touching in absence of sight. As he says, 'We see *what there is*, but we see what there is *from here*' (ibid., 84). Now, as the reciprocity of construing the sense of an interaction becomes clearer on screen, from here to there simultaneously means from there to here. We know what the others are seeing of us, but we do not know how the others are making up for the absent part of us. This would and does happen also in actual presence, yet, it is only on screen that this lack in presence becomes explicit.

Our eyes work as two hands that poke and probe and explore the object and make sense of it, imagining its entirety or its actuality, or its meaning, or its use. René Descartes, in *Dioptrics*, had already envisaged some sort of virtual touch being placed in the optic machine of the human eye, as according to his famous image of the blind man with two sticks—we do not represent things in a pictorial bidimensional space, but we explore their 3D quality as if we were touching what presents itself to us.

Similarly, Noe's enactive theory considers sight secondary to touch and action. I would add then that the effort we make in grasping a digital environment that appears on a screen restores the predominance of touch over sight. Although observation guides experimentation in scientific research on the physical world, it is the sense of touch that receives a deeper impact in cyberspace and, therefore, in ordinary conversation and understanding. Being deprived of the supportive sense of touch, in the absence of any contact surface that defines the picture, or a background onto which it becomes clear and distinct, it is to the sense of touch that we resort in the effort to cross and penetrate space.

In the threshold condition generating ubiquity (we are here and there; we occupy a space that is empty and full), identification is an interface, a systemic coupling that depends on our mutual construction of our selves. Our identities lose substance and take on temporary intermittent appearances.

Augmented space means increased distance and its dissolution; we are slowly modifying our physiological system to make it fit for touch at a distance, to touch through an augmented contact surface that captures and holds an environment whose real instability is now recognized and respected.

When a surface is at hand but untouchable, muscles make more of an effort to reach it and contract. When the visible object is far away, the eye muscle relaxes not focusing on anything particular and embracing a whole. In a situation of digital contact, our eyes have a surface at hand, which is the screen itself, but the destination of the sight is far away.

The eye muscle remains contracted despite the distance of the object. Our cognitive physio-psychological reaction consists of complementing the two spaces to give the perceptual target a sense of lived place. We see less and we imagine more; we react with contracted eyes but we retroact more; that is, while acting, thinking and conversing, we belittle sight and look for embodied strategies that restore tactile space and identification.

THE SENSE OF TOUCH AS LYNCHPIN OF THE *REAL*

An empiricist philosopher, heir of the Enlightenment, or an *idéologue*, Antoine-Louis-Claude Destutt de Tracy, published in 1825 *Elements d'idéologie*, a treatise clearly inspired by David Hume, and aimed at retrieving empirical cognition in opposition to the mentalist *philosophes* of the previous generation. Philosophy is a kind of zoology, he stated, in which touch is considered to be the ground of all cognition and the origin of the other senses—all sensations have a tactile quality (Destutt de Tracy, 126), in that, however distinct, sight, hearing, smell, and taste have to touch a surface to be activated (not to talk about the proprioceptors and us feeling our organs). Touch is a continuous sense, being displayed all over the skin which constantly touches the air. Its activity consists of pressure; perceiving means to move and to be stopped by some obstacle; the resistance that results from the mutual pressure is the basic information we constantly exchange with the environment, through a double sensation—one of movement and one of its cessation (Destutt de Tracy, 225). As the first property detected in other bodies is a quantity of inertia, tactile sensations exist at the moment in which they are hindered in their inertial force.

Touch is the unique path to ontological proof: 'Sensing something that resists our utmost volitional actions invincibly proves to us the reality of the existence of something other than our sentient capacity' (Destutt de Tracy, 227–8).

But the sense of reality it induces is one of partiality; it is a small-scale perception. When we touch, so much remains beyond the scope of the actual stimulus, which keeps dividing space into parts to be detected step by step. As Noe noted, when seeing an object, I evaluate how I could touch it, how it could stop my action. Paradoxically, touch, the most intimate of the senses, conveys the most virtual of realities; it occurs through actual pressure. As David Hume had already argued one century before Destutt de Tracy, pressing a stone does not relate to any other reality than solidity; and, as solidity necessarily supposes two bodies (Hume, Book I, Part IV, Section IV, 364), reality is the interface between them. Even freedom can be reduced to a natural sensation of being activated and disactivated depending on the pressure exerted between two surfaces—I freely act until I find a stopping resistance. If I move to test the pressure of something on myself, reality occurs in between.

Now, by sensing presence through a screen, we do not know where we can get stopped in our movements. It is the indefinite transparency of the screen that makes us fail at meeting the other in a way of resistance. The flatness of the 2D surface opens up a space that is at the same time a selected environment—a built scene of self-definition and communication—and random (what appears is just what the camera can take).

We are bounced back to ourselves. The muscles of the eye contract and, missing the grasp with depth, never relax.

CONVERSATION AS A WORK OF ART

An endless sensation cannot exist. If sensation means hitting a surface, no surface corresponds to no sensation. But we might—or the next generations will, being increasingly exposed to digital environments and communications—develop an augmented touch, or a new sensorium which will learn to contact presence in absence.

As humans learned to expand a sense of time, when printing entered their cognition and they could keep track of the remote past through documents, so now we will introduce into our cognitive apparatuses the capability to correct the narrowness of the indefinite cage with no walls but no exit, which is the screen, and turn it into an expanded touchable place. It will be the very absence of clues that will compel us to transform the indefinite into an in-built obstacle, a ludic theatre of possible feedbacks, a sympoiesis in which what we are in our eyes is immediately shared with what we are in the others' eyes; and individual identity, though fragmented, shows to be a painlessly mobile interface. The lack of an immediate material obstacle will conceive of a second-order matter that, far from providing for a contact surface, will be artificially posed to be shaped as a quasi-work of art.

One example of an augmented tactile activity that might become a model for the new sensorium for cyberspace is artist Stelarc's decades-long project culminating in the work presented at the 2020 Adelaide Biennial, called *Reclining Stickman*, which consists of a remote touchscreen that elicits sensations and motion of a distant body. A body proves to be capable of being moved as much as it moves other bodies through an electronic device that literally uses touch to build a super-organism composed by many individual organisms in cyberspace (Stelarc 2020).

A TENTATIVE CONCLUSION: TOWARDS A NEW SENSORIUM?

> No-one has yet determined what a body can do…
>
> —Baruch Spinoza, E. III. n. 2

What kind of strategies will we find then? Enhancing the theatrical quality of conversation?

Planning colour, background, a certain way to move our bodies, maybe more emphatic gestures, a *mise-en-scène* suitable for the new sensorium? Will there be a new performative art that will use public speaking on a solitary but shared self-built stage? Simulation of a tangible place will be naturalized, added to environments as another expression of nature. After all, what we used to call virtual reality is already a memory (Lister et al. 2009, 105); the real reveals its intrinsically virtual quality, given its dynamic, social and technological character, or, following

Destutt de Tracy, its relational character. If gestures are the first marks of space (Destutt de Tracy, 355), we will invent a new gesture language in order to transmit the potential of one's own body in motion. And these distributed gestures on networks will develop a sense of the self that is closer to the performative and to a rhapsody of perceptions that give us a sensation of being ourselves in the absence of a fixed 'identity' (quite in line with Hume's deconstruction of personal identity). This contingent self is constantly re-shaped by the successive performances and mutual adjustments, it is public and flexible, devoid of essential traits and determined by the intermittence of augmented tactile perceptions.

This new self that emerges from a new sensorium was described in a diary that Francisco Varela kept a few months before dying, after undergoing liver transplantation. The title of the text is *Intimate Distances* and states:

> My life in its contingency mirrors the history of techniques, the growing know-how about human bodies, which knows nothing about the lived-bodies that can and will come from it. Technology, as always, stands as the mediation that reveals the inter-relatedness of our lives.

As having someone else's organ makes one a hybrid distributed identity, so does talking on screen challenge a human body to become one that touches what is not tangible—it fosters an idea of the 'real' that is reduced to pressure and resistance and gets rid of the visual model. As stated by Varela:

> The touch afforded by the extended surface of one hand over the other, or over other sensitive skin, leads us directly to the experience of the darkened side of the corps propre, the innards, the viscera.

As we 'touch' parts of our dark body inside, invisible and unknown, now we will touch our dark side in the distance, where we *appear* not to be. As we touch only one part at a time of ourselves, we will touch only one part at a time of that super-organism made of us *with* the others.

The touch retrieves a gesture of utmost intimacy and utmost

humility—touching oneself as another, touching one hand with the other. We become increasingly aware that in touching 'the alterity is constitutive' and we witness 'a push and counterpull between depth and imaginary surfaces' (Varela 2001). We expand a sense of self that does not claim individuality the way we used to.

After cyber-reality has become a matter of fact in human lives, after the global condition of the lockdown has made humans aware of the deep change they undergo in social interactions, we are learning to 'embody' the others in a new kind of endosymbiosis and to retroact to that through forms of art or *tèchnai* (the Greek word *tèchne* includes invention of machines, tools, and artworks).

The dramatization of space as stage enhances a kind of 'aptic' imagination, an aptic resistance between surfaces that do not touch, which will endow humans with a sense of symbiotic self that does not feel torn apart but liberated from the claim of having an 'essence' to be found. The absent-mindedness envisaged by Benjamin marks the end without tears of the artificial closure that each selfhood had to hold fast to. The continuity of an augmented touch can result in a slow but steady adjustment to one another in global harmony. This, however, may sound utopian.

DISCOURSE, CRISIS AND CORONA: SOME ETHICAL IMPLICATIONS OF THE GERMAN DEBATE ON THE COVID-19 PANDEMIC

Ernest W.B. Hess-Lüttich

PRELIMINARY NOTE

On 12 September 2020, the Johns Hopkins University in Baltimore and the Robert Koch Institute (RKI) in Germany reported almost 4.66 million people infected with SARS-CoV-2 in India. Despite a hard and long-lasting lockdown, India moved into second place after the US (approximately 6.45 million infected persons), ahead of Brazil (4.28 million infected persons).[1] With 77,472 deaths caused by the infection, India was in the third place behind the US, where the mark of 200,000 COVID-19 deaths was expected to be exceeded, and was in fact exceeded, soon; Brazil had recorded over 130,000 deaths. The media in Europe reported about the growing psychological stress among the Indian population and about the rising suicide figures ('COVID-19 Blues'). When 122 million Indians suddenly lost their jobs in April 2020, this understandably triggered not only health worries but also social fears. The pressure is growing, and the daily reporting in the Indian media increases the concerns; but not reporting is not an option. The *Indian Journal of Medical Research* reported, according to a report of the German newspaper *Süddeutsche Zeitung*, that the number of undetected cases is likely to be much higher than what the official bodies have announced.[2] India is a country with

1. COVID-19 Dashboard by the Center for Systems Science and Engineering (CSSE) at Johns Hopkins University. (See https://www.arcgis.com/apps/opsdashboard/index.html#/bda7594740fd40299423467b48e9ecf6)

2. See 'Second lockdown in Israel', *Süddeutsche Zeitung*, 14 September 2020 (https://www.sueddeutsche.de/politik/coronavirus-weltweit-mallorca-inzidenzwert-1.5023075).

the fastest growing number of infections in the world. At the same time, hygiene discipline is declining and Corona fatigue is spreading.

The same applies to Europe, and especially Germany, where hardly a week passed after the lifting of the (comparatively liberal) lockdown without demonstrations against the preventive hygiene measures imposed by the federal government and the sixteen state governments. Approximately 80 per cent of the German people supported these measures, but the number of opponents steadily grew, with the demands of the heterogeneous protest marches becoming louder, and the slogans becoming more diffuse. How did this development come about? Looking back on the first half of 2020, I would like to report out of discourse-ethical interest in the public debate on the COVID-19 pandemic in Germany and embed it in the larger context of crisis communication. This is not so much about the currently known biological-epidemiological facts and mathematical-statistical data—on which I am reporting in collaboration with a microbiologist and a mathematician elsewhere (see Hess-Lüttich et al. 2020)—but rather about the scientific, political, and moral responsibility of the actors in this exceptional global situation, the economic and ecological causes and consequences, as well as the consequences that would have to be extrapolated for crisis management.

INTERIM BALANCE OF AN EPOCHAL CRISIS

In the first quarter of 2020, the entire world was hit by a catastrophe named the 'Corona Pandemic' by the World Health Organization (WHO). Since then, it has dominated public communication to a great extent. For weeks, the media focused on a topic that affects people in almost all countries, in one way or another. Every day in Germany, we follow the speeches of experts from a plurality of disciplines whose scholarly and concerned polyphony makes some people dizzy. Intensive-care physicians, virologists, and epidemiologists show the tables of deaths on televised news and warn of exponentially rising infection rates. They calculate incubation periods and distance requirements, mortality rates, lethality rates, and reproduction figures. They seek to stabilize the number of people infected by a person carrying the disease per day to below one (Rt< 1), because the German health system is unable to cope with more and could become as overburdened as the healthcare systems in Italy or Spain, Alsace, Great Britain, or the US. Microbiologists report from their laboratories and provide us with vivid pictures of the structure of the coronavirus; pharmacologists stir up (in applications for research grants) or dampen (in the media) hopes for drugs and vaccines; engineers and technicians try to convert production plants for the production of respirators or protective masks.

In TV talk shows, economists hold their statistics and projections up to each other, none of them optimistic. Ecologists conjure up the danger of multiple crises and create dystopian scenarios if politicians should lose sight of environmental and climate crises that are no less pressing. Lawyers argue about the limits of serious restrictions on fundamental rights or the delicate issue of generational separation. Sociologists explore the consequences of the lockdown for society in view of the resulting increase in social inequality. Criminologists add up the damage caused by criminal crisis profiteers. Psychologists warn of the increasing risk of domestic violence, loneliness, and depression. Political scientists note the failure of populist leaders, who have no conception of how to solve the problem, but who once again smell conflict issues ('open everything but boundaries') to sow discord. Ethics councils present cleverly balanced papers, and scientific societies offer advice from their representatives. Young people report on Facebook and Twitter how they experienced the almost deserted streets and squares, the ghost stations, the buses or trains with only a few passengers like in a surreal film, or as if they were characters in a dystopian thriller like that of the South African author Deon Meyer, in whose eerily prophetic bestseller *Fever*, first published in Afrikaans in 2017 and in English in 2018, a large part of humanity is infected by a coronavirus.

Keeping track of this public and multimedia babble of voices is an intellectual challenge of its own as well as a fascinating subject of discourse research.

Let us summarize the development of the crisis in the first half of 2020 (in Germany and to some extent in Europe) in a brief sketch, based on the reporting in leading media in Germany such as *Die Zeit*, *Der Spiegel*, *Die Welt*, *Süddeutsche Zeitung*, *Frankfurter Allgemeine Zeitung* and public TV programmes, and use this to derive the central discourse-ethical questions that have shaped the social debate since then.

In mid-November 2019, a young man, let us call him 'Patient Zero', had presumably been infected with a pathogen at the Huanan animal and fish market in the Chinese metropolis of Wuhan, causing symptoms such as fever, cough, and shortness of breath. Within a very short time, the number of cases with the same symptoms increased, reminding doctors of the SARS epidemic of 2002/2003. Then, the ophthalmologist Dr Li Wenliang realizes that danger is imminent, and on 30 December, he reports his observation of a new type of respiratory disease to a group of colleagues. The very next day, he is summoned by the municipal health commission and condemned to strict silence. At the same time, the Chinese government informs the WHO about the virus and closes the animal and fish market in Wuhan.

But it is already too late. On 7 January 2020, the pathogen identified as the 'coronavirus' had already crossed the country's borders and began its rapid march across the globe. On 13 January, the first case outside China was reported from Thailand, and on 27 January, the first case in Germany is confirmed. Borders are closed and air traffic is reduced to a minimum. On 30 January, the WHO identifies a health emergency of international proportions and publishes the corresponding procedural rules: 'Procedures concerning public health emergencies of international concern' (PHEIC). On 11 March, it declares the outbreak of this new viral disease a pandemic (Auswärtiges Amt [Federal Foreign Office] 2020).

While populist politicians in the Western world such as Boris

Johnson, Donald Trump, or Jair Messias Bolsonaro speak of a 'minor flu' or of the 'Chinese virus', which 'will miraculously disappear by itself' (Trump), medical professionals in the affected countries cannot remember anything comparable in their professional lives—medicines, materials, and disinfectants are running out; intensive care units, even entire clinics are crowded with patients who all have an identical diagnosis; up to a third of medical staff will soon receive the same diagnosis; there are not enough test kits for statistical screening; the respirators do not provide for all those who need them; a term from war medicine ('triage') suddenly becomes horribly topical again.

Dr Li Wenliang receives no more help despite an apology from the health authorities; he dies from the consequences of the infection he reported on 7 February. After initial hesitation, the German government also took action in Germany. In the following weeks (until the beginning of April), more than 200,000 Germans were flown back home in special planes from the countries most severely affected by the pandemic in an unprecedented recall operation. At the same time, the closure of kindergartens, schools, universities and other educational facilities not regarded as relevant to basic services was ordered. From 23 March, the restrictions on contact would be further tightened: people would only be allowed to go out into the streets alone, in pairs or with relatives living in their own households; they would have to observe hygiene regulations and keep their distance from other people. Restaurants, clubs, and pubs would be closed, along with various service businesses. Regulatory authorities monitor compliance with the regulations. In neighbouring countries, especially in Southern Europe, much stricter measures are often applied, curfews imposed, and compliance monitored by the police and military. Elderly people are interviewed and confirm that there has not been such a thing since the end of World War II. The fundamental rights of a free society are temporarily suspended.

> The Corona crisis today plunges everyone into an ethical dilemma, no matter who is in charge. Two of the highest

> goods can hardly be reconciled, the protection of life and the freedom of society. The virus calls for a decision on what should weigh more heavily, the danger to the life of individuals or the death of public life. (Bartsch et al. 2020, 29)

'The world stands still' is the title of an article by Giovanni di Lorenzo, editor-in-chief of the renowned Hamburg weekly *Die Zeit*, in its leading article in the issue of 19 March 2020, and describes what triggers the ubiquitously felt threat in people—empathy, creativity, and solidarity in some, and selfishness, greed, and criminal energy in others. Conspiracy myths are discussed in the forums of the networks that cast doubt on 'whether the superstition of the people has changed significantly since the Middle Ages' (di Lorenzo 2020, 1). Breathing masks, disinfectants and protective clothing for hospital staff are not available in sufficient quantities, and the disastrous consequences of the neoliberal economization of the healthcare system and the almost complete dependence on global supply chains are now coming to light in all severity. Crisis profiteers sell inferior or unsuitable protective and consumable materials at a hundred times the current market price, while more and more people fall ill and struggle to survive. Are we prepared to accept these machinations when human lives depend on them?

A tiny virus brings the world's overheated gearbox to an abrupt halt. Economic life comes to a standstill; the social distortions in the wake of it are hardly quantifiable worldwide. What will the crisis cost us, leading economists ask; can we even afford a longer lockdown? Which weighs more—the lives of a few particularly vulnerable people or the social crash of large parts of society? The economic wing of the conservative party Christian Democratic Union (CDU) is quick to call for an end to the restrictions in order not to bring the economy to a complete standstill. What is more important to us—victory over the virus or social life as we knew it? Economy or health? Money or life?

But perhaps the crisis is also an impulse to reorder our priorities. To rethink unquestioned certainties and established habits. Will it have the effect—after the crisis—that the adjective 'systemically relevant' gets a new meaning and is no longer associated only with bosses and bankers, but with the many at the lower end of the income scale who 'keep things running'? Can a virus dampen the mantra of the trinity of growth, prosperity, and value creation?

> How addicted to work and growth have we become that even in matters of life and death the first thought is how to stop the fall in stock prices and help the economy? The question we are confronted with is of magical purity: money or life? (Minkmar 2020, 78)

We will have to come back to such fundamental questions and ethical dilemmas, but any discourse-ethical debate first assures itself of the facts and figures in situations of diverging interests and potential for social conflict. Similar to the environmental, climate, or world financial crises, pandemics are global structural problems of the present that affect every individual. Such key problems, that affect both the individual and society as a whole, are 'typical of the epoch' in the sense of Wolfgang Klafki, in so far as they are 'a canon of problems that may change the future', that they have the potential to change our life and our society in the long term (Klafki 1996, 60). They are global in so far as they affect the (technically, economically, socially) complex networked societies as a whole; they are interdisciplinary in so far as they can only be understood and researched from the plurality of perspectives of different disciplines; they are ethical in so far as they determine maxims of morally correct action (cf. Hess-Lüttich 2020).

ZOONOSES AND HUMAN RESPONSIBILITY

Zoonoses (Greek: ζῷον = zoon = living creature and νόσος = nosos = disease, epidemic) are infectious diseases caused by viruses, but also bacteria, parasites, fungi, or prions that can be mutually transmitted between animals and humans (cf. BfR 2020). Many types of viruses that have spread from bats to humans cause dangerous diseases such as mumps, measles, rabies, Marburg fever, etc. But animals (pigs, cattle, chickens, birds) are also increasingly becoming victims of such epidemics caused by viral infections (and those caused by prions in the case of cattle). Dangerous diseases like the West African Ebola fever (since 2014), the acquired immunodeficiency syndrome (AIDS, since 1959; Zhu et al. 1998) and the severe acute respiratory syndrome (SARS, since 2003) could be attributed to the trade with and consumption of wild animals.

The new head of the UN Environment Programme, Inger Andersen, holds humans, their destruction of the environment and threat to biodiversity, overpopulation, and archaic rituals responsible for zoonoses occurring at ever shorter intervals. When people and animals live closer and closer together, natural habitats of the latter become smaller and barriers to contact disappear. Zika viruses, dengue fever, schistosomiasis, yellow fever, chikungunya, malaria, etc., all have their roots here. Despite all the evidence, Chinese, Southeast Asian, and African governments are apparently unable (or unwilling) to curb wildlife markets, wildlife consumption, and illegal trade of protected species. In April 2020, WWF International and GlobeScan presented current studies and background papers with overwhelming evidence and illustrative diagrams (WWF 2020a, 2020b).

WHAT DOES 'EXPONENTIAL PROPAGATION' MEAN?

While an *epidemic* simultaneously affects a very large number of people in a region, one speaks of a *pandemic* when the epidemic spreads transnationally or worldwide. A distinction must be made between an epidemic disease, which is always present but generally only occurs in a few cases in a population. Historically, there have been many pandemics, and political attempts have been made to identify the culprits. The polemic of the US president ('yet another virus from China'), for example, is applauded on social media as common knowledge: pandemics come from China. However, the 'Spanish flu' (> fifty million dead, lethality < ten per cent) came from Kansas, US (cf. Spinney 2018); HIV and Ebola came from Africa; the cholera epidemic in the 1960s from Indonesia; MERS 2012 from Saudi Arabia; the pig flu or swine influenza from Mexico, etc. The number of mammalian or avian viruses that can jump to humans is estimated at around 700,000, over 260 of which have already done so and can be expected to do so again at any time. A list prepared by the Robert Koch Institute has more than two dozen pathogens that can be particularly dangerous to humans, from AIDS to hepatitis, measles, tuberculosis, and Zika. The history of medicine is one of threats to humans from microbes and their sometimes successful fight against them (cf. Grolle 2020). Interestingly enough, in modern times, an accumulation of pandemics caused by influenza viruses is striking (cf. Rengeling 2017).

The COVID-19 pandemic probably began in mid-November 2019 in the Chinese city of Wuhan in Hubei province, where it initially spread rapidly as an epidemic. The first case of Corona in the US was reported from Seattle on 20 January—the same day as in South Korea. Due to the particular infectiousness of the pathogen, the WHO was forced to speak of an international health emergency as early as 30 January 2020. On 11 March, the WHO finally declared the epidemic a pandemic, the first since the 2009/2010 influenza pandemic (WHO 2020a). Following the outbreak in China, cases were quickly reported from Thailand, the US, and the Philippines. These cases were initially explained by Chinese citizens travelling to or from Wuhan. The first European case was registered in France and was also due to the travel of a Chinese citizen.

In March 2020, the number of new infections in Germany doubled every five days. Only if the reproduction rate is $Rt<1$ should steps to ease the situation be considered, given that a low absolute number of infections also allows health authorities to follow up contacts (the benchmark being 50 cases per 100,000 inhabitants). In fact, the number of infections or deaths worldwide increased dramatically in a short period: the limit of three million infected persons was quickly exceeded, and the number of people dying from the infection had exceeded 230,000 by the beginning of May 2020 (Worldometers 2020;

WHO 2020 b; Gisand data 2020). By the end of March, 192 countries and territories were already affected (depending on the source), including 21 in Asia, 22 in the Middle East, 39 in Africa, 57 in Europe, 46 in the US, and 7 in Australia and Oceania. The WHO counted the most cases in mid-April to be in the US, Spain, Italy, Germany, France, China, Iran, Great Britain, Turkey, Belgium, Switzerland, and the Netherlands (WHO 2020c; Johns Hopkins 2020), while in mid-September the picture had changed considerably—now the list of almost 30 million people infected worldwide was being led by the US (6.52 million), India (4.85 million), Brazil (4.33 million), and Russia (1.06 [?] million), and the number of global deaths was approaching the one million mark (Johns Hopkins 2020).

TAKING MEASURES: CONTAINMENT OR MITIGATION?

In a paper published by the OECD on 20 March 2020 entitled 'Flattening the COVID-19 peak: Containment and mitigation policies' (OECD 2020), the authors summarized the main factors that have contributed to the rapid increase in the number of COVID-19 cases worldwide (the number of reproductive, asymptomatic, and incubation cases) and the measures taken to reduce them (early detection, follow-up of contact with infected persons, hygiene, social distance or keeping distance, school closures, protection of vulnerable groups, travel restrictions, compulsory use of masks).

Until effective vaccines and medicines would become available, countries had to rely on non-medical counter measures to contain the epidemic. Various policy options were being discussed, and in some cases, already implemented to mitigate the COVID-19 pandemic. Suppression models (according to studies by the London Imperial College) aim to stop the spread of the virus through strict measures, while mitigation models aim to keep the number of cases and capacity limits of the healthcare system in balance. Despite efforts by scientists, it seemed unlikely that vaccines would be available in time to prevent the second wave of the pandemic expected in autumn and winter 2020/21. Hopes, therefore, rested for the time being on testing the potential effectiveness of drugs. In terms of vaccines, earlier progress in research and development of emerging coronaviruses formed the basis for current development. SARS-CoV-2 is 80 per cent similar to SARS-CoV-1, the coronavirus that triggered the SARS pandemic in 2002/03.

Research was pursuing three main possible approaches: i) the development of vector vaccines using attenuated vector viruses to introduce hereditary information from SARS-CoV-2 into human cells to stimulate the immune response; ii) virus building blocks produced artificially or separated from the virus by molecular scissors (restriction enzymes), resulting in fewer side-effects but a weaker immune response; iii) the patient being injected only with nucleic acids from the laboratory, which in the cells serve as a blueprint for an antigen that activates immune cells on the cell membrane and stimulates the production of antibodies. Although this technology would enable the rapid production of vaccines in sufficient quantities, it has not yet been approved against any pathogen (cf. Hackenbroch et al. 2020). Unfortunately, which of these three approaches would lead most quickly to a vaccine that could be used globally depended not only on the success of the researchers but also on economic interests.

The (economic) race to a functioning vaccine, therefore, not only touched on medical but also on ethical questions, because researchers and pharmaceutical companies, politicians, and authorities were taking risks that are hardly calculable. At a WHO meeting in mid-February, representatives of public research institutions and pharmaceutical companies agreed that human trials should begin before all animal studies are completed. The decision immediately triggered a discussion in the scientific magazine *Nature*, because animal testing is normally a prerequisite for determining whether a potential vaccine has dangerous side-effects. Vaccine researcher Peter Hotez, for example, was quoted in *Der Spiegel* (21 March 2020) asking whether some companies were trying to use the coronavirus to 'push their experimental technology onto the market' (Hackenbroch et al. 2020, 103). Klaus Cichutek, president of the Paul Ehrlich Institute, which is responsible for vaccine approval, pointed out that there are a number of flexible options for speeding up the approval process, even when due care is taken (ibid.).

Another ethical problem was linked to the question of who benefited from the drugs when they become available. Will they be made available to all countries affected by the pandemic or initially only to those who can pay the most? Will new knowledge be generally available or will it be withheld in national or economic interest? For example, the decision by the US pharmaceutical company Gilead Sciences to exercise its patent rights in full was criticized. Its pricing policy in previous cases (e.g. Sovaldi for Hepatitis C) is obviously more profit-oriented than geared towards the welfare of patients, most of whom cannot afford the drug. The proposal to make materials, drugs, or vaccines available to the WHO for the purpose of fair distribution was also unlikely to be successful at a time when the US President had withdrawn his country's contributions to the organization. The Chairman of the Munich Security Conference, Wolfgang Ischinger, confirmed that insufficient resources (equipment, protective clothing, masks, drugs, vaccines) and the question of their distribution remained, for the time being, an 'ethical, economic and political problem that remains unsolved' (quoted in Kohlenberg et al. 2020, 29).

WARNINGS

Scientists' warnings following the SARS and MERS epidemics, including the speech by Bill Gates in 2015 predicting a Corona pandemic for which the world is not prepared, were ignored by most governments. The Swiss cardiologist Paul Robert Vogt pointed to several such concrete warnings (Vogt 2020). In March 2019, for example, the Chinese epidemiologist Peng Zhou from Wuhan made a concrete forecast in a study that a new Corona pandemic, which originates in China, could be expected to break out at any time. At least after the SARS and MERS epidemics, precautions should have been taken and vaccines developed, criticized the renowned medical historian Frank Snowden in an interview with the news magazine *Der Spiegel* (25 April 2020), recalling the periodically recurring debates on the conflict between humanity and economy, which was mostly decided in favour of the economy, costing countless lives (Snowden 2020).

Germany could also have been better prepared, because the information was available and was not only being discussed in expert circles but officially in the German Bundestag. At the beginning of 2013, a report on risk analysis in civil protection was presented there in *Bundesdrucksache* 17/12051, a federal paper, which anticipated the current pandemic event in a surprisingly realistic scenario. The report presented a risk analysis on the 'pandemic caused by the Modi-SARS virus'. The scenario developed under the leadership of the RKI and with the participation of other federal authorities described in great detail a possible epidemic event that occurred almost exactly as it did a few years later (Deutscher Bundestag 2013, 5). Meanwhile, many critics consider the study to be proof of lack of political action in the conflict of maxims of public welfare and lobby interests. By publishing the results in the Federal Gazette, the RKI fulfilled its ethical responsibility to warn decision-makers and the public in case of imminent danger. But why did the political decision-makers not recognize the explosive nature of this warning at the time and take appropriate precautions?

MORAL DILEMMAS

Unlike in Taiwan, Japan, Singapore, Hong Kong, or South Korea, many governments in Europe, the Americas, and in Russia have allowed valuable time to pass before recognizing the full gravity of the situation and starting to act on their responsibilities. National differences in approaches give food for thought. Some countries—in addition to those already mentioned, such as Great Britain, Brazil, and the US—initially classified the pandemic as an ordinary wave of influenza and relied on the automatic infestation of society ('herd immunity'), which would help to avoid economically unpleasant cuts. The empirical-statistical findings on infectivity and mortality have freely and emphatically refuted this utilitarian risk strategy.

The respective ethical responsibility of decision-makers cannot be delegated to statisticians, stochastics, and epidemiologists. Whether the lethality rate was 0.37% and the mortality rate 0.06%,[3] as the Heinsberg study by Bonn virologist Hendrick Streek suggested, or significantly higher, as the graphs of the RKI or Johns Hopkins University suggested, it would be likely to seem much less important to those affected than the question of whether they will survive the infection. For them, the curve is less important than the area below it, because it represents the number of deaths. This touches on central moral questions that are currently the subject of controversial discourse-ethical debate in public. Should society, as a whole, be held liable for the protection of what may only be a comparatively small proportion of the particularly vulnerable? Is it permissible to offset an individual human life against the damage that the lockdown will cause to many? Should we not sacrifice the particularly vulnerable groups of old and frail people who are no longer in the labour force for the benefit of the young and working people, because they are the ones who generate our prosperity?

Yes, answered the London philosopher Roger Crisp, who defines himself as a representative of the utilitarian school of moral philosophy, in *Der Spiegel* (28 March 2020, 90). He negated the question of whether the individual identifiability of misery should play a role at all in ethical considerations. Rather, one should act in such a way that maximum happiness can be achieved for a maximum number of people. Therefore, it is not only justifiable but rationally necessary to sacrifice a manageable number of human lives of elderly patients,

---

3. Lethality ≠ mortality. Lethality refers to the ratio of the number of deaths from COVID-19 to the number of new cases; mortality refers to the ratio of the number of deaths to the average population.

because this could benefit society as a whole in the end. The German Federal Constitutional Court, referring to Article 1 of the German Constitution and the relevant fundamental rulings derived from it, would probably clearly contradict this. The quoted Swiss physician Vogt also emphatically warns against any eugenic temptation, albeit less for reasons of legal ethics than because of the medical risks of mutation potentials that cannot be predicted with active infestation (Vogt 2020).

Nevertheless, doctors must consider in each case when they put an individual on an available respirator, for example, if two or more patients in need of ventilation are competing for it. This is the classic decision dilemma of *triage*, which in practice is usually solved by a probabilistic approach to the chances of recovery. The recommendations of the German Ethics Council (Deutscher Ethikrat 2020), which claims to provide assistance in the crisis situation of the pandemic, including the principles of solidarity and responsibility, to weigh competing moral goods, also aim in this direction. Considering the core conflict between the human right to life or the fundamental right to physical integrity (pursuant to Article 2 of the German Constitution) on the one hand and the stability of the healthcare system on the other, the Ethics Council sees a need for ethical guidance. In its hand-out, the Council warns, for example, that such 'conflict scenarios should also be understood as normative problems' (Deutscher Ethikrat 2020, 3) and that political decisions in question should not be based solely on scientific recommendations. The representatives of the medical professional associations are also aware of this, and in their statements on such decisions affecting the fundamental rights of patients and which raise questions of prioritization in access to crucial medical resources, they also propose corridors of action, prioritization algorithms, and decision-making aids that would, of course, themselves have to be ethically and juridically safeguarded. This could well lead to collisions between fundamental standards of ethics and law, which 'could turn out to be almost insoluble dilemmas' (ibid.).

In fact, both the Constitution (*Grundgesetz*) and the

catalogue of human rights explicitly do not hierarchize or prioritize fundamental rights. Wolfgang Schäuble, the President of the Bundestag, the German federal parliament, reminded us of this when he warned in the Berlin *Tagesspiegel* (Schäuble 2020) that the right to life should not be given absolute priority. The sentence triggered a lively debate. It is true that the basic rights to life, to freedom, and to equality are absolutely valid as *principles*, but they cannot be absolutely realized without restricting each other. That is why, in social practice, they must be weighed against each other with reasons. The justification structure of such argumentation is complex, especially when individual rights of freedom and collective protection collide and both run counter to the principle of equality, which is considered a condition for the possibility of 'justice'.

In concrete terms, do doctors who are committed to the principle of 'indifference in the value of life', i.e. who are not allowed to make any differentiations or classifications (according to age, gender, ethnic origin, sexual orientation, social role, health prognosis, etc.), but then have to do so in *triage* constellations, feel freed from the dilemma of relying on algorithms and flowcharts in decision-making? In such constellations, the Ethics Council distinguishes between *triage in ex-ante* competition, where the number of respirators is insufficient for those in need, and *triage in ex-post* competition, where life-support measures are terminated for one patient to clear the space at the respiratory care unit for another. In the first case, the decision should be taken based on transparent and uniform criteria; in the second case, the decision conflicts with existing law that explicitly prohibits the active termination of an indicated treatment to save a third party.

Given the sheer number of people affected, decisions concerning the lockdown and the consequences thereof are, therefore, correspondingly controversial in the public debate. According to the German Ethics Council, the necessary protection of human life is not absolute either, i.e. by no means should all other rights of freedom and participation, economic, social, and cultural rights be unconditionally subordinated to it (ibid., 5). It remains to be seen what resources of solidarity our society has at its disposal and what risks the State is allowed to take and responsibilities it is allowed to assume to ensure that the idea of 'secur[ing] the elementary functional conditions of social life' (ibid.) is accepted by the broad majority. The approval can in fact quickly be relativized over time. Even now, demands are being made for the separation of defined risk groups (similar to the separation of homosexual men at the beginning of the HIV/AIDS pandemic) so that younger people who are supposedly less vulnerable can return to work.

Apart from the fact that such demands presuppose strong assumptions that have yet to be medically proven, they are subject to the obligation to justify themselves, as is the case with any restriction of fundamental rights. For example, it should be asked what role utilitarian arguments may play in weighing moral legitimacy and political-administrative legality, or perhaps even should play in avoiding threats to the system. If the central societal functional areas of economy and culture, education, and science are permanently affected by the lockdown, a constant review of the restrictions or their relaxation with regard to appropriateness, effectiveness, and proportionality is required. Prerequisites for this are: i) assured knowledge (provided by science) and ii) democratically mandated decision-making bodies (parliaments).

The political authorities had to make decisions based on fuzzy decision-making premises. As long as there was a lack of fundamental data for reliable information, the process of opening the shutdown remained a dance on the razor blade. As of summer 2020, there was no clear indication whether an infection that had been suffered and overcome guarantees of immunity (reports from South Korea of second infections sowed doubt); and if so, how long it lasts (months, years, a lifetime?); the possibility that, as the virus spreads, mutations of the SARS-CoV-2 type will generate new infections to which there is no immunity could not be ruled out; the hope that summer temperatures would prevent the virus from surviving had proved to be as premature in Europe as it was during the

MARS epidemic in hot Saudi Arabia; how long the SARS-CoV-2 virus can survive on which materials had been as much in dispute as the duration of its infectivity on contact with such surfaces (smear infection); it was unclear how heavily bio-aerosols could be contaminated with particles of SARS-CoV-2 (i.e. transmitted via the air as in influenza, tuberculosis, measles) and what was the minimum infectious dose that leads to infection; speculation also differed regarding the exact role of nitric oxide concentration in the regions with the most severe occurrence of the disease; there were no calculations as to when, with a reproduction rate Rt<1, a minimum 66% (herd immunity) will be reached; far too little was known about the long-term effects of the infection, except that they may affect practically all internal organs; we did not know when drugs would be developed that would be able to defeat the virus with acceptable side-effects; we did not know whether the vaccine registered in Russia as 'Sputnik V' as early as August 2020 would be medically effective at all, or whether it was just used for political propaganda; when and if a vaccine suitable for mass production would ever be available to the general public at all (the often proclaimed prognosis that it will be available by the end of 2020 could have turned out to be wishful thinking, given the failures to date in the development of vaccines against other coronaviruses or HIV). In the meantime, we remained involuntarily witness to and participants in a global experiment.

THE LIMITS OF RESPONSIBLE CARING IN THE COVID-19 PANDEMIC[1]

Joan Tronto

A caring democracy is a democratic state in which engaged citizens understand that the most vital questions faced by government concern the proper allocation of resources and responsibilities so that people can care—that is, be cared for, care for other people and care for their world—and thereby live in the world as well as possible (Tronto 2013). The United States, from where I write, is very far from a caring democracy. From the standpoint of the ideal, the unfolding tragedies of the COVID-19 pandemic provide a sliver of hope that people will suddenly realize and face the horrible situation for caring on a global scale. The optimistic story to tell ourselves about the outcome of the COVID-19 pandemic would run something like this:

Faced with a nefarious new pathogen, humans working to defeat it came to an awareness about the limits of their destructive ways of life. As health officials insisted that 'a virus has no politics', people realized that the pandemic was a kind of 'stress test' for a global way of neo-liberalized, capitalistic life (Tronto 2017).Thus, they saw the limits of organizing the world in a manner that devalued care and the lives of ordinary people for the sake of the accumulation of ever more, unlimited, wealth. Given how unpredictably the virus affected people, leaving some without symptoms and quickly killing others, humans could not deny their mortality and the sense of vulnerability this knowledge produced. Yet from this mutual vulnerability came another revelation, i.e. the profound awareness of the fact that not all people were equally

1. My thanks to Inge van Nistelrooij, University for Humanistic Studies, the Netherlands, for helpful comments on an earlier draft of this essay.

vulnerable. Some are at much greater risk. With this realization came also shame, and from that shame, a desire to act to mitigate the injustice. Hence, throughout the world, people began to press their governments to seriously make provisions for all people to take care of their nearest and dearest, to provide adequate support to all types of essential workers, to reinvest in public institutions such as public health and public transit and public schools. Workers everywhere became treated with dignity and paid adequately, and unpaid care work became as important as waged work. And something else changed as well. Citizens in their own communities and nations began to recognize that what contemporary politics essentially does is to use public resources and frameworks to allocate capacities to care. As the skewed ways in which care is now provided became visible, more and more people demanded of their states that they become caring democracies. As that demand became more firmly entrenched in national politics, the global issues of unequal care in the world became a central political issue. And so, with due attention to cultural and geographic differences, care became the global framework for thinking about what is good, politically.

As much as I wish it were so, this is not going to happen. Not only will this pandemic not usher in a new wave of human solidarity, despite the bland claim that a virus has no politics, here in the United States the politics of dealing with the virus has already provided a way to enlarge and deepen disputes among people and magnify their hatreds. From people who refuse to wear masks as restricting their freedoms to people who race-bait Asian people, the realities of the pandemic are no different from those of other viral infections throughout human history: they provide another pretext to sharpen fears of others.

The question that I want to think through in this essay is why this is so. What makes the scenario of continued ignorance, hatred, and division seemingly more plausible? To answer this question, I want to provide an analysis of what in current American politics limits our capacity to see the alternative world of caring democracy as a possible reality. Three pieces seem to fuel the current vicious circles: the ignorance-responsibility nexus, how hatred and fear of loss fit together, and the destruction of solidarity and trust. After exploring each of these in turn, we can perhaps search more realistically for that sliver of hope.

IGNORANCE AND IRRESPONSIBILITY

> When you know, you're responsible.
>
> —Kate Millett, *Flying* (1974)

One of the strangest phenomena of the present moment is an incapacity to separate fact from fiction and therefore to make analytical judgements. Why? Some attribute this decline in faith to scientific knowledge, to the growth of the internet and the spread of multiple competing claims for authority in providing knowledge and 'information'. New technologies always disrupt human patterns of interaction; the ready availability of many different realities and kinds of opinions seemingly creates a free-for-all. I think there is, however, another, deeper, and equally compelling, explanation. It has to do with the nexus of knowledge and responsibility. Responsibility grows out of a response to something or someone. If one is ignorant about the existence of the other and one's relationship to them, then one cannot be held accountable for not solving a problem they have. One cannot exercise responsibility, that is, use one's power to respond, in the face of ignorance of the fact that a response is called for. Denying the existence of white supremacy, for example, absolves a white person of being the beneficiary of the many ways in which whiteness functions to give one an advantage.[2] Saying 'I didn't know' is the first defence for inaction. And because one doesn't know what knowledge might lead one to a new kind of responsibility, being ignorant is a form of protection against any kind of undesired action. Hence, the

2. Among the burgeoning literature on this topic, see Harris (1995), Lipsitz (2006), Katznelson (2005), Merritt (2017).

eager acceptance of Donald Trump's pronouncements that 'It's all a hoax...' or the denial that face masks protect oneself and others from the coronavirus. From this perspective, ignorance, as a method for abjuring responsibility, becomes something else again. It becomes a way to avoid change; it becomes an important form of self-protection, of self-care.

What can we do about such ignorance? Famously, Socrates posed this as one of the limits of philosophy in the opening lines of *The Republic*: His colleagues ask him, 'How can you persuade us if we refuse to listen?' Despite Socrates's acknowledgement that there is nothing one can do in the face of such an unwillingness to listen, it is still worth pointing out why such ignorance is so harmful. Blanket ignorance requires a thoughtless approach to one's responsibilities. So how can one know which responsibilities are appropriately one's own? Being able to make such judgements requires capacities for thought, action, and self-reflection. It requires discussions with those whom one is connected to decide which are proper, and which improper, requests for responsibility (Walker 2007). Simple denial of the reality of one's interconnections with others makes it easy to avoid not just responsibility but even the need to consider that one might be responsible.

Thus, in a perverse way, ignorance becomes a form of self-care. If, for example, white Americans remain ignorant of the ways in which they benefit from various forms of white privilege, and if they believe that African Americans are simply lazy, then they can absolve themselves of any blame for the wealth and income gaps in the United States. Indeed, when we listen to the resentment expressed by white Americans against 'lazy' African Americans, we can also hear the grounding of their view that African Americans are themselves responsible for their fate.[3]

Avoiding responsibility through ignorance is a risky strategy because it leaves one in a state of ignorance. It makes it dangerous

3. On white Americans' views of African Americans as lazy, and the opposing reality, see Gilens (1999), Jones and Wilson (2017).

to live in a world where one does, in fact, need to know some things about how the world operates. The alternative is to become fatalistic and to avoid one's responsibility by denying that one has any power to enact change. So the task is to persuade people that their pursuit of ignorance is a *perverse* form of caring for oneself. But how to accomplish this end? This is not only difficult because people do not want to be persuaded of it, but also because anyone else who tries to persuade them of it will be viewed with suspicion simply because they are saying it is not a good thing to be ignorant. The ease of saying 'fake news' to anything that challenges one's worldview is a very effective way to reduce cognitive dissonance, to remain ignorant, and to continue to believe that one is right. It provides a blanket answer to all challenges, and it only deepens itself over time. After all, wilful ignorance is a passive way to exist. It turns citizens into passive recipients of others' views, claims, and ways of thinking. In such a state, the way not to appear passive is to become ferociously active and aggressive in the defence of one's ignorance.

Hence, ignorance becomes interlaced with fear and hatred. This hatred and fear is not the opposite of love, though. I would describe it as a perverse kind of care for the self or care for the in-group[4] that grows out of a fear of being asked to take on responsibilities for one's past action. Simply to accuse people with whom one disagrees of being 'haters' cannot persuade them. To their minds, they are acting out of love for what is familiar to them, not out of hatred. This is the key lesson to learn, for example, from Arlie Hochschild's account of *Strangers in their Own Land* (Hochschild 2016). The discussion is not between love and hate, but between different ways to understand collective responsibility. What then becomes complicated is when responses to consider responsibilities differently are met with hatred and fear.

4. Although I do not find sociobiological arguments so persuasive, Daniel Engster (2015) makes the case for them as limiting care to in-groups.

HATE-FILLED HEARTS AND THE EXISTENTIAL FEARS OF 'OTHERS'

> You've got to be taught / To hate / And fear…
>
> —Richard Rodgers, 'You Have To Be Carefully Taught', *South Pacific* (1958)

Ironically, those with hate-filled hearts rationalize their hatred by describing their actions and beliefs as care. These beliefs are often saturated with a view about masculinist protection; as Iris Young argued nearly twenty years ago, security discourses often hinge on the protection of the vulnerable, especially of women and children, not from all men, but from bad men, who are always framed as those 'others' (Young 2003). While Young cast this form of protection as 'masculinist', it also applies to other forms of protective care; one needs protection from those others who lurk outside of the family, community, religious or ethnic group, or nation. It is easy to believe that they are the threat to the 'good' people who are deserving of protection, who just happen to overlap almost entirely with 'us', whoever 'we' are. In this way, insisting of the need to care for 'us' becomes an 'inoculation against insight' as W.O. Brown described a rationalization (Brown 1933). It becomes a justification for hateful attitudes towards others, and for action to separate them from us. In this way, justice and care become intertwined: those others are literally beyond our care because they deserve hatred, not care.

For some people, the proper way to care for themselves and those closest to them is to hate or fear 'others' and to teach their children to hate or fear those same others as well. Such hatred justifies segregation and thus, behind the gap in experience of knowing those others, there is nothing to undo the view that those others are as they are imagined. Such hatred and its subsequent forms of separation thus produce profound ignorance about the others which also generates fear of them, shame about the ignorance, and so forth.

DESTROYING SOLIDARITY AND TRUST

From this way of looking at the world, denying that one shares any responsibility to those others becomes an easy act, fed not only by ignorance but also by hatred, disgust, and distaste. Something more happens, though, than simply losing the capacity for empathy. Since showing empathy for the other would now be seen as betrayal of those to whom one is close, one must now defend one's hateful views ever more forcefully and ignore evidence for compassion in front of one. Such hatred becomes self-reinforcing.

Adding economic pressures to this toxic stew only makes it worse. If one thinks of the amount of care, and the stock of resources for care in the world, as limited, then one needs to be able to limit others from taking from one's own share of such care resources. Before long, one's desire to care for one's own has become the limit to recognizing the legitimate claims of others. And because one is doing it for the right reasons, it becomes difficult to dislodge such views. Imagine: if one cares for their own and leaves others to do the same, can one not say that this is good care? Too bad for the other if they are simply not very good at taking care of their own, another reason to disparage them.

Indeed, if such hate-filled hearts also donate to charity, they can convince themselves that their charity is a sufficient form of care for others. The problem is that while acts of charity are generous and praiseworthy, they are no way to solve inadequate care in a democratic society. Charity requires people to make judgements and to distinguish the worthy from the unworthy. In a democratic society, we should treat each other as equals. Reducing others to charity cases diminishes them as our equals.

Here is another problem with the one-off nature of charitable care: Care needs not only to be timely (White 2020), it also needs to be reliable over time. While caring well for one other through one crisis is a kind of care deserving of gratitude, once we try to scale-up care to the social and political level more is required than acts of occasional charity. After all, in order to make care politically meaningful, we must expect that care will reoccur throughout any particular person's life and throughout the life-cycle. At any moment in every society, there are infants, children, teens, adults who work at jobs away from home, people with some kinds of disabilities, elderly people, and people with illnesses. All of these caring needs have to be met at once; no one person or family can meet them all. So a society requires care on a more permanent and reliable level. People need to know that all of those types of care will be available for them when they need them. This ability to rely upon ongoing care, 'caring with' (Tronto 2013), requires the virtues of solidarity and trust. Here, solidarity refers to a kind of fellow feeling that one shares with others who are in a similar situation or for whom one can have empathy; for example, all of the parents in a school share a sense of solidarity about the education their children receive; members of Amnesty International feel solidarity with political prisoners. Trust refers to a relationship with caregivers or others responsible for care that good care will be provided; for example, the parents feel trust towards the school's staff and the school district's administrators. Both trust and solidarity are vital elements of this democratic political form of caring-with and they reinforce each other.

Ignorance breeds distrust and dissolves solidarity. People who are trying to remain ignorant—to avoid assuming responsibilities—are also likely to become distrustful of the institutions with which they interact, because they do not understand what is happening in those institutions. Hatred of others makes it difficult to feel solidarity with them. So if one cannot extend care beyond one's narrow circle it becomes more difficult to experience solidarity with others who are similarly placed, or to trust institutions or experts who are not within one's immediate circles of care.

Thus, ignorance, hate-filled hearts, distrust and the absence of solidarity join to create a situation in which people come to think that the best thing they can hope for is caring for their own selves and narrow circles of care. This is precisely the wrong way to tame a pandemic.

PANDEMIC EXPECTATIONS

A pandemic affects everyone but it does not affect everyone in the same way. The coronavirus pandemic has seemed to expose the limits to good care in the USA. People of colour and the poor have been disproportionately affected by the virus. Supply chains have broken down and nurses have demonstrated to receive proper personal protective equipment (PPE). The scandalous lack of standards to ensure that nursing homes provide adequate care has been exposed to the public at large. And the kinds of distrust borne of hatred and ignorance wrecked the ability of public health officials to get people to protect themselves and others in an epidemic by wearing a mask, quarantining, and practising social distancing. Before we can escape from this vicious circle, there is one more complication to consider: how power interacts with responsibility, ignorance, hatred and the absence of trust and solidarity.

Arguments eschewing responsibility through ignorance leave the structures of responsibility in place as they are. Those in positions of relative power therefore get to keep their power. Claims to justify caring through existing hate-filled paths also constitute an argument to leave things as they are, and even roll back recent forms of democratic inclusion. Those who claim to be hateful protectors thereby maintain and perhaps enhance their power. Raising questions about whether responsibilities are properly allocated in a democracy potentially upsets this balance of power. From the standpoint of the powerful, it is better to leave such questions about responsibilities for care unasked.

What democratic caring requires, though, is precisely the opposite; it requires asking who should have which caring responsibilities for whom, who should be called upon to make which sacrifices.[5] Philosophical arguments about how to act justly almost always include some account of reciprocity:

5. On allocating responsibilities for care, see Tronto (2013). On allocating sacrifices, see the important analysis by Danielle Allen (2004).

put yourself in the place of others and see what would you do, or how you would react to your actions from that other position. But this task of putting oneself in someone else's shoes is perhaps one of the most difficult and challenging of intellectual and emotional tasks. It requires curiosity, deep knowledge of oneself and others, a willingness to set one's own views, existential threats, etc. aside, and a capacity for self-reflection. Ironically, I would argue that rather than it being one of the marks of the most civilized among us, it seems to be a skill about which the truly powerful and rich have trained themselves to be incapable.[6] Reading Adam Hochschild's account of the British military at the outset of World War I, it is clear that much of the tragic outcomes arose because those generals had simply become complacent in their belief that they knew everything that there was to know about military science (Hochschild 2011), or Robert Putnam's account of the dysfunction of Southern Italian culture where no one would tell the padrone the truth (Putnam 1993).

People in positions of great power often cannot gauge how frustrated and angry the people beneath them are: hence, the collapse of the Soviet Union and its satellite states, perhaps what unfolds at the present moment in Belarus, perhaps the fate of white racists in the United States. This incapacity to know the world does not always produce this outcome, but at some critical moments, the misjudgement that comes from dismissing others' experience of care comes at an immense cost. Ignorance may keep people from drawing connections about justice to their own lives, fear-mongering may keep people from recognizing others as equally in need of, and capable and willing to provide, care. But at some point, the advantages that elites gain from keeping these structures of destructive erosion among people may dissipate. At that moment, people will be ready to act together, in concert, to see how more caring democracies may function.

6. Indeed, some accounts of Hegel on the master-bondsman relationship also argue that the master is the more ignorant one. For constraints of space we shall refrain from fully engaging this idea here.

Yet, sadly, there is also a limit to this form of learning. Unjust elites motivate their base to fear to hold on to their power. They do so by projecting their own motives onto others: they project onto those they have oppressed their own greedy and biased motives. They fear, out of their ignorance, that if they let go of the unjust power they have wielded, they will be crushed in the same way that they have tried to crush their inferiors. But, as Kimberly Latrice Jones, a protester in Minneapolis, made the point shortly after the murder of George Floyd, this is not what protesters seek. Speaking to those who feared that the loss of property meant danger to themselves, she remarked, 'And they are lucky that what Black people are looking for is equality and not revenge' (Jones 2020).

Limits to our abilities to understand the experiences, desires, aspirations, of others are, however, a fairly abstract concern. The real task is to bring the discussion down to more concrete levels, to discuss the actual practices of care that are being disrupted. For example, the absence of personal protective equipment in hospitals is a real danger. The inability to pay one's rent or to feed one's family are real problems. In situations of unequal power, of unequal knowledge, of co-morbidities, when we may need others' care, where we are standing at the outset will have a profound effect on what happens to us. From the standpoint of those who would guide us more safely and humanely through a pandemic, this becomes a question of trust. Who can be trusted, and how?

How might we learn about the limits of using care as a way to speak about public life? It requires that we take true measures of care. How much care is needed, in what forms, to maintain a system of public schools where work schedules and school schedules do not match each other? How much care is needed to provide adequate PPE and medical treatment for all, when some are afraid to call doctors? How much should people's desires to open their businesses supersede the needs of public health? These are the kinds of questions that need to be hashed through by using a concern for care as the guidance for democratic engagement. To do so also requires being knowledgeable and informed about all of these issues and avoiding ignorance about them.

Not all human societies have been subject to the unmitigated greed of the contemporary global ruling class, and many societies in the past had various means to mitigate the effects of inequality. Many religious practices limit the harms that can be inflicted on the lesser people within the society. Redress for the accumulated greed of the modern world would require revolutionary changes. It would require a huge tax on wealth, a reckoning with colonialism, forgiveness of the debts of lower-income countries. It would require redrawing property boundaries and giving back, redistributing, public and private resources. Imagine thinking about creating a limit to systems of injustice.

It is important to become curious about how many practices for justice, which restore conditions for better care, exist within our vast intellectual traditions. And new practices might come from our imaginations were we set free from the limitations of hatred and fear and protecting only our own. It is daunting to think about what we would have to do in order to live up to the responsibilities of our capacities to limit a pandemic, provide enough food, stop global warming, and make the world a better place. But the fear of taking such action are the real limits that this pandemic has exposed.

PANDEMIC: PHILOSOPHY AND PUBLIC POLICY

Sebastiano Maffettone

1

My book, entitled *Il Quarto Shock* (*The Fourth Shock: How a Virus Changed the World*),[1] published in the summer of 2020, at the height of the first wave of the COVID-19 pandemic, poses a mystery to be solved right upfront: the choice of title. What do I mean by a 'Fourth Shock'? The conceit is that humanity—in a time of pandemic—is experiencing a massive shock. This due to a microscopic virus that has exposed humans in all their impermanence. It has rendered us from one day to the next more insecure and fragile. A similar shock wave took place but three other times in the past: when intellectual giants such as Copernicus, Darwin, and Freud begrudged us our sense of being masters of our creation, our destiny. Suddenly, we have found ourselves acutely aware of how the globalized society we had constructed could find itself faced with a fatal threat, all from natural causes; at the hands of Mother Nature, who we believed to have been domesticated and controllable. A nature that revealed itself to be far more stubborn than we could have ever imagined—and just as social—bound as we were to our human capacity for technological and economic innovation.

Throughout 2020, in an effort to gain understanding, we listened to and learned from scientists, physicians, journalists, and politicians. At first, we were terrified over COVID-19; after all, our lives were at stake, and those of our loved ones, not to mention that of so many human beings. Then, we started

---

1. The book was published in Italian by Luiss University Press, first in digital format (May 2020) and then in print (June). As far as I can tell, it was one of first 'philosophical' books published on the COVID-19 pandemic.

fretting over the economic crisis that followed. We barricaded ourselves in our homes, physically isolated, and, for the first time in our existence, we engaged with the outside world almost entirely through digital means. In short, we were living through, and still are living in, an unprecedented crisis.

To take things seriously, an all-encompassing vision was called for: one that went beyond the various specializations or particulars. We needed a narrative that allowed us to pick up right back where the train of our thoughts and feelings had been derailed. Ever since childhood, we've been conditioned to conquer our fears and accept real-world challenges through the telling of fables, the tales of our youth. Like the story of Simba, the Lion King, my grandchild's favourite book. Simba's story is an exemplary tale of death (of his father), loss, and surrender, and in the end, a return to the majesty that awaits him. My book offers a similar narrative arc, albeit in spirit, if not in substance. It tells the story of an epic crisis, of a person who takes stock of himself when confronted with a mortal danger—to himself and his community—and extends an invitation to reflect upon the various means of escape. Just like in the best of fairy tales.

Approaching this from a bird's-eye view, as I've defined it, means first and foremost compiling various perspectives on the pandemic, starting with ethical and economic considerations. With regard to ethics, especially if drawing upon its Kantian origins, life holds a certain priceless 'dignity'. I would like to own a safe car, for example, but I'm not willing to spend any amount for it. The same goes for the entrepreneur who wants workers to work at a company that doesn't take excessive risk, or the train company that strives to avoid accidents. Although it may seem strange at first glance, such issues often come up when it comes to healthcare and the healthcare system. With the latter, predominantly a public service (in Italy), it's hard to imagine there being no limit of expense when it comes to saving the life of a single patient. Usually, the question gets resolved, so to say, by splicing the argument in two: Hospitals and nursing homes have limited resources subject to government budgets and they must operate within the confines of said budget.

A pandemic unleashed confounds the typical structure in place, however. In fact, the pandemic forces a correction, demanding a commensurate increase in healthcare provisions, as was the case when the northern Italian region of Lombardy was hard hit by a raging epidemic. On the other hand, another way of looking at it comes into play; one that's not based on a simple cost-benefit analysis: an emergency-based model, that of 'rescue'. In a rescue model, calculations aren't made. You stage an immediate intervention, and that's it. If you're an Allied soldier arriving in Auschwitz in 1945, you don't take time out for reasoning—instead, you try to reach all the victims as quickly as you can. The same goes if you see someone drowning, or, perhaps you come across a submarine on the ocean floor. The question, then, is: In what way, in the throes of a pandemic, must we apply the rescue model?

The answer is not simple. Once again, we're tempted to state that, morally speaking, we must undoubtedly strive to save as many lives as possible, at any cost. Politically speaking, however, that may not be the case. Policy must be determined after weighing all of the options on the table, not just those moral considerations. And it's here that perspective is called for, to reiterate: If something were missing from Italian policy-making during this pandemic—and truthfully, not only in Italy—it was the weighing out of all the various available options in terms of determining a proper response. Often, we had the sense that the position taken, in light of the triumvirate of Experts-Policy-makers-Media, meant that the rescue model would prevail, if only because it was far easier to communicate and it paid off in terms of garnering immediate consensus. But the body politic, as difficult as it may be, must task itself with mediating between the two models in order to arrive at the optimal solution that, yes, protects public health, but does not at the cost of wreaking inordinate damage to the economy. Obviously, considerations such as these are easier said than done.

Posing questions over what the repercussions brought on by the pandemic will be for individuals, and what they will hold for society as a whole, are inescapable. And should the current crisis offer unequivocal lessons for the future, what are they? Are there any outcomes we need to ward off? In response to these queries, *Il Quarto Shock* is an attempt towards guiding the reader to frame a current philosophy surrounding the COVID-19 pandemic; a philosophy that can provide analysis as well as advance proposals by means of public ethics and critical thinking.

~

Il Quarto Shock starts off with an undertaking of the notion of public ethics, leading into a deconstruction of the purely clinical treatment of the pandemic. It's presented as an environmental reaction resulting from a mismatch between technological and socio-economic growth on one hand and our emotional and genetic response on the other. It presumes the current theory that the pandemic appears to be fundamentally an environmental crisis. The question is complicated by the fact that the separation between society and nature, as traditionally thought of, is perhaps no longer valid. The social sphere is quite dependent on the natural world, starting with the fact that it is populated by various non-humanoid actors, bacteria, and viruses among them. At the same time, the natural world is ever more imbued within the social arena, in an era which, not by chance, is labelled the 'Anthropocene'—literally, 'the era of Humankind'.

It is my belief that this pandemic has served to expose yet another example of human impotence. This example can be classified under an even more general category. Biologists refer to this overall classification of cases as 'evo-devo', whereby 'evo' stands for evolution and 'devo' for development. Generally speaking, evolutionary developmental biology (evo-devo) can be defined as a field of research that explores natural history from the perspective of the mechanisms presiding over the biological evolution. This field has led us to discover that, in nature, it is possible to modify gene regulation to draw out new functions or to co-opt a form so it may adopt an adaptation different from what was originally intended. There exist genetic mechanisms that activate or suppress the switches and regulatory genes that, in turn, determine the form, positioning, and dimensions of each structure.

It's here that we preach the existence of a mismatch: On one side, slow human evolution, requiring great lengths of time measured in hundreds of thousands (if not millions) of years, while on the other side, technological and economic growth, often measured in just dozens of years. When something occurs, it may come with a lapse in time. In this instance, humans aren't able to allot, both genetically and psychologically, the necessary time for external growth (technological and otherwise). During this time lapse, we, as individuals and as a species, may sustain enormous damages; and ones that prove not (easily) countered. And it's for this very reason that human beings become acutely aware of their own impotence.

In this field of research, some of the most interesting hypotheses advanced are those coming from epigenetics. Simply stated, epigenetics is the discipline of studying alterations in an organism caused by modifications in gene expression, and not from modifications found in the actual genetic code. This implies a certain plasticity of development that acts through environmental interactions between the *genotype* and (via induction) the *phenotype*.

Modifications that occur epigenetically can be passed down even if they don't mutate actual genetic information or genotype. From here, it's not difficult to imagine that the changes in question may be elicited by environmental disturbances provoked by human beings; the kinds of failures, as we are all aware, that place the entire equilibrium of the planet at risk. The human propensity to disrupt the universe depends on the capacity to modify its own ecological niche in its own image and likeness through the use of technologies.

This capability is without a doubt unique and truly extraordinary. But it comes with a downside, one that could have grave consequences for human health. We are more and more presented with evidence showing how pollution may influence the epigenome. So much so that it's given rise to a new therapeutic approach called 'clinical epigenetics' which looks into the impact on the individual resulting from environmental pollutants and the possibility that they can be passed down to subsequent generations.

To this, one can effectively add the theoretical hypothesis—confident in empirical data derived from experimentation—that viral infections such as SARS-CoV-2 can also be regulated epigenetically. As a result, one can surmise that we should be moving in this direction, even from a clinical standpoint. This is already under way at the COVID-19 Open Research Dataset (CORD-19), in fact, as announced by the White House Office of Science and Technology Policy in partnership with organizations such as the Chan Zuckerberg Initiative, Microsoft Research, Allen Institute for Artificial Intelligence, National Institutes of Health National Library of Medicine, Georgetown University Center for Security and Emerging Technology, Cold Spring Harbor Laboratory and Google's Kaggle AI platform.

Epigenetics, as stated above, is usually described as the study of those genetic and non-genetic factors that can control some variations of the phenotype. These variations are generally influenced by our relationship with the outside environment, interactions that modify gene performance without necessarily changing the makeup of the DNA structure. Viruses like SARS-CoV-2 aren't able to mutate DNA structures but can alter that of the epigenome by permitting it to weaken the immune system response, for example, thereby facilitating the spread of disease. Over the last ten years, an immense body of study has been dedicated to providing an explanation for the correlation between autoimmune disorders and their evolution and epigenetic alterations. The basic premise being that environment can play a heavy hand in determining and modulating modifications that alter—not our genetic code—but the expression or repression of certain genes. This does not signify that Darwin was wrong and Lamarck was right: we nonetheless pass down *our* own genome to descendants, not a different one. It can signify that some genes alter their response, and in doing so, also alter the risk of contracting one disease or another.

Various forms of epigenetic alterations are found in the pathogenesis of the immune system. So it is not out of the question that a similar occurrence could be seen in the transmission of a virus like SARS-CoV-2, even though this is just a hypothesis. As we've learned, the coronaviruses are all part of a wide family of animal and human pathogens that include SARS-CoV, MERS-CoV, and so forth. The pathogenesis of the COVID-19 virus in these cases is complex, but what they all have in common is the capability to involve entry into the phenotype; resulting in its ability to replicate and thereby control one's pre-existent immune system.

Epigenetic research can investigate environmental pathogens that alter phenotype makeup (causing disease), without undermining the underlying genotype. The problem with the group of viruses mentioned above, and COVID-19 in particular, is that they have developed a huge ability to keep the host epigenome at bay, and by doing so, control the immune system response and the defensive barriers overall, leading to a replication of the virus and, in short, the pathogenesis of it.

The current pandemic can be classified as one of those paradigm cases in which the spillover from technological and economic-social growth to humans was not as yet constrained. Spillover in these cases means that a virus like COVID-19 can nest inside animals, finding its way to invade humans in only a few and unfortunate circumstances, ultimately giving rise to pathogens that are epigenetic in nature, as described above.

Industrial agricultural, mining, progressive urbanization, deforestation, air pollution, desertification, and in general, the transformation of habitats are destroying our once uncontaminated nature. The level of planetary biodiversity is at risk, and more and more animal species are learning to cohabitate with humans or are consumed as food. The viruses that flagellate us time and again come directly from nature, at one time in the wild, but now expropriated from animals with which we are in direct contact. David Quammen, in his prophetic novel *Spillover: Animal Infections and the Next Human Pandemic* tackled this very notion.

The 'World of Life' rebels against the pace of undefined economic and technological progress. What follows is a dark regurgitation of evils that run the gamut from pollution to epidemics. With this current global pandemic, it's been theorized that the disease attacks our species via epigenetics. In such cases, the rationality behind each single case—taken individually—is insufficient to contain the perverse 'evo-devo' effects, as we refer to them. Proposed solutions in terms of public morals, at the end of the day, are in line with what Yuval N. Harari proposed in an article published in the *Financial Times* (20 March 2020): Encouraging individuals to take ownership is better than spying on them, and global cooperation proves indispensable. Though at the same time, it calls for vastly different means of getting there.

In terms of public morals, the long-term solution means encouraging personal responsibility, both from an individual and a collective point of view; enhancing cognitive and critical thinking, so they may prove to be more responsive and strive for the good of others.

~

The next chapter of *Il Quarto Shock* takes up what could be the most delicate question of all: How can we profoundly change our own selves?

I take a two-pronged approach to answer this. In the first section, I emphasize the fundamental rapport between science and economics on one side and the individual on the other, in order to close a destructive gap. In the second part, instead, I present the necessity to create a sense of limitation, an effort to apply the brakes on our presumptuous and dangerous feeling of omnipotence. Here, I bring up various practices extending from psychoanalysis to meditation that can assist in raising the necessary consciousness. The chapter closes with an *abrégée* version of the theory of value.

In my opinion, there exists a sense of our own limitations

that emerges from deep within contemporary culture. This is evident, for example, in the latest developments in bioethics or in psychoanalytic reflections on omnipotence and the rampant narcissism that underpin our technological and capitalistic society. The significance of these criticisms raised against progress lies in the assumption that not everything based on technology has to be done in the name of economic and ethical-political prospects. Allowing oneself to be carried away by the rapid pace of technology and capitalism can result in both a perverse unravelling of our natural world as well as a loss of the sense of our human experience (caused by an incapacity to rely on the profound demands of an abandoned naturalness, for example). This vision is interesting because it does not rely upon the (un)sustainable world of metaphysics of being or on the laws of God, but rather, leans on a sort of categorical, modernized imperative; in other words, on a moral wedge that asserts limits to the exploitation of our environment and resources.

The concept of our sense of limitation is in a way, wholly original, even though it draws from some of the concepts advanced by Foucault on morals and self-care. I consider it novel if for no other reason than, after having pondered public ethics in the wake of authors such as Habermas and Rawls, I usually gave scant attention to ideas behind personal transformation. But this concept runs in concert with a more general trend: The fact that, these days, our perspectives of the world rely predominantly on scientific underpinnings, obfuscating the complex inner workings of our individual character; thereby rejecting any animistic, totemistic or analogistic notions (as various cultural anthropologists have observed, among them Philippe Descola), despite these very characteristics being innate to each of us.

On the other hand, a similar occurrence burst onto the scene in the history of Western thought, for example, during the Renaissance. Around the end of the sixteenth century, alternative thinkers such as Giordano Bruno raised a certain qualitative ontology as juxtaposed with the quantitative thinking of Galilei. In other words, they were only recuperating the abandonment of animistic philosophy addressed by Descola. And the '*eroici furori*'—the 'heroic raptures' of Brunian thinkers—to follow were but a regurgitation of the vitality that had been overshadowed by the dominant physical-mathematical models and in the process, hyper-objectifying the external world, thereby discarding its affinity to us.

The sense of limitation, as referenced above, has to do with the recouping of a lost awareness which the prevalent mind-set typically attempts to reject. The impossibilities that a reliance on technology has forced us to reckon with tend to coincide with finding new ways to think outside the box in terms of our sense of identity. From this perspective, one may say that a sense of limitation offers a prospect for sustainable policies (the argument addressed in Chapter 3 of *Il Quarto Shock*). Aligning ourselves with the paradigm of sustainability, means accepting our own innate limitations that we heretofore had cast from our collective consciousness.

In this way, the fact that sustainability touches on both the limits of individual morals by virtue of creating an ad hoc responsibility, as well as on the equilibrium of the entire system, it appears more or less as a promising signal from a philosophical vantage point. The most interesting aspect of a social psychology hinged upon a concept of limitation consists, however, in the capacity of a similar model to explain market and consumer behaviours. For the 'limitation model' to be sound, consumer choices must be oriented in a different way, towards being substantially sustainable. Consumers, over time, will exhibit their preferences for businesses with a proven capacity to offer sustainable products in the marketplace.

The increase over time of the market share of those so-called 'fair trade and equitable' products, along with the financial success of sustainable markets will open the doors to other options as well. This means that businesses with more sustainable business practices (in general, operating from non-economic means of accounting), will ultimately make a profound impact even on financial markets.

In other words, the social-psychological implications of being aware of our own limitations as discussed above, correspond to a subjective introjection of those physical barriers to growth that the sustainable development paradigm strives to yield upon the very foundations of economic theory.

~

Chapter 3 of *Il Quarto Shock* is based on premises made in the first two, addressing, as already anticipated, a global programme of environmental, economic and social sustainability. It seeks to provide an answer to the pressing possibilities of a dystopian future comprised of ecological crises and global inequities. I start out with questioning the destiny of democracy and capitalism: Will they be able to make the radical changes that fully respond to what is required of them? Won't this usher in new forms of egoism and authoritarian risks?

~

The final and fourth chapter looks to draw some conclusions based on all that preceded it; seeking to avoid any ambiguity in interpretation, by reiterating the normative nature in a philosophic sense of my vision serving to clarify the political aspirations for a liberal and social democracy.

The final meditation on death is an invitation to reflect on the end of life and the afterlife, thoughts that have certainly accompanied this tragic period of loss and mourning. Even for those who don't believe in an individual's life after biological death, the concept—induced by the pandemic—that humanity could, sometime in the future, vanish, renders our most vivid and true desires senseless. This line of thinking seems to confirm the previous stance regarding value: that value depends on the relationship between us and others. A thesis that may hold weight as a philosophic conclusion of an undoubtedly philosophic tome, but one written to explain oneself to any ready and willing reader. At least, one hopes.

2

This next section tackles the implicit philosophical underpinnings of *Il Quarto Shock*. Overwhelmed by a tidal wave of emotion, terrified of death, shocked by an unexpected and truly devastating event, we're forced to reflect. In effect, culture, art and sciences are all facing epic challenges. The COVID-19 pandemic isn't a crisis like any other. It represents the apex of a curve marking the end of an era. In other words, the pandemic has, in effect, ushered in a paradigm shift. It's from this perspective that I would like to present my interpretation, by emphasizing three philosophic aspects that characterize this paradigm shift:

1) First, central to the new paradigm will be a rediscovery of complexity.
2) Second, philosophy can play a role in this new paradigm, based on its complexity and capacity to be 'inter-linear' and critical.
3) Finally, one must reflect upon the role that the notion of value and normativity plays in this new paradigm as I have illustrated.

I will start out clarifying what I mean by these three assumptions, as follows: The past counts when it comes to cultural evolution, as historians teach us, but in a different way than by way of natural evolution. Culturally speaking, change comes far more rapidly. I was born a Catholic, but if I wanted to, I could become a Buddhist without experiencing any real delays in terms of evolution. Biological evolution, instead, requires an enormous environmental pressure for it to transpire. Cultural changes, far less. Traditionally, it was thought that biological evolution occurred purely by chance. But more recently, we have gained greater systemic insights, leading one to believe—as previously asserted—that perhaps epigenetic changes can influence evolution by way of changes in the environmental context.

One could venture moreover that the same thing applies to cultural evolution. The COVID-19 pandemic should signal that it's time to renovate our collective house; or rather, our ecological niche. Philosophy plays a role in this by learning to take into greater consideration the systemic complexities of the realm in which we operate. Systemic complexities that, on one hand, obligate us to think and act in terms of collective intelligence, while on the other, to favour the robust resilience of nature.

Collective intelligence means that the vast problems we face today can't be solved in a vacuum. If a Leonardo da Vinci were to come into this world in today's day and age, he wouldn't be an individual but a group of persons. An interdisciplinary and multitasking group. The traditional—and on the whole sensible—imprint of academic specialization is no longer viable. In the sense that it's no longer equipped to solve the tremendous issues of our day, from environment to finance, from poverty to epidemics. This does not signify we should abandon pursuing individual competencies, but rather we must learn to integrate them with other areas. That is what's meant by collective intelligence.

The COVID-19 pandemic brought all of this to light. Healthcare issues are just the tip of the iceberg. Beneath the surface lie ecological, economic, political issues and our response to them. Only through teamwork can we even begin to confront the entirety of such intricate issues. Today, we boast widespread potential in processing Big Data. But what's still missing from the equation and what we are tasked with contributing is the building of a collective cultural capacity to interpret it properly.

An analogous argument can be made for what I call the 'resilience of nature'. That same nature that we have violated repeatedly in the name of economic success and technological progress. As I attempted to do in my book, one can link the discussion over public health with that of protecting nature. While very different, the more we progress, the more we see they are two sides of the same coin. It no longer makes sense to continue butting up against the environment with the myopia of immediate returns. The time in which we could act this way, if it ever really existed, has long passed.

In 2020, we witnessed the blooming of flora and fauna in places where they had been long forgotten. They simply were filling the void left by our partial absence from the scenery. Animals and plant varieties remade their entrance onto the world stage, without us. The premise of the resilience of nature signifies that this should occur all the same; but not in our absence, in our presence. In a much more harmonious ontology of living creatures, culture should accompany us along this way as we search for a new systemic sustainability.

With a little bit of fantasy, we can imagine that this is how we apply the art of hermeneutics—like a philologist critiquing ancient tomes, but applied to the interpretation of Big Data. One can discuss the resilience of nature in much the same way as Darwin, by putting biology through the lens of a historian. To see to it that economists base their forecasts not only on formulaic notions, but also with the classic literature in mind. And while our youth continues seeing the world through their screens, they'll filter it through the visual arts. With a flowering of transversal detours like psycho-geographic paths, alternative linguistic tools, sound visualizations, concerts, poetry, and on and on it goes.

In *Il Quarto Shock*, I maintained that if we want to understand ourselves and that which we do, we must pay attention to two schisms that are emerging in profound ways; one practical, the other theoretical. In the former, the question we pose ourselves relies on the possibility of thinking of ourselves in two distinct parts: one purely rational and a maximizer in the pursuit of self-interest, the other emotional and empathetic. We tend to employ that vision, quite implausibly, in much the same way that (generally) economists and ethicists conceive of the basis of the choices we make.

In the latter, the schism surrounds instead two aspects of awareness. The question being, in what way does objective awareness bring about a transformation of a conscious individual? It's an age-old question posed time and again and to which we have often taken pains to respond, starting with Foucault's 'self care' and running counter to the Cartesian tradition of modern thought.

My premise, as previously discussed, is that these two schisms are surmountable within the context of a theory of value. That theory implies a continuation of being self-serving when making practical choices, while at the same time regarding self-transformation as a consequence of a serious epistemological commitment. And it's precisely this union of the two aspects of a person—the rational and reasonable, the cognitive alongside the ascetic—that can ascribe value as I have described it. And in turn, this possibility exists in that it is by virtue of being in relationship with others that we render possible authentically knowing oneself.

The philosophic origins my vision of value stem from the conception of value as an organic unit. It's a tradition holding an illustrious pedigree, from Aristotle, Confucius, Al-Farabi or the more recent philosophies of Kant, Hegel, Aurobindo, John Stuart Mill and even George Edward Moore and Robert Nozick, among others. It is no easy task to clearly establish what, precisely, is meant by *value consisting in the pursuit of the organic unit*. First off, the concept of value as an organic unit signifies conceiving of the existence of ways in which diversity is reconfigured under a specific unit, capable of conferring a value that is greater than the sum of its parts. In short, the theory of value as an organic unit signifies that one can gain a surplus of value when, in whichever way it gets defined, the value of the whole surpasses the aggregate of the single parts of which it is made. One can visualize value in terms of: a large family, a successful soccer team, a virtuous orchestra, a physics theory such as relativity, an artistic masterpiece. Each of these things exemplify in their own way value as an organic unit.

The vision of value as an organic unit runs certainly contrary to purely subjective theories, in that it predicates an objective and intrinsic value of certain behaviours and states of things. At the same time, however, value as an organic unit appears as though it can integrate a subjective element with an objective one. One can easily find examples of this: Messi on the Barcelona soccer team, Muti and a grand symphonic orchestra, and so forth. The fact that we speak of an 'objective and intrinsic' value holds a certain theoretic option that's anything but innocent, and rather undoubtedly controversial. Nonetheless, it's not the only challenge a vision such as this presents.

A theory surrounding value as an organic unit runs counter to the analytic bent of breaking up the whole into its component parts. And it's precisely this operation, deconstructing value into its component parts, that gets blocked by the theory of value as an organic unit. From this perspective, the theory is not only up against other theories such as utilitarianism, whereby component parts are aggregated and summed up in the name of the whole, but is also in conflict with one of the cardinal principles of analytic theory: the principle of monotonicity, that often takes on meaning when seen through the lens of value.

According to this principle, there potentially exists a neutral vector upon which one can measure rises and falls in value by means of the increases and reductions of the largeness expressed by the vector itself. Pleasure is the inherent largeness of this type of vector in classic utilitarian terms. But monotonicity expresses an even more generalized criterion such as: 'the more you have, the better off you are' (e.g. in richness, beauty, etc.). This criterion is usually dissected or deconstructed into the parts that have value in its state of things or in its actions.

Once one understands the nature of value as an organic unit—naturally nothing prevents one from doing so—we are extended an invitation to reconstruct it in analytic terms. In the history of philosophic thought, Kant's *Critique of Judgment* represents an attempt to overcome the schism of pure reason/reason/practice or phenomena/noumena in order to arrive at a conclusion uniting the two particular visions. And by doing so, offering the abstract possibility to overcome the potential rift between assigning value and analytical thought when it comes to the natural realm.

In the case at hand, the idea of value as an organic unit is of interest because it could consent to the conjoining in a single paradigm, economic and cognitive choices on one hand, and moral obstacles on the other. This means, in my opinion, implicating that the economy, science and ethics can be rejoined towards sustainability, and more precisely, what we usually refer to as 'sustainable development'. Sustainable development presupposes, in fact, a vision whereby economic growth is commensurate to biological, emotional and, more generally, ethical limits that have been addressed prior.

I close this section with one elucidation: From the onset, I have asserted that public morals as defined, albeit purely fact-based and reflective of current ideas, are by nature, normative. In short, it's Neverland: Being in the world we'd like to have. One based perhaps even on rationale, but still remaining but a fantasy and somewhat out of reach.

I am, in other words, well aware that calling for collective and individual changes such as these are not an easy enterprise. It could very well be that we humans will never be able to improve our standards of public ethics, even after this tragic pandemic we are living through has come to pass.

Why, then, observe or indulge in such an exercise? Personally, I can think of two reasons. One, prior to embarking on a trip, it's important to have an idea of where you're headed; a map of how we'd like our journey to go, and its end destination, in short. Two, a normative vision, projected as the version of what things could look like, can induce us indirectly into thinking of what it is we *don't* want to have happen in the future. I have in mind post-crisis a dystopian future that contemplates the twilight of liberal democracy, the spread of egotistical individual personality, and the affirmation of political-totalitarian regimes. The gap between aspiration and reality—implicit in normative thought—could in this way help us give full meaning to those famous, and somewhat hackneyed, words of poet Eugenio Montale: '*Only this is what we can tell you today, that which we are not, that which we do not want.*'

3

The COVID-19 pandemic has unleashed a planetary crisis. It thus comes as no surprise that great crises spur social and political consequences of equal measure. And which, truthfully, can't be considered negative or positive. The crisis of 1929 ushered in Nazism and WWII, but along with it, the New Deal and ultimately, the end of colonialism. More recently, the fading of communism at the end of the 1980s and the financial and economic crises of 2007–08, brought about in the former a shift in the world order and in the latter, a rebirth of populism and nationalistic tendencies. Naturally, it's difficult to foresee in real time what consequences may stem from the current crisis; we will only be capable of evaluating them with a measure of balance in hindsight. Certainly, the current crisis will carry misery and desperation across the globe, and especially in those countries already at the limit of subsistence living. This, in all probability, will give rise to popular unrest, with the accompanying risk that demagogues will look to fill the vacuum through popular consent and rise to power. New mass migrations from the poorest of countries will spur hostilities and widespread rage, sentiments that usher in authoritarian governments. As a result, the liberal-democratic system, the one which we've all grown up in, and in which, by and large we believe, can—as a number of commentators remark—put at risk the very liberties we enjoy, that went repressed as a response to control the pandemic at hand.

Building upon this premise, what follows is a discussion on the topic 'Pandemic and Democracy' as a critique of the COVID-19 pandemic, six months post publication of *Il Quarto Shock*.

Six months on, we have lived through a number of vastly different experiences, from the first horrifying deaths at the onset, followed by a summer reprieve and now, well into the second wave of the epidemic, with social unrest on the rise, a reaction to the psychological stress and economic crisis that has been visited upon us. In terms of politics, the pandemic risks upsetting the stability of liberal-democratic systems, already under threat prior to the crisis. This stems from a variety of motives that the urgency of the moment has consolidated, namely: i) the necessity to make decisions in a state of emergency, favouring a concentration of executive decisions which in turn unleashes fears of weakening individual liberties, ii) the difficulty in getting voters to accept sustainable policies which in turn makes a shift towards more 'sustainable' policy-making more difficult (as detailed in *Il Quarto Shock*), and iii) increasing social unrest that transforms uncertainty into instability.

In effect, democratic regimes have over the past decade undergone what the political scientist, Larry Diamond, called a 'global recession'. From this perspective, negative outcomes resulting from the pandemic are easily imaginable. Attacks on liberal-democratic regimes—already underway over the years by populists and nationalists—would be accelerated.

Unscrupulous leaders, such as Hungary's Orban or Duterte in the Philippines, are already profiting from the situation by conferring extraordinary emergency powers on themselves. Other countries, such as China, El Salvador and Uganda have taken similar measures that carry them further from liberal-democratic systems. Everywhere, barriers to immigration are being erected, and often one is under the impression that while invoking a 'state of exception', they're busy whittling away at liberties and democracy, a process we've come to know since the Weimar Republic.

The fact is, more or less everywhere, policies to counter COVID-19 have been implemented under emergency measures. Even in countries with strong liberal-democratic traditions, this was 'the hour of the Executive'. The implicit risk being that the emergency, protracted well beyond certain limits, can amount to a progressive erosion of liberal-democratic institutions. The risk facing us is reinforced by the already widespread scepticism of the workings of liberal democracies. Naturally, the erosion of liberal democracies threatens those countries that were already witnessing the weakening of such institutions, as seen in Eastern Europe or Latin America.

Yuval Noah Harari, in the article previously referenced, makes the assertion that there are greater authoritarian risks associated with controlling the pandemic. We're fearful of contagion and measures to keep it at bay are necessary. Before one can benefit from herd immunity, in tandem with a discovery and administration of a valid vaccine, controls by way of electronic instruments (such as cell phone apps) have proven to be effective.

This signifies that the State or Big Tech (such as Google or Apple) will systematically violate our privacy. The *Economist*, in its 28 March 2020 edition, published a piece aptly entitled, 'Creating the Coronopticon'—a clear nod to the Foucauldian interpretation of the 'Panopticon' and its ready surveillance and ultimate control over a populace—comparing anti-contagion measures taken across a number of countries.

This isn't in the extreme something new; that we already lived under a surveillance and control society we were well aware. But this is quite a different form of surveillance from that direct, profit-motivated kind on offer by widespread capitalism, as addressed by Zuboff in his tome *The Capitalism of Surveillance*. This time, it would be a moral and political control, and in all probability, with public opinion fully on board with it.

If, in fact, we offer people the cut and dry choice between security and freedom—as Thomas Hobbes teaches us—they will consistently choose security, whatever the cost may be. The same goes for those who have to choose between health and privacy. Harari offers a response in terms of resistance, based on the empowerment of citizens, stating, inasmuch, when we give them greater awareness and information, they'll be more equipped to resist creeping authoritarianism. So then they'll be able to fend for themselves, without appealing to the Leviathan of the authorities. My rebuttal, similar in scope, differs in substance.

There exists thus a strict relationship between the search for security and the risk of authoritarianism. The pandemic reinforces our fears, and with it, suspicion of 'the other'. It thus becomes even more complicated to integrate those who are different; foreigners, migrants. Fear is essentially reactionary and only by starting from fear can we fully understand emotions such as fury and disgust: the emotions at the heart of populist and anti-liberal waves of contemporary politics. In fact, it's *fear* which is the motivating factor in widespread efforts of 'othering', whereby we wind up excluding, rather than including those who differ from us.

Franklin Delano Roosevelt was correct when he stated, 'We have nothing to fear, but fear itself.' Fear, as defined by the great psychoanalyst and paediatrician, Donald Winnicott, depends on the loss of control over one's surroundings and stems from an infantile instinct. It consists in obsessing over the course of a lifetime in what amounts to a nightmare—originating with a fear of abandonment by one's parents—of a newborn incapable of taking care of itself. In short, every fear is fear of death, a permanent status of our awareness of being both ultimately ephemeral and vulnerable.

The problem is that fear is not only psychological; it's also social and generates reckless emotional reactions in the masses, which then find expression in racism and revolt. Narcissism implicit to fear becomes, in short, the foundation for moral anti-democratic grievances. And from fear comes fury unleashed on others, with the subsequent drive to punish those who have caused it. From fear also comes the rejection of diversity, such as against Blacks or Jews. It stems from the sensation of having 'suffered' unjustified damages at the hands of others. Deep down, there's a need for reassurance. How could one, armed with an understanding of the genesis of these negative feelings, try to avoid the subsequent undesirable and nasty effects?

First and foremost, looking to frame our existence in places that help and facilitate better responses, perhaps by way of 'transitional' objects (Winnicott), such as the blanket of Linus. But more generally, transforming blind rage into civic protest, without aiming for vendettas or punishment. In the final analysis, the democratic order should be an agent for setting aside one's negative feelings such as rage and disregard, leaving space to more positive feelings. There exist a number of life values worth pursuing, such as those that allow for love of those near and dear to us, or the pursuit of goals tied to our work. In short, it would be a good and positive thing to transform fury in 'hope practices' such as these (Nussbaum 2018), thus avoiding the more nefarious consequences spurred on by fear.

The normative political theory serves at this point to unmask the implicit errors of rage, reminding us that rancour is often unjustified. That anxiousness over one's status is oftentimes overly excessive, and at the end of the day, seeking vendettas is senseless. In this way, public morals serve as indirect empowerment for the citizenry, as a way of partially conferring on persons the ability to control the pandemic phenomenon.

Putting aside the fact that a competent and more well-informed populace would be more autonomous, as Harari asserted, I believe that we should not dismiss the role of public ethics outright. Public ethics amounts to a highly important asset when there is relative trust between governments and the governed. The hypothesis is that citizens will take government directives such as 'stay at home orders' seriously only when they regard their government as trustworthy. When that's the case, there is no need for authoritarianism. Furthermore, authoritarianism doesn't work without public trust. Trust is based on public opinion with regard to the credibility and capacity in their government. Just to be overly explicit: If American citizens do not abide by the anti-contagion norms, it's because someone like Trump has little credibility.

In the same way, if Italians don't follow government decrees, it's because they have no faith in the competency of the governing class. Both examples signify that governments are unable to generate trust. Governments that earn their citizens' trust are able to maintain—for a relatively longer period of time—a situation such as a lockdown.

This does not signify that a liberal-democratic power delegates the execution of directives to its citizens. On the contrary, during a state of emergency, no regime can afford to delegate the power of the Executive. As we've learned from a tradition that extends from Hume to Rawls, there are 'circumstances of justice' within which we must think about institutional choices: When it comes to maintaining a minimum of public welfare, the usual considerations or rules of justice do not apply. In practice, this means that all governments, when faced with a crisis like the present health crisis, will opt for certain measures that implicate a reduction in civil liberties. The difference then, between liberal-democratic regimes and authoritarian ones, lies in maintaining the equilibrium between coercion and freedom of choice. Authoritarian states allow for very little individual freedom, while democratic ones aim to balance this out. Up until now, there did not seem to be a direct correlation between the kind of regime and the efficacy of an anti-pandemic response, although countries like China and Singapore (authoritarian regimes) showed decidedly better results than Great Britain and the USA (democracies).

Given the context, it's decidedly difficult to say which type of response comes from an authoritarian government and which from a democratic one. The general impression shared by many is that, globally, distribution of power continues its march eastward; a trend that has been going on for quite a while. As we know, things in the USA have not been going very well. This, in part due to a disgrace of a president as is Trump, has cost it considerably in international prestige, especially due to the government response in times of crisis. It goes without saying that China, on the other hand, faced down the pandemic crisis—despite its originating right in China—better than either the USA or Europe. In short, China has fared relatively better during this crisis. If for no other reason than the fact that its government took immediate control of the situation and the economy began growing again sooner.

It is most probable that these kinds of outcomes depend in large part on the traditional culture of a place: South Korea, for example, started tracing credit cards, employing GPS systems and closed circuit video surveillance cameras, and releasing the data in the public sphere in order to dissuade any possible close contacts. Overall, this strategy worked, but in the West, it would have been viewed as a totally intolerable suppression of civil liberties. China, on the other hand, placed nearly a million people in quarantine, unleashing its full authoritarian powers, which, in the end, proved effective. This is not to negate that

European countries (Italy, France, Spain, and Great Britain) imposed massive lockdowns of their entire populace thereafter.

In any case, it appears that the Asian model has produced a more positive result in combating the pandemic versus that of the West. Various Asian countries such as Japan, S. Korea, China, Hong Kong, and Singapore are more inclined to accept paternalism and authority; if for no other reason than a Confucian inheritance (S. Maffettone, *Politica*, October 2019), resulting in a greater tendency to obey the State. This tendency allowed these countries to tackle the virus by means of digital vigilance. Data experts backed up virologists and epidemiologists while clearly enforcing limits to civil liberties. And in doing so, they did not unleash any particular sense of resistance, as would have occurred in the West. The result: Big Data works to counter epidemics, but only if the populace is ready and willing to accept an invasion of privacy.

The pandemic has carried with it a heretofore unthinkable opportunity to make comparisons between citizenry reactions across nations; their capacity for social acceptance and discipline. Government responses to it were widely diverse, extending from countries that went into lockdown (China, Italy), to ones taking a more passive approach (Sweden, Brazil). Even the way the media covered COVID-19 varied from country to country (as tracked by the Johns Hopkins Coronavirus Resource Center).

The more time passes, the more knowledge we gain about COVID-19 and its consequences. And the more we realize that the current crisis will be a lengthy one, playing out in a matter of years, not months. This stems from the very nature of the virus that is, certainly, less deadly than others (such as Ebola), but far more contagious. Its long-term forecast implicates a far greater challenge for attaining sustained growth of the economy and a V-shaped economic recovery seems as of this writing, far more improbable, especially in the short term.

Il Quarto Shock asserts that public policy over sustainability needs to be pursued by States especially in light of a pandemic response. But there exists a sort of natural tension between sustainability and democracy. This is particularly the case when questions of environmental sustainability are in play, but it also seems to extend generally as well. Sustainability has to do with making a commitment—not only today but for the future. And it's not easy for a 'sovereign people' to vote for long-term goals that transcend their current interests. There exists, in short, a certain myopia on the part of the average electorate often referred to as 'short-termism'. Short-termism signifies 'giving priority to immediate benefits at the expense of sacrificing future gains'. Short-termism wreaks havoc whenever policies are being decided over long-term gains, typical when addressing issues posed by environmental sustainability (and global warming, per se).

In such cases, one must sacrifice their current interests; paying higher taxes, for example, for future gains. And voting for such an option does not come easily. Calls for making these sorts of sacrifices often work to the advantage of those representatives of what we would call 'future generations', further adding to challenges faced. In short, going up against the natural instinct of favouring one's present benefits over future ones, one must consider that they also come with a relative uncertainty as to what future damages we are attempting to ward off. A real outcome is falling for the temptation of kicking any costs associated with policies down the road that could otherwise provide for a more general sustainability.

The above is what occurs in a democracy, albeit for no other reason than considerations replicate politically the current prejudices of citizens to opt for momentary benefits. Naturally, this does not imply that it would be impossible to guard against these prejudices. Liberal democracies can protect themselves towards this end by implementing anti-majority policies; for example, adopting constitutional norms in favour of sustainability. But this signifies that the issue remains and anti-majority strategies risk creating serious legitimacy crises. And, if consistently adopted, even the danger of creeping authoritarianism.

All of this is reinforced by the non-correspondence of electoral cycles, usually quite short, versus those substantial sustainability issues which are associated with long-term effects. As a result, politicians, who are simply aiming for re-election in the next cycle, do not think of generations to come and thereby don't easily gamble on the future. An additional challenge stems from the fact that generous choices made today in the name of future sustainability could prove to be ill-thought, when the time comes. Or perhaps not fully appreciated by those who, in theory, would have the most to gain from said policies. And finally, when it comes to imagining 'worst case scenarios' such as global warming, we often tend to ignore the probability that these are subject to verification, another impetus for the inadequate responses to real dangers we face (given that the response may be too weak, or even contrary to the desired effects).

From a logical perspective, it's important to make a distinction between risk and uncertainty. Risk is when one doesn't know whether an event shall occur, but is aware of the probability of it happening (such as a number coming out on the roulette wheel). Uncertainty, instead, is when not only does one not know if the event will take place, but they also do not know the future probability of its occurrence (a meteorite crashing to earth, for example). How great our risk is in terms of the sustainability of our planet is filled with uncertainty. This signifies that it's ever more complex to forge an adequate response. Every cost-benefit analysis becomes an arduous task, especially if we consider the eventual risks that the future may hold for upcoming generations.

This kind of situation lends itself to what are called 'veto-players'. Veto-players are those actors who, although in the minority, throw up obstacles to public policy implementation. As is noted, veto-players aren't in themselves a bad thing; they can sometimes impede rash political decisions from going forward that could ultimately prove dangerous. When it comes to sustainability, however, veto-players can cause some damage, for example blocking any initiatives towards policies geared towards countering global warming. Perhaps the greatest evidence of veto-players having a negative impact on the general equilibrium is seen in the prospect of ethical-economic sustainability in terms of equality. Extreme economic disparities across the entire planet, and in the United States in particular, serve as confirmation of the tremendous difficulties in trying to change the status quo. Blocking any steps to counter this tendency becomes a 'tyranny of the minority' (the wealthy class being in the minority). This highlights two principle defects—one in opposition, the other complementary—to democracy, when seen through a sustainable lens: Tyranny by majority leads to short-termism while tyranny by minority renders impossible any such measure that might bring about greater social-economic equity.

Traditionally, a way around these democratic deficits comes by appealing to experts; persons to whom liberal-democracies generally turn to encourage acceptance and implementation of 'difficult' political decisions. This was the case in Italy for the formation of the CTS (Technical Scientific Committee) in order to provide an adequate response to the pandemic.

At the end of the day, the crisis could bear some positive fruit. We come from a period in which demagoguery and mass incompetence have prevailed over expertise and professionalism. So much so that the term 'death of expertise' is now bandied about. The pandemic, from this vantage point, could have a beneficial effect whereby expert opinions are respected again, and allow above all for the evaluation of political decisions on the merits of actions taken and results attained. The pandemic, in short, acts as a benchmark for political evaluation. Anti-pandemic strategies like those implemented by people like Bolsonaro, Trump and Johnson would not otherwise be appreciated from this perspective. Even Putin, who claimed to have things well under control, will come out the other side of the pandemic partly delegitimized by the experience. And in the final analysis, perhaps this will swing the pendulum in favour of liberal-democratic institutions.

Despite what's stated above, counter trends are in full force. As we are well aware, intellectual expertise is not prized in democracies, save for exceptional instances in which it proves effective for making one's case. After all, in democracy, large numbers can outperform the truth. We have seen this played out in the example of the anti-vax movement: Its basic premise relies on the additional onus that a 'sovereign people' don't trust in experts. Nowadays, these viewpoints are reinforced across the internet. The web, we have seen, has rendered all viewpoints qualitatively equal; flattening, if you will, the value of expertise. Compounding this is the fact that web algorithms seem to favour disagreement over baseline factual notions, while reinforcing prejudices or seeking consensus for one's viewpoint, independent of the truth. Popular campaigns defying vaccines, or denying global warming, give credence to this description. And we find ourselves once again not heading in the direction of taking action on sustainability.

The COVID-19 pandemic has undoubtedly brought with it an enormous challenge to liberal democracies around the world. From the start, governments came out stronger, while parliaments were weakened. During this initial phase, individual rights of citizens were often violated in the name of emergency measures. The socio-economic gap between classes of society and individuals was widened. And lately, we've seen how this gap has catalysed revolts stemming from widespread misery and frustration. Searching for an understanding of these phenomena becomes essential and all the more urgent for a liberal democracy, both in terms of theory and practice. Taken as a whole, we are left with the general impression that the crisis has unleashed forces and events in complex ways, if not wholly contradictory.

Without a doubt, the pandemic has revealed weaknesses of liberal democracies that we already knew existed, but which are now much more apparent. The most evident failures for now have come about in those liberal democracies that were already fragile. It's as if the cracks that were already there, widened, while in strong and mature liberal democracies, we did not witness structures give way altogether. At the same time, we saw almost everywhere a return to greater State authority. The decidedly emergency situation highlighted the fact that it is indeed the State that has the ultimate authority and is the only entity capable of finding plausible solutions at the source to tackle such a pervasive crisis. Now more than ever, ultra-liberal recipes—already shaken by the 2007–08 financial crisis—seem totally unacceptable. We only need look at the damage caused by the policies implemented as a remedy, with their accompanying death tolls, just to take stock of it all.

The pandemic crisis, as usually transpires, has widened the chasm that was already far too excessive between the haves and have-nots. All of this, in my opinion, should serve to provoke a wave of solidarity along with the impetus to find common solutions to protect the most economically and socially disadvantaged among us. The proposition set forth in *Il Quarto Shock* on attaining a sustainable system responds to this need. We have seen how difficult it is to reconcile it in a democracy, especially if this democracy appears weakened and shaken. But the liberal democracy itself could be mortally wounded if the objectives of solidarity are not pursued.

One possibility, however abstract or remote, could be found in the recovery of a certain transcendence. The last two Encyclicals released by Pope Francis emphasize the sustainability of the system as a whole. Here, 'transcendence' is taken to mean a particular religious belief (which could, nonetheless, be classified under it). Instead, I intend transcendence as a form of widespread spirituality that allows one to overcome the hardships brought on by short-termism, and in the name of a more expansive vision that encompasses the significance and value of life. Or perhaps to conceive of a sense of limitation that permits us to maintain a balance in a system heading towards sustainability just on the horizon. In philosophic terms, one can theorize that there could be thus a recouping of a tradition at the crossroads of knowledge and spirituality.

It's not easy to be optimistic. We are currently on the cusp—as many political scientists recognize—of an evident weakening of the rational potential of public discourse, and as a result, of the capacity for understanding on the part of society at large. For complex reasons, including the omnipresence of social networks, media alarmism and populist uprisings in general, the rapport between public policies and scientific and professional expertise has been greatly diminished over the last few years. As has been said, the current health crisis may spur a return to faith in science, but we must remain cognizant that it is still an uphill battle.

The reinforcement of the State—by way of the knee-jerk response to the pandemic along with the political climate in general—was a direct response to the shutdowns of national borders; the paradox being that a global problem, which the pandemic undoubtedly is, was transformed into a conglomerate of single-nation responses. Even though there were instances of international solidarity, such as the donation of equipment and services from one country to another, the general rule proved to be 'the revival of territories' (Casaglia et al. 2020). This carries grave repercussions for the general intelligence surrounding the pandemic phenomenon and eventual remedies, but also, even more explicitly, for those who may hold an uncertain status in terms of citizenship: refugees or stateless individuals.

All of these issues raise the call for more global justice, as stressed in *Il Quarto Shock*. Some of the brighter responses witnessed during the pandemic, such as those (partially) experienced after the first reciprocal closings across the EU, are a positive sign that we may be headed in the right direction. Nonetheless, we are going down what should prove to be a long and arduous path.

COVID-19 AND THE 'RETURN OF THE NORMATIVE' IN ECONOMIC POLICY[1]

Sanjay G. Reddy

1. THE NORMATIVE ELEMENT IN ECONOMIC POLICY: IN 'NORMAL' TIMES AND IN CRISES

All economic policy must have objectives, and in this sense, is always 'normative'. But the need for judgements based on values in order to develop coherent and defensible policies is often buried, causing the role of the normative to be hidden and leading economic debates to focus on truncated questions rather than on the relative significance and role of diverse values.

In 'normal' times, questions about *which* values should guide economic policy have often been pushed to the edges of attention, or even treated as the province of malcontents and cranks. Mainstream discussions in a capitalist market economy typically have assumed a consensus in favour of specific goals that are presumed to be shared—for instance, economic growth. Fetishism of the economic and resulting obscurantism in relation to normative ends is a feature of everyday economic policy-making, especially in a 'capitalist' system, and in this sense, economic policy-making masquerades as 'non-normative'. In 'normal times', hard choices are often obscured or evaded because consensus goals are assumed to accommodate various subsequent possibilities, deferred to some 'later' stage of decision-making. For instance, assuming the separability of the policy choices needed to bring about economic 'efficiency' and 'equity' has allowed output to be

1. This paper is based on the keynote lecture for the seminar on 'Normative Economic Policy' at the Research Centre on Normative Orders, Goethe University of Frankfurt, given on 11 December 2020.

considered a proximate goal, with distributional goals taken to be subsequently implementable through suitable transfers (Scitovsky 1941; Bhagwati et al. 1969). Even 'non-economic' environmental and social goals are regarded achievable through suitable ex-post expenditures, if they are mentioned at all.[2] The working assumptions of economic policy in 'normal times', therefore, permit a degree, even a high degree, of deferral or obscurantism concerning what is ultimately to be valued and pursued.[3]

In contrast, crises can bring to fuller visibility the truth that is often hidden from view, however obvious it may appear to be: which economic policy choices 'should' be made depends on societal values. As a result, framing an economic policy requires the recognition of the range of possible ends that may be affected by the choices made, including those that are 'non-economic'. This imperative requires economic policy choices to be rooted in democratic legitimacy, facing all of the consequent demands and risks.

2. THE CRISIS AND THE INELUCTABLE NORMATIVE

Crises generate specific situational dynamics that 'bring back' the normative. We consider here three ways in which the normative has been foregrounded in the current crisis (see also Reddy 2020a).

2. This premise may help to explain the famous remark of Peter Mandelson, chief strategist of New Labour, that 'I am intensely relaxed about people getting filthy rich, as long as they pay their taxes'. This was also the premise behind arguments made by prominent economists and policy-makers against including labour and environmental standards considerations in the rules governing the international trading system (Barry and Reddy 2008).

3. I recall one memorable—because so unmemorable—occasion in the 1990s when the then Finance Secretary of the Government of India made an after-dinner speech at a major conference on India's economic reforms, disappointing controversialists, that could be boiled down to the following: 'Some say that we can achieve an eight per cent growth rate. I, too, think we can.'

2.1 The Economy as a 'Sub-System'? The Return of the Repressed

In 'normal times', the economy may be imagined, especially by those inclined towards market-centric thinking, to possess aspects of automaticity, returning to an 'equilibrium' path after being subjected to shocks. The features of normality that are imagined to be restored 'automatically' through the economy's built-in stabilizers may be conceived, for instance, in terms of utilization of capacity, full-employment, or other features. In contrast, an alternative tradition conceives of non-automaticity of desired conditions as being central to the description of an economy. In this alternative understanding, there are at least two major strands. The first, prominently identified with Keynesianism, sees a need for economic intervention to achieve desired economic outcomes, viewing the solution as being within the same realm as the problem—the economic. The second, associated with classical political economy and traditions as diverse as feminism, Marxism, and ordo-liberalism, sees economic activity as existing in a context that needs safeguarding and care. Economic activity may even be viewed as actively undermining the social and ecological integument of the 'economy', leading to 'contradictions', such as between the individualism of the market economy and the shared societal character of its non-market preconditions. The solution thus is no longer in the same realm as the problem, as the economic possesses non-economic conditions—social, ecological, or biological. In a crisis, the idea that the economic is a sub-system with its own sovereign rules and prerogatives is challenged by reality.

The current pandemic has enforced recognition of the empirical interdependence between two 'spheres' in particular—the economic and the epidemiological—and as a result demanded the intervention of a third sphere, the political. The presumed ethic of care underlying political interventions to manage disease risk, even at the cost of the 'economy', concedes the normative priority of the human which is otherwise often overlooked, especially when the human is viewed primarily in instrumental terms as an economic actor (e.g. a worker possessing 'human capital', manager, or 'entrepreneur'). This brings out a truth that is otherwise contested—what is good for the 'economy' is simply what is good for human beings.[4] The response to the pandemic falsifies the idea of the economic as a subsystem, and hence, also undermines the separatist presumption underlying the typical discourses of 'everyday' economics in capitalist societies (see Godelier 1972; Polanyi 1944; Tribe 1978).

The crisis has brought to the fore expressly normative considerations originating in the non-economic sphere—centred on the protection of public health—but has also raised questions of the scope of legitimate political authority and of what economic and social consequences of policies, often distributed in a highly unequal fashion, can be reasonably accepted. Given the unprecedented governmental intrusions into everyday life and massive economic and social consequences with unequal distributional impact, the crisis has made it simply untenable to form policies without recognizing their effects in these dimensions. But this, in turn, has meant pushing aside the 'truncated normativity' of the economic sphere, at least temporarily, in favour of an 'expanded normativity' that recognizes the central role of normative commitments in offering justification for policies and guiding their design. Sen (2020) has argued that the often-used simile that likens fighting a pandemic to fighting a war is misleading. But a pandemic *is* like war in at least one respect—in both cases, the imperative to achieve specific non-economic objectives gives a persuasive basis for the subordination or at least the moderation of the economic—disenthroning it from its customary position of priority in a capitalist society.

4. This is, of course, the point of view of the human development approach, and related criticisms of income-centric societal evaluation: see e.g. United Nations Development Programme (1990), Sen (1999) or Stiglitz et al. (2009).

2.2 Hard Choices: Valuation's Complex and Plural Landscape

The crisis has brought to the fore the need to overthrow the 'normal rules' of economic policy-making in capitalist societies in more than one sense. One way in which it has done so is by leading to the disavowal of constraints previously thought of as sacrosanct—with previous guardians of fiscal probity urging increases in spending to achieve more urgent societal ends ('Spend as Much as You Can', 2021). This has underlined that a 'constraint' in the social world is in fact a consequence of a specific causal theory or order of priority, which can be revised when these are revised (Reddy 2005). Another way in which the crisis has caused the 'normal rules' to be overthrown is by underlining that all of the available choices favour the interests of some persons over others, and that policy-making cannot therefore shirk from comparing them. Of course, this is always true to some degree, but is often obscured in everyday policy talk (or in its journalistic counterparts, which focus on what is good for the 'economy', as if that meant one thing). In particular, mainstream economic policy analysis typically sidesteps such comparisons to focus instead on guidance as to how to achieve 'efficiency', presumptively benefiting all. Famously, Robbins (1932) derided such choices as involving balancing 'Thy Blood or Mine' and unsuitable for a scientific economics to address—even if unavoidable in public life. But, contrary to Robbins, policy choice that is not a mere exercise of power requires arriving at choices through a disciplined weighing of concerns based on the application of principles. This process of thought must be reasoned and reflective, whether or not it qualifies as 'scientific'.

In the context of COVID-19, policy choices have been made around the world that have favoured the interests of some at the expense of others. Consider for instance government actions that have sought especially to protect the old, who face very much higher mortality risks from contracting COVID-19, but have used instruments toward that end which have caused sizable harms to the young (specifically, undifferentiated 'lockdowns' which have caused massive disruption of economic security, schooling, social relationships, personal mobility, and mental or physical health). Those who argue that these measures have had justification undertake implicit (or explicit) interpersonal comparisons. Those who argue against these policies argue, contrarily, that the harms to some, whether conceived in terms of outcomes or loss of liberties, outweigh the benefits to others. The weighing that is involved involves persons in different circumstances (e.g. the young and the old) facing harms and benefits of diverse kinds. This weighing is therefore intra-personal as well as inter-personal, bringing in diverse values which have distinct and irreducible significance in a life (e.g. education vs. health, or the opportunity to live a normal life vs. the opportunity to live a longer life).

The exercise of valuation which is necessary to arrive at or defend policies involving such interpersonal comparisons is both plural and complex: it involves multiple dimensions—bringing in train ethical considerations that are diverse in nature—*and* multiple, unequally situated, persons. While there is some evidence of public authorities and politicians justifying the choices made in terms of the sacrifices which are appropriate to ask of some in order to benefit others, it does not seem that there have been many efforts to undertake a disciplined exercise of evaluative judgement based on a comprehensive accounting. The problem of 'management' of the response to the pandemic seems often to have been handed instead to subsidiary authorities (e.g. of public health) obscuring the wide scope of the evaluation involved.

In order to make headway in a problem of this kind, it is necessary to adopt an evaluative framework that encompasses both freedom and outcome concerns. But concerns of each of these kinds can also be internally complex. For instance, positive freedoms—freedoms effectively to attain valuable ends[5]—might,

5. See, for example, Sen (1995) and prior literature, most famously Berlin (1958).

in some causal circumstances, be expanded through limitations on negative freedoms (freedoms from obstruction). If the causal premise is satisfied, the control of a contagious disease through limitations on personal movement or interaction provides an example. In such a case, the argument for limited restrictions on freedom can also be viewed as being 'freedom-based'—accepting necessary restraints on freedom to expand freedoms *in toto*. This can be either because the freedoms lost (e.g. freedom of association) are accompanied by—presumptively 'greater'—gains in other freedoms (e.g. freedom to live healthily) for the very same persons, or because losses of freedom of some are deemed to be adequately compensated by gains of freedom by others (freedom being the same 'currency' in both cases).[6] The complex and plural nature of the exercise—determining the acceptability of trade-offs between freedoms of different kinds and as experienced by different persons—is, again, unavoidable. The conclusions derived will depend on diverse values and the weights attached to them, as well as on the facts of the case.

While freedom and outcome arguments (e.g. liberty and efficiency) are often run together in 'neoliberal', even if not in 'neoclassical', economics, where market economies are seen as advancing both together (see Friedman and Friedman 1980) it is quite clear that in the context of a pandemic there *may* be inescapable trade-offs.

All told, it is quite clear that a narrowly consequentialist framework of evaluation is not adequate. Process and outcome considerations must be integrated together, while also recognizing the internal complexity present in each of these categories.[7] The resulting complex and plural exercise requires weighing of objectives, and therefore, normative policy-making.

---

6. Liberals and even libertarians have at times accepted arguments along these lines in favour of public health based restrictions on liberties. See e.g. 'Public Health Ethics', Stanford Encyclopedia of Philosophy (https://plato.stanford.edu/entries/publichealth-ethics/).

7. Sen (1982) presents, under the heading of 'goal-rights systems' one way of integrating such diverse values.

The hard choices involved have not always been made explicit, as might be demanded in a context of democratic justification. How to provide adequate processes for such justification, in 'real time', as required in a crisis, is both a theoretical and a practical challenge, which by any measure has not been met during the current crisis.

2.3 Dilemmas of Expertise

The crisis has given rise to heavy reliance on expertise for guidance and for legitimation, in a historical moment in which claims to expertise are already severely challenged, and with some good reason (see Babones 2018). In the case of epidemiology, legitimate questions have been raised about the evidence basis and modelling framework employed in the frameworks most frequently applied as a basis for policy advice (see Collier 2020). What is the *form* of expertise adequate to such a crisis?

First, the available expertise must be suitable to the purpose at hand. This requires that its predictive or explanatory capacities must be oriented toward providing the contribution required from it to underpinning effective public decisions. Second, the available expertise must illuminate what choices there are and their implications. The role of expertise is to provide the knowledge necessary to achieve desired goals—making transparent both what alternatives exist and the practical as well as value judgements needed to select among them. This requires, *inter alia*, describing what trade-offs may exist, what uncertainties are present, and how they may be delimited (e.g. by even roughly characterizing the likelihoods of outcomes). Expertise is a tool for public decision-making, but not a substitute for it.

All of this seems exceedingly obvious, and yet it, apparently, isn't. Consider, for instance, that few countries in the world appear to have anticipated, or integrated into their decisions as to how to respond to the pandemic, the various spillover consequences that quite predictably resulted. These include trade-offs between the health outcomes being safeguarded through societal 'lockdowns' and *other* health consequences (see Reddy 2020b) as well as between health and non-health concerns (e.g. education, or employment and income security). There is little evidence that pandemic planning extended to such causal linkages, or that they were taken into account in emergency decision-making (for instance, by making provisions to address these knock-on consequences, even if the public health measures taken remained the same).

When such spillovers are involved, the resulting inescapable normative demand for weighing makes deference to experts (a policy prominently proclaimed by various leaders) a disavowal of responsibility—both because the experts generally have at best fragmentary knowledge—an effect of the very disciplinary division of labour that makes them experts—and because the weighing of diverse concerns is a public prerogative, that should appropriately be informed by democratic values (Ramakrishnan 2020).

The crisis has underlined that a more adequate framework for tapping expertise ('expertise on tap and not on top' [Spivak 2021]) is greatly needed. Indeed, developing such a framework is a central unaddressed challenge of contemporary democracy, necessary to weave a course between two opposite dangers. The first danger is a focus of 'populist' suspicion: that purportedly democratic institutions do not function democratically, because of the influence of alleged 'experts' whose opinions substitute for the normative values that should properly govern decisions, and which ought to emerge from a societal context. The second danger is that expertise is not employed even when it ought to be. The avoidance of the first danger requires avoiding the use of expertise as an alibi for the repression of legitimate normative concerns in the decision-making processes of a society. The avoidance of the second danger requires avoiding the use of legitimate normative concerns as an alibi for the repression of expertise in the decision-making processes of a society. To avoid both dangers, it is necessary to give normative values their due while keeping them in their place. What features would a suitable synthesis between the claims of democracy and of expertise have? The COVID-19 pandemic experience suggests that such a synthesis should:

- *Bridge domains.* A more adequate framework for policy-making requires a more expansive yet disciplined form of thought bridging domains, so as to recognize the relevant causal inter-linkages. This is needed both to recognize and face possible trade-offs (e.g. lockdown impact on output and employment) and what opportunities may exist to avoid them. In addition to hard choices there may be 'Paretian' opportunities for mitigating or even avoiding such choices—but arriving at these possibilities (for instance, to ensure the continued delivery of other health services, the provision of schooling, or the maintenance of employment while also limiting the transmission of the disease) requires understanding what causal linkages are present, and what enabling supports or incentives may make a difference.[8] The disciplinary division of labour is a device for the production of knowledge, but also of ignorance. An expansive 'new science' which seeks to overcome the resulting acquired blindness and to bridge the prevailing gaps is needed.
- *Anticipate scenarios.* Despite the presence of fundamental uncertainty, it can be possible to sketch and prepare for possible outcomes. Efforts to do so occupy the space between reason and imagination. They represent a form of extended realism, as contrasted with the myopic realism that sees only the 'now'. Such scenario-building is inherently difficult. It must recognize that a problem such as pandemic management is in the nature of a 'wicked problem', contending with causal complexity, pervasive fundamental uncertainty, and valuational plurality all *together*. Nevertheless, some scenario-building is better than none. More often than not, the current pandemic has placed an uncomfortable spotlight on a lack of even obvious precautions, and even

8. The evolving understanding of whether schools play an important role in the transmission of COVID-19, leading to revised guidance, provides an example. See WHO, UNESCO and UNICEF (2020).

the systematic undermining of precautionary efforts. (Consider, for instance, how the pursuit of short-term efficiency over resilience or stability of supply chains, which has led in a number of countries to international outsourcing and a lack of domestic capacity to produce health commodities that have been needed: tests, drugs, and vaccines).

- *Enlarge options.* 'Expertise' that confines itself to a few preconceived possibilities risks limiting our consideration of the available options. For instance, the policy options were more than merely having on and off generalized 'lockdowns' as anticipated in much of the policy literature and focused on by policy-makers in many countries, including India. (Indeed, in India, the stringent lockdown adopted early on seems to have had little impact on the subsequent progression of the disease.) The East Asian countries, which have achieved better disease control with less adverse economic impact, show that interventions applied in a focused manner may make generalized lockdowns unnecessary. Under the exigencies of the crisis, there has been considerable innovation in social welfare systems—for instance leading to the adoption of a version of the German '*Kurzarbeit*' wage subsidy model so as to maintain employment and avoid business closures, in the UK and elsewhere; temporary income supports along the lines of a universal basic income, etc. These innovations also underline the importance of considering the range of possible interventions. The role of 'experts' should be to propose options and not to limit them.
- *Make sense of motivations.* Much of the 'expertise' that has been applied has assumed that human beings act nearly mechanically,[9] but a more sophisticated portrait of human motivation is of great importance

9. The influential models of Prof Neil Ferguson and his Imperial College group are cases in point (see Collier 2020; Reddy 2020b).

to enacting successful public interventions and policies. Understanding by agents of why they are being asked to act is essential for motivating them. Moreover, they are likely to be motivated not merely by narrowly 'self-interested' instrumental calculations but also by considerations of extended or enlightened self-interest, by procedural regard for 'doing the right thing' and by concern for others.[10] Public interventions must be grounded in a recognition of these diverse motivations and their inter linkages. (For instance, it may be easier to do what is right if it is also easy.) Alleviating constraints and providing incentives through policies can enable and encourage people to act in pro-social ways, but it is their internal motivation to do so which is tapped. Individual rational agency cannot be detached from nor reduced to moral sensibilities, and responses to public interventions are likely to reflect this complexity. Neither 'behavioural insights'[11] nor arbitrary presumptions (e.g. of how long a lockdown is likely to be socially sustainable) since the success of interventions depends ultimately on their acceptance by citizens who act as independent reasoning agents.

- *Span levels of action.* The pandemic has shown the limited extent of regional and global cooperation (with some notable exceptions, such as in Africa, where the African Union has played an important role in collective vaccine procurement and in framing the response to COVID-19 generally). 'Nationalism' in policy-making has led to a failure to make use of many opportunities for productive international coordination, in relation

10. This might help explain the finding of higher compliance with public health guidance for COVID-19 than anticipated in prior modelling exercises (Reddy 2020b).

11. A 'Behavioural Insights Team' played a role in particular in shaping the UK government response (https://www.bi.team/blogs/behavioural-insights-the-who-and-covid-19/).

to disease prevention and control, data sharing, development and production of health commodities such as tests and vaccines, and many other areas. This is a colossal failure of collective rationality that has been inadequately recognized as such.[12] A capacious expertise at the service of democratic values should avoid the explanatory and prescriptive self-limitation of a fetishist concern with nation-state policy. Expertise gains relevance from a link to the 'reason of state' but also risks relevance if it does not confront that link. A democratic form of expertise is at the service of society rather than state.

3. CONCLUSIONS: DEMOCRACY, EXPERTISE, AND POLICIES

Normative goals and principles (e.g. as to what trade-offs should be made) are a necessary reference point in social choices. Nevertheless, there is pervasive obscurantism about when and how the normative enters policy-making—especially economic policy-making—in ordinary times. A crisis, such as a pandemic, brings the normative to the fore. The current 'moment' of the (relative) foregrounding of the normative may go on for some time, as a result of the many health, social, and economic effects of the crisis, and the questions it has raised concerning the appropriate distribution of burdens and benefits. These questions are as diverse as how to respond to the accumulation of debt by firms and countries (as a result of the output contractions brought about by closures), how long and on what scale to pursue stimulus policies to restore output, what to do to ensure universal access to vaccines or other health 'commodities', etc. The dimensions of the crisis in each of these areas raise questions of a fundamental kind concerning

12. The formula for a vaccine provides an example of a (global) public good that is best cooperatively produced and freely shared. See Acharya and Reddy (2020).

the adequacy of existing institutions and norms as well as the priorities and political economy revealed by societal choices.

The COVID-19 crisis has underlined a number of challenges to public decision-making. These have included how to deal with pervasive and profound uncertainty, resulting in part from complex causal relations; what role to give to expertise that is both indispensable and inadequate; how to generate and employ bridging knowledge that takes note of causal spillovers; how best to make sense of the irreducible plurality of evaluative concerns—values of different kinds at stake for distinctly situated people. Our acknowledgement of these difficulties has been at best partial, even as the normative has 'come back in'. But the lack in our institutions, procedures, and ways of thinking and speaking—highlighted by the crisis, but not confined to the crisis—points to the elements of a solution. We must reinvent them to ensure that the normative stays where it should be—at the centre of public life.

THE 'GREAT RESET'? YES, PLEASE—BUT A REAL ONE!

Slavoj Žižek

Back in April 2020, reacting to the COVID-19 explosion, Jürgen Habermas observed that '*existentielle Unsicherheit verbreitet sich jetzt global und gleichzeitig, und zwar in den Köpfen der medial vernetzten Individuen selbst*' (existential uncertainty is now spreading globally and simultaneously, in the heads of medially-wired individuals themselves). He also added, '*So viel Wissen über unser Nichtwissen und über den Zwang, unter Unsicherheit handeln und leben zu müssen, gab es noch nie*' (There never was so much knowing about our not-knowing and about the constraint to act and live in uncertainty) (Schwering 2020). And he is right to claim that this not-knowing does not concern only the pandemic—we at least have experts there—but even more its economic, social, and psychic consequences. Note his precise formulation: it is not simply that we don't know what goes on; we *know* that we don't know, and this not-knowing is itself a social fact, inscribed into how our institutions act. We now know that in, say, medieval times or early modernity they knew much less—but they didn't know this because they relied on some stable ideological foundation which guaranteed that our universe is a meaningful totality. The same holds for some visions of Communism, even for Fukuyama's idea of the end of history—they all assumed to know where history is moving. Plus Habermas is right to locate the uncertainty into 'the heads of medially-wired individuals': our link to the wired universe tremendously expands our knowledge, but at the same time it throws us into radical uncertainty (Are we hacked? Who controls our access? Are what we read there fake news?). The ongoing discoveries about a foreign (Russian?) hacking of the US government institutions and big companies exemplify this uncertainty—Americans are now discovering that they cannot determine even the scope and ways of the ongoing hacking. The irony is that virus now struck in both meanings of the term, biological and digital.

When we try to guess how our societies will look after the pandemic will be over, the trap to avoid is futurology—futurology by definition ignores our not-knowing. Futurology is defined as a systematic forecasting of the future from the present trends in society—and therein resides the problem: futurology mostly extrapolates what will come from the present tendencies. However, what futurology doesn't take into account are historical 'miracles', radical breaks which can only be explained retroactively, once they happen. We should perhaps mobilize here the distinction that works in French between *futur* and *avenir*: '*Futur*' is whatever will come after the present while 'avenir' points towards a radical change. When a president wins re-election, he is 'the present and future president', but he is not the president 'to come'—the president to come is a different president. So will the post-Corona universe be just another future or something new 'to come'?

It depends not only on science but on our *political* decisions. Now the time has come to say that we should have no illusions about the 'happy' outcome of the US elections which brought such a relief among the liberals all around the world. John Carpenter's *They Live* (1988), one of the neglected masterpieces of the Hollywood Left, tells the story of John Nada—Spanish for 'nothing'—a homeless labourer who accidentally stumbles upon a pile of boxes full of sunglasses in an abandoned church. When he puts on a pair of these glasses while walking on a street, he notices that a colourful publicity billboard soliciting us to enjoy chocolate bars now simply displays the word 'OBEY', while another billboard with a glamorous couple in a tight embrace, seen through the glasses, orders the viewer to 'MARRY AND REPRODUCE'. He also sees that paper money bears the words 'THIS IS YOUR GOD'. Additionally, he soon discovers that many people who look charming are actually monstrous aliens with metal heads. What circulates now on the web is an image which restages the scene from *They Live* apropos Biden and Harris: seen directly, the image shows the two of them smiling with the message 'TIME TO HEAL'; seen through the glasses, they are two alien monsters and the message is 'TIME TO HEEL'.

This is, of course, part of the Trump propaganda to discredit Biden and Harris as masks of anonymous corporate machines that control our lives, but there is (more than) a grain of truth in it. Biden's victory means 'future' as the continuation of the pre-Trump 'normality'—that's why there was such a sigh of relief after his victory. But this 'normality' means the rule of anonymous global capital which is the true alien in our midst. I remember from my youth the desire for 'Socialism with a human face' against USSR type 'bureaucratic' socialism—Biden too promises global capitalism with a human face, while behind the face the same reality will remain. In education, this 'human face' assumed the form of our obsession with 'well-being': pupils and students should live in bubbles that will save them from the horrors of external reality, protected by Politically Correct rules. Education is no longer intended to have a sobering effect of allowing us to confront social reality, and when we are told that this safety will prevent mental breakdowns, we should counter it with exactly the opposite claim—such false safety opens us up to mental crises when we have to confront our social reality. What 'well-being activity' does is that it merely provides a false 'human face' to our reality instead of enabling us to change this reality itself. Biden is the ultimate well-being president.

So why is Biden still better than Trump? Critics point out that Biden also lies and represents big capital, only in a more polite form—but, unfortunately, this form matters. With his vulgarization of public speech, Trump was corroding the ethical substance of our lives, what Hegel called *Sitten* (as opposed to individual morality). This vulgarization is a worldwide process. Here is a European example: Szilard Demeter, a ministerial commissioner and head of the Petofi Literary Museum in Budapest. He wrote in an op-ed in November 2020: *'Europe is George Soros' gas chamber. Poison gas flows from the capsule of a multicultural open society, which is deadly to the European way of life'* (Hungarian Cultural Commissioner 2020). Demeter went on to characterize Soros as *'the liberal Fuhrer'*, insisting that his *'liber-aryan army deifies him more than did Hitler's own'*. If asked, Demeter would probably dismiss these statements as rhetorical exaggeration; this, however, in no way dismisses their terrifying implications. The comparison between Soros and Hitler is deeply anti-Semitic: it puts Soros on a level with Hitler, claiming that the multicultural open society promoted by Soros is not only as perilous as the holocaust and the Aryan racism that sustained it ('liber-aryan') but even worse, more perilous to the 'European way of life'.

So, is there an alternative to this terrifying vision, other than Biden's 'human face'? Greta Thunberg recently resumed three positive lessons of the pandemic: 'It is possible to treat a crisis like a crisis, it is possible to put people's health above economic interests, and it is possible to listen to the science' (Thunberg 2020). Yes, but these are possibilities—it's also possible to treat a crisis in such a way that one uses it to obfuscate other crises (like: because of the pandemic we should forget about global warming); it's also possible to use the crisis to make the rich richer and the poor poorer (which effectively happened in 2020 with an unprecedented speed); and it's also possible to ignore or compartmentalize science (just recall those who refuse to take vaccines, the explosive rise of conspiracy theories, etc.). Scott Galloway (2020) gives a more or less accurate image of things in our Corona-ridden time:

> We are barrelling towards a nation with three million lords being served by 350 million serfs. We don't like to say this out loud, but I feel as if this pandemic has largely been invented for taking the top 10% into the top 1%, and taking the rest of the 90% downward. We have decided to protect corporations, not people. Capitalism is literally collapsing on itself unless it rebuilds that pillar of empathy. We have decided that capitalism means being loving and empathetic to corporations, and Darwinist and harsh towards individuals.

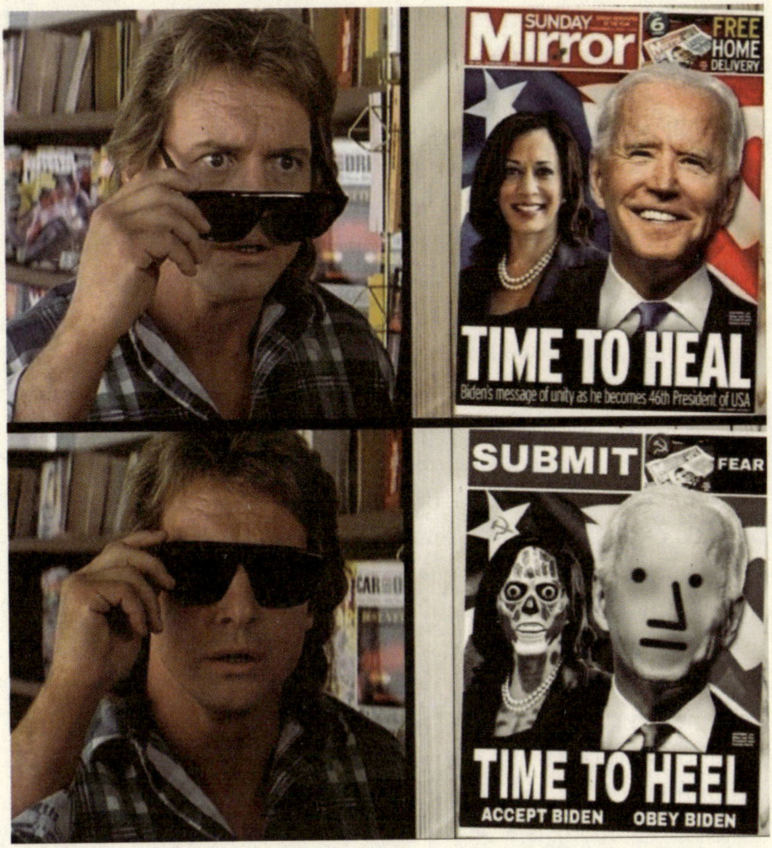
SUNDAY
Mirror
FREE HOME DELIVERY
TIME TO HEAL
Biden's message of unity as he becomes 46th President of USA
SUBMIT
FEAR
TIME TO HEEL
ACCEPT BIDEN
OBEY BIDEN

So, which is Galloway's way out, how should we prevent social collapse? His answer is that 'capitalism will collapse on itself without more empathy and love': 'We're entering the Great Reset, and it's happening quickly. Many companies will tragically be lost to the economic fallout of the pandemic, and those that do survive will exist in a different form. Organizations will be far more adaptable and resilient. Distributed teams currently thriving with less oversight will crave that same autonomy going forward. Employees will expect executives to continue leading with transparency, authenticity, and humanity' (Baer, 2020). But, again, how will this be done? Galloway proposes creative destruction that lets failing business fail while protecting people who lose jobs: '*We* let people get fired so that

Apple can emerge and put Sun Microsystems out of business, and then *we* take that incredible prosperity and we're more empathetic with people.'[1]

The problem is, of course, who is the mysterious 'we' in the last quoted sentence, i.e. how, exactly, is the redistribution done. Do we just tax the winners (Apple, in this case) more while allowing them to maintain their monopolist position? Galloway's idea has a certain dialectical flair: the only way to reduce inequality and poverty is to allow the market competition to do its cruel job (we let people get fired), and then...what? Do we expect market mechanisms themselves to create new jobs? Or the state? How are 'love' and 'empathy' operationalized? Or do we count on the winners' empathy and expect they will all behave like Gates and Buffett? I find this supplementation of market mechanisms by morality, love, and empathy utterly problematic—instead of enabling us to get the best of both worlds (market egotism and moral empathy), it is much more probable that we'll get the worst of both worlds.

The human face of this 'leading with transparency, authenticity, and humanity' are Gates, Bezos, Zuckerberg, the faces of authoritarian corporate capitalism who all pose as humanitarian heroes, as our new aristocracy celebrated in our media and quoted as wise humanitarians. Gates gives billions for charities, but we should remember how he opposed Elizabeth Warren's plan for a small rise in taxes. He praised Piketty and once almost proclaimed himself a Socialist—true, but in a very specific twisted sense: his wealth comes from privatizing what Marx called our 'commons', our shared social space in which we move and communicate. Gates's wealth has nothing to do with the production costs of the products Microsoft is selling (one can even argue that Microsoft is paying its intellectual workers a relatively high salary), i.e. Gates's wealth is not the result of his success in producing good software for lower prices than his competitors, or in higher 'exploitation' of his

1. Galloway as quoted in Shapiro (2020). 'Capitalism "will collapse on itself" without more empathy and love.

hired intellectual workers. Gates became one of the richest men in the world through appropriating the rent for allowing millions of us to communicate through the medium that he privatized and controls. And in the same way that Microsoft privatized the software most of us use, personal contacts are privatized by Facebook, buying books by Amazon, search by Google. The new mega-corporations that emerge through the privatization of commons justify (to some degree, at least) the idea that we are witnessing today the rise of neo-feudalism, of feudal capitalism. By way of controlling our commons, the new masters (Bill Gates, Elon Musk) effectively act in a way similar to feudal masters. To quote Jodi Dean:

> Unlike the capitalist whose profit rests on the surplus value generated by waged workers through the production of commodities, the lord extracts value through monopoly, coercion, and rent. ... Digital platforms are the new watermills, their billionaire owners the new lords, and their thousands of workers and billions of users the new peasants. (2020)

This is how Apple, Amazon, Microsoft, Facebook, and Google function. We retain the freedom of our personal choice, but the scope of this choice is determined by the corporation which privatized a part of our commons: you buy whichever book you want *through Amazon*; you freely determine your public identity *through Facebook*, etc. These mega-corporations recently tried to colonize our future (Bill Gates regularly proposes projects on how our future lives should be organized) and even the outer space (Musk owns many satellites and plans settlements on Mars).

There is thus a grain of truth in the Trump 'rebellion' against digital corporate powers. It is worth watching the War Room podcasts of Steve Bannon, the greatest ideologist of Trump's populism: one cannot but be fascinated by how many partial truths he combines into an overall lie. Yes, under Obama the gap that separates wealthy from poor grew immensely, big corporations grew stronger... But under Trump this process just went on, plus Trump lowered taxes, printed money mostly to save big companies, etc. We are thus facing a horrible false alternative: big corporate reset or nationalist populism which turns out to be the same. 'The great reset' is the formula of how to change some things (even many things) so that things will basically remain the same.

So, is there a third way, outside the space of the two extremes of restoring the old normality and a Great Reset? Yes, a true great reset. It is no secret what needs to be done—Greta Thunberg made it clear. First, we should finally recognize the pandemic crisis as what it is, part of a global crisis of our entire way of life, from ecology to new social tensions. Second, we should establish social control and regulation over economy. Third, we should rely on science—rely on but not simply accept it as the agency which makes decisions. Why not? Let's return to Habermas with whom we began: our predicament is that we are compelled to act while we know we don't know the full coordinates of the situation we are in, and non-acting would itself function as an act. But is this not the basic situation of every action?

Our great advantage is that we *know* how much we don't know, and this knowing about our not-knowing opens up the space of freedom. We act when we don't know the whole situation, but this is not simply our limitation: what gives us freedom is that the situation—in our social sphere, at least—is in itself open, not fully (pre)determined. And our situation in the pandemic is certainly open. We learned the first lesson now: 'shutdown light' is not enough. They tell us 'we' (our economy) cannot afford another hard lockdown—so let's change the economy. Lockdown is the most radical negative gesture *within* the existing order. The way beyond, to a new positive order, leads through politics, not science. What has to be done is changing our economic life so that it will be able to survive lockdowns and emergencies that are for sure awaiting us, in the same way that a war compels us to ignore market limitations and find a way to do what is 'impossible' in a free-market economy.

Back in March 2003, Donald Rumsfeld, then the US Secretary of Defence, engaged in a little bit of amateur philosophizing about the relationship between the known and the unknown: 'There are known knowns. These are things we know that we know. There are known unknowns. That is to say, there are things that we know we don't know. But there are also unknown unknowns. There are things we don't know we don't know.'[2] What he forgot to add was the crucial fourth term: the 'unknown knowns', things we don't know that we know—which is precisely the Freudian unconscious, the 'knowledge which doesn't know itself', as Lacan used to say. If Rumsfeld thought that the main dangers in the confrontation with Iraq were the 'unknown unknowns', the threats from Saddam about which we do not even suspect what they may be, what we should reply is that the main dangers are, on the contrary, the 'unknown knowns', the disavowed beliefs and suppositions we are not even aware of adhering to ourselves. We should read Habermas's claim that we never knew so much about what we don't know through these four categories: the pandemic shook what we (thought we) knew that we knew, it made us aware of what we didn't know that we didn't know, and, in the way we confronted it, we relied on what we didn't know that we know (all our presumptions and prejudices which determine our acting although we are not even aware of them). We are not dealing here with the simple passage from not-knowing to knowing but with the much more subtle passage from not-knowing to knowing what we don't know—our positive knowing remains the same in this passage, but we gain a free space for action.

It is with regard to what we don't know that we know, our presumptions and prejudices, that we must admit China (and Taiwan and Vietnam) did so much better than Europe and the US. I am getting tired of the eternally repeated claim 'Yes, the Chinese contained the virus, but at what price...' I agree that we need a Chinese Assange to let us know what really went on there, the whole story, but the fact is that, when the epidemic exploded in Wuhan, they immediately imposed

2. I used this example many times in my work, most extensively in Chapter 9 of *Defense of Lost Causes*.

lockdown and put on a standstill the majority of production in the entire country, clearly giving priority to human lives over the economy. With some delay, true, they took the crisis extremely seriously. Now they are reaping the reward, even in the economy. And let's be clear, this was only possible because the Communist Party is still able to control and regulate the economy: there is social control over market mechanisms, although a 'totalitarian' one. But, again, the question is not how they did it in China but how should *we* do it. The Chinese way is not the only effective way, it is not 'objectively necessary' in the sense that, if you analyse all the data, you have to do it the Chinese way. The epidemic is not just a viral process, it is a process that takes place within certain economic, social, and ideological coordinates which are open to change.

Now we live in a crazy time in which the hope that vaccines will work is mixed by the growing depression, despair even, due to the growing number of infections and the almost daily discoveries of the new unknowns about the virus. In principle the answer to 'What is to be done?' is easy here: we have the means and resources to restructure healthcare so that it serves the needs of the people in a time of crisis, etc. However, to quote the last line of Brecht's 'In Praise of Communism' from his play *The Mother*: 'Er ist das Einfache, das schwer zu machen ist' (It is the simple thing that is so hard to do). There are many obstacles that make it so hard to do, above all the global capitalist order and its ideological hegemony. Do we then need a new Communism? Yes, but what I am tempted to call a *moderately conservative Communism*: all the steps that are necessary, from global mobilization against viral and other threats to establishing procedures which will constrain market mechanisms and socialize economy, but done in a way which is conservative (in the sense of an effort to conserve the conditions of human life—and the paradox is that we will have to change things precisely to maintain these conditions) and moderate (in the sense of carefully taking into account unpredictable side-effects of our measures).

As Emmanuel Renault pointed out, the key Marxian

category that introduces class struggle into the very heart of the critique of political economy is that of the so-called 'tendential laws', the laws which describe a necessary tendency in capitalist development, like the tendency of the falling profit rate.[3] Describing this 'tendency', Marx himself uses the term *antagonism*: the falling rate of profit is a tendency which pushes capitalists to strengthen workers' exploitation, and workers to resist it, so that the outcome is not predetermined but depends on the struggle—say, in some welfare states, organized workers forced the capitalists to make considerable concessions. The Communism I am speaking about is exactly such a tendency: reasons for it are obvious (we need global action to fight health and environmental threats, economy will have to be somehow socialized...), and we should read the way global capitalism is reacting to the pandemic precisely as *a set of reactions to the Communist tendency*: the fake Great Reset, nationalist populism, solidarity reduced to empathy.

So how will the Communist tendency prevail? A sad answer: through more repeated crises. Let's put it clearly: the virus is atheist in the strongest sense of the term. Yes, it should be analysed how the pandemic is socially conditioned, but it is basically a product of meaningless contingency, there is no 'deeper message' in it (just as there wasn't when they interpreted the plague as God's punishment in medieval times). Before choosing the famous line by Virgil '*acheronta movebo*' as the motto of his *Interpretation of Dreams*, Freud considered another candidate, Satan's words from Milton's *Paradise Lost*: 'What reinforcement we may gain from Hope, / If not what resolution from despair'. If we cannot get any reinforcement from hope, if we are compelled to admit that our situation is hopeless, we should gain resolution from despair. This is how we, contemporary Satans who are destroying our Earth, should react to the viral and ecological threats: instead of

3. As Renault noted, it was already Adorno who has insisted on these dimensions of Marx's concept of '*Tendenz*' which makes it irreducible to a simple 'trend' (see Adorno 2008, 37–40).

looking vainly for reinforcement in some hope, we should accept that our situation is desperate, and act resolutely upon it. To quote Greta Thunberg again, 'Doing our best is no longer good enough. Now we need to do the seemingly impossible.' Futurology deals with what is possible, we need to do what is (from the standpoint of the existing global order) *impossible.*

PART II

EXPERIENTIAL REFLECTIONS, NARRATIVES AND STRATEGIES

Reflections on Health and Wellness

A NARRATIVE GROUP PROJECT FROM TURKEY: EXPLORING DIVERSE RESPONSES TO COVID-19

İclal Eskioğlu Aydın

INTRODUCTION

In Turkey, COVID-19 started in March 2020. From March to June, the country went under lockdown only for two to four days per week. With June, the lockdown days came to an end. In these six months, some people started to work at home. The psychotherapy centre that I work at also moved to online sessions until June. However, in Turkey, doing therapy sessions online was still a new idea. Most people prefer to have face-to-face sessions. Most therapists were also unaccustomed to online sessions. So, it was an adaptation period both for the therapists and the people consulting the therapists. With the emergence of the pandemic, we (my master's students and I) made a group project that was guided with narrative ideas. In this paper, the story of the project, the guiding narrative ideas, and group processes are explored.

STORY OF THE PROJECT

The project came about in response to the difficulties that popped up in our lives because of COVID-19. I work at the Ibn Haldun University Center for Psychotherapy Research in Turkey as a narrative therapist. I also supervise the master's students of clinical psychology at the university who are doing their internships. Because of the pandemic, their internships were left half-finished. Their academic dissertation processes were also affected. Some of them had to go back to their homes, out of İstanbul. So, they found themselves in a very uncertain place full of anxiety and disappointments and stressed out with the emergence of the pandemic.

The centre was planning to announce that people who were experiencing difficulties could call for help for free. As the students were willing to help other people, the therapists at the centre were expected to guide the students in approaching those who wanted support. During our session with the students, in which I was proposing a narrative framework in supporting applicants, they revealed that they were experiencing great hardship during those pandemic days, and they did not know how to help other people when they did not feel well enough themselves. I offered to arrange narrative group work for them to talk about the difficulties they experienced and find some ways that may help them respond to these difficulties. In addition, they could use the ideas they would learn from this group work. However, since there were 18 students who wanted to attend the group work, I offered to split them into four groups, thereby making it easier to work.

NARRATIVE PERSPECTIVES THAT GUIDED THE GROUP WORK

COVID-19 came into our lives suddenly, with no end in sight. Because of the pandemic, our lifestyles have changed dramatically, with social distancing separating us from each other. We have lost the warmth of our loved ones, leading us to face isolation and causing depressive feelings. Because the future is blurred, and our plans were cancelled or postponed for an indefinite period of time, uncertainty and anxiety appeared in our lives in different forms. While some people have to stay home with a violent partner, others face the risk of death. Due to such drastic changes, some narrative ideas may help us reconsider the conditions we live in.

Trauma

The shape of the coronavirus made me think about trauma. We may say that it is collective trauma because lots of people experienced the intrusive and unexpected emergence of the effects of the virus. In narrative therapy, Michael White (2006) claimed, 'no-one is a passive recipient of trauma'. White asserts that everyone does something in order to prevent or modify the trauma or its effects because people try to protect what is precious in their lives. Therefore, we should evaluate both the effects of the trauma and the responses to trauma. However, trauma generally tries to convince us to see only its effects and ignore the responses to trauma. Thus, in a narrative approach, 'listening doubly' refers to listening to both the effects of and the responses to trauma, which in therapy enables 'double-storied' conversations. The double-storied conversations assist people to add a new dimension to their story, that of their responses to trauma, rather than having single-storied (only the trauma story) conversations (White, 2006).

In the group work, listening doubly helped me find out things that helped group members cope during the pandemic. We could thus discover their skills, areas of knowledge, and the values that they cling to in the face of difficulties. With listening doubly, I assisted them in strengthening their stories of responses to trauma.

Liminal Phase

A liminal phase is a period of the 'rite of passage' in life and it is described as a phase 'in which one's familiar sense of being in the world is absent, and where nothing means quite what it did before. This phase is invariably characterized by periods of disorientation and confusion, and times of significant despair' (White 2020). It is possible to think of the pandemic days as a liminal phase in life. Before the pandemic, we were working at workplaces; going outside; making holiday plans; cultivating relations and participating in social activities, etc. However, with the emergence of the pandemic, our 'sense of being in the world' became unfamiliar, and we started to face disorientation, uncertainty, and hopelessness.

In the group work, we discussed this period of time as a liminal phase. In addition, we also talked about previous such liminal phases in their lives. These conversations made it possible to see that what we experience is a phase. Hence, feelings of disorientation changed to those of 'it is a phase in life that I will go through and it will end like the other liminal phases I have experienced before and overcome'. When we know that we are going through a liminal phase, it is easier to focus on the things that help us cope in this process.

Sustaining Rather Than Solving

When we consider the situation as an overwhelming problem that should be solved, we can try to find solutions to end it, change it, escape from it. That may tire and exhaust us. However, when we accept the situation as a process, it may invite a sustaining and surviving position. A sustaining position may allow us to look at what we have in our hands—the things that help us endure, to continue in the process.

GROUP WORK PROCESSES AND NARRATIVE PRACTICES

The group works were conducted online in three sessions for all the four groups, each of which lasted about two and a half hours. The first session involved some guiding questions that aimed to understand the difficulties they experienced and discover the sustaining stories of the group members. In order to do that, some narrative ideas and practices guided us. The second meeting focused on generating collective documents. The third meeting was held to evaluate the process.

First Meeting: Discovering the Skills, Knowledge, and Values

In the first meeting, we talked about both the difficulties that they experienced in the pandemic days and the responses that they had to this hardship. I prepared some guiding questions for the conversations in the first meeting. However, during the group processes, I tried to take a de-centred position which, in narrative therapy, refers to bringing to the centre of the therapeutic conversations areas of knowledge and skill of the people consulted to therapy, not of the therapist (White 2011). These were our guiding questions:

- How do you evaluate the coronavirus period? What kind of anxiety or distress do you experience? Could you specify your anxiety/distress?
- Could you name the anxiety/distress? What kind of an image do you have in your mind when you think about this anxiety/distress?
- What are the effects of this anxiety/distress in your life?
- Are there any places, times, people, circumstances that increase the anxiety/distress?
- Are there any places, times, people, circumstances that decrease the anxiety/distress?
- Do you remember a difficult time previously when you found a way for sustaining?
- In that difficult time, what kind of a skill/knowledge/value helped you to sustain?
- Could you tell a story about how this skill/knowledge/value made a difference in a difficult time?
- What is the history of this skill/knowledge/value? How did you learn it? Who did you learn it from?
- Is this skill or value linked in some way to collective traditions (familial/community) and/or cultural traditions? Are there proverbs, sayings, stories, songs, images from your family, community and/or culture with which these skills and knowledge are linked?
- Could you share your feedback? What do you think about how this conversation went?

These questions were developed to benefit from some of the narrative ideas and practices discussed below.

Specification and Externalization of the Problem

The pandemic has a very pervasive form that affects many areas of our lives. When we see a problem as pervasive, we may feel uncertainty. Therefore, if we narrow our conversation and choose a specific starting point, it is possible to feel a bit more certain, as an antidote to the uncertainty of the pandemic. So, I tried to specify the problem in the group conversations. For example, talking about 'anxiety' is a very big task; we may get lost in it because there are many types of anxiety. However, when we talk about the 'anxiety of losing our loved one', the territory of the conversation may be more certain. So, I preferred to stay in this specific area.

One of the helpful practices were externalization conversations. In relation to Michael White's (2007) statement, 'the person is not the problem; the problem is the problem', we talked about the difficulties that they experienced in a concrete way. In other words, I asked them to externalize and name the problem/difficulty that they experienced. They found an image to describe their problem as an 'experience-near' description (White 2007). For example, one of them identified the feeling of loneliness/isolation as that of being 'drawn into a black hole that is trying to strangle through silence and make us lonely'. Through externalization, we were able to discuss the problems separately from the person's identity. After identifying the problem, they were asked questions of 'the statement of position map' (Russell and Carey 2004). In relation to these questions, we searched for the effects of the identified problem in their lives. In addition, we talked about the places, times, circumstances when the effects of the problem increase and decrease. The latter helped us figure out what works for them in these times, that is, what skills, values, knowledge help them reduce the effects of the problem.

Unique Outcomes and Double-Storied Conversations

Externalization of conversations made it possible to separate the person from the 'problem-saturated story' which enables them to feel a sense of 'personal agency', which means they have a participation in their own lives (White and Epston 1990). The question which aimed at searching for the times, circumstances, and places when the effects of the problem decreased revealed the 'unique outcomes'. Unique outcomes refer to 'those aspects of lived experience that fall outside of the dominant problem story' (White and Epston 1990). Finding out the unique outcomes made it possible to discover the skills, values, and knowledge which helped them see the experiences that 'fall outside of the dominant problem story'.

Each group member found their own sustaining skills in which we discovered the stories, histories, and broader connections of these skills and knowledge. When we were talking about stories of their skills, I encouraged them to find a time where these skills and knowledge made a difference. In this frame, I used the questions that David Denborough mentioned in his book *Collective Narrative Practice* (Denborough 2008).

To trace the stories of these skills, knowledge, and values that they found helpful for sustaining in these days, I asked them whether these sustaining skills had made a difference during another liminal phase in the past. They were surprised to see that they used the same skills and knowledge in two different liminal phases in their lives. It was like a bridge that they discovered, something special for them, coming from experiences acquired through hardship and having been kept for a long time. One of them expressed her discovery with these words: 'I realized that this skill was helping me for many years. However, now I could know it and name it. This awareness made me feel strong and hopeful.' Some of them said that with the discoveries of skills and knowledge, they felt that 'the control of their lives' is in their hands; not in the problem's hands.

Revealing the skills and knowledge led us to engage in double-storied conversations. In other words, at the beginning of the first meeting, they came with a dominant problem story (single story). However, after talking about the skills and knowledge, they developed double-stories (both the story of the difficulties they experienced and that of the responses they had to these difficulties) at the end of the first meeting.

Discovering the History and the Connections of Skills and Knowledge

In the conversations where we were searching for what sustained them in the process of the pandemic, I asked them to discover the history of their skills, knowledge, and values with the following questions proposed by David Denborough, 'How did you learn this? Who did you learn it from?' (Denborough 2008). They found some important, precious people in their lives that they had learned these skills from. The moments that the connections were established between these people were very powerful. They indicated that these people were a strong support in their lives.

Then I inquired about the broader connections of these skills and knowledge with the following questions: 'Is this skill or value linked in some way to collective traditions (familial/community) and/or cultural traditions? Are there proverbs, sayings, stories, songs, images from your family, community and/or culture with which these skills and knowledge are linked?' With this question, skills and knowledge were described in a collective context (Denborough 2008).

SECOND MEETING: GENERATING COLLECTIVE DOCUMENTS

Denborough (2008) mentioned the aim of 'collective documents' as 'collectively convey[ing] a range of hard-won skills and knowledge, in parallel with a rich acknowledgement of the circumstances in which these have been hard-won'. After the first meeting, group members wrote their own discoveries of their sustaining skills, knowledge, and values. However, the stories were still individual. In order to tell stories in a collective way, in the second meeting, we collected all the writings and read them aloud in the group. Each group read and edited the writings together. Before reading, we decided on these guiding tips to gather them in a collective way:

1) *Selecting phrases, metaphors, images.* They focused on selecting the words, phrases, sentences that may attract the attention of the people who will read/watch the collective documents. They tried to find impressive phrases, literary descriptions, metaphoric expressions that may help evoke the imagination and feelings of the audiences.
2) *Collective expressions.* The group members tried to eliminate the individual statements and pick out the collective expressions.
3) *Double-storied telling.* Each document focused on both the shared difficulties that they experienced in the pandemic and the skills, knowledge and values that helped them to survive in these days.

At the end of the first editions, I asked the following questions:

1) What do you want to do with these expressions?
2) Do you want to write a poem, or make a video, or draw a painting or something else?
3) How do you want to convey these documents to the audiences?

Each group responded in a different way. The first group wanted to write paragraphs, the second group chose to write a poem, the other group wanted to make a video, and the last group decided to develop a formula. So, each collective document went through very creative and unique processes.

Sharing the Collective Documents and Enabling Contributions

'Once we begin to acknowledge people's responses to trauma and what it is they give value to, we can start sharing our survival skills and making contributions to one another' (Denborough 2014). It is really important to share our skills, knowledge, and values with other people who have similar difficulties in their lives. Denborough (2014) stated that, on television, newspapers, and online news, we watch/read only trauma stories (violence, abuse, disasters, etc.); however, we don't read/watch/listen stories of surviving skills that include the steps people take in order to protect themselves or others, to create safety.

After they developed collective documents, I asked them with whom they wanted to share these documents. All of them decided to share the documents with people in Turkey and the people around the world who experience difficulties. Thus, they wrote the documents in Turkish and then translated them into English. The collective documents were put on the Ibn Haldun University's website in Turkish;[1] and the Re-authoring Teaching website in English.[2]

For receiving responses, they prepared some questions which they hope would be helpful for the audiences. The questions were formed for the sake of establishing a connection with the audience, evoking the contributions of other people, and adding a new layer to the sustaining stories. Here are some examples from the questions:

'When you watched the video, which expression(s) caught your attention?'

'What did the expressions which caught your attention remind you about your life?'

'Does the poem contribute in any way to your sustaining in this process?'

'If you wanted to write one more stanza to this poem, what could it be?'

'Do you think that you can also develop your own formula of your stories (both with the effects of difficulties and the ways in which you can survive against these difficulties)?'

'Did our stories remind you of anything that assists you in surviving in the face of the pandemic?'

---

1. See 'Different Ways of Coping in the Corona Virus Process', Ibn Haldun University website (https://ipam.ihu.edu.tr/narrative-grup-projesi-corona-virus-surecinde-farkli-bas-etme-yollari/).

2. See 'Re-authoring Confinement: Inspirational sparkling moments in everyday life' (https://reauthoringteaching.com/resources/re-authoring-confinement-inspirational-sparkling-moments-in-everyday-life/).

THIRD MEETING: DEFINITIONAL CEREMONY AND EVALUATING THE PROCESS

After the editing of the collective documents, we met again for definitional ceremonies so that 'the process [could] move from the written word to an oral ritual' (Denborough 2008). Each group read out aloud or watched the collective documents together. When they read/watched again in a ceremonial frame, they had the chance to give voice to a double-storied re-telling, and they gathered around their stories of survival. Afterwards, we evaluated the group process and received feedback for the project. Some of the feedback has been quote below:

'Actually I noticed that this skill has been in my life for many years; however, I recognized it in this meeting. This makes me feel stronger and hopeful.'

'I see that the control of my life has been in my hands in the face of difficulties since I was a child.'

'Sometimes we cannot think what can help us when we face hardship in life. However, I now know and I can use this skill in the future instead of trying to find it.'

'This awareness says to me, "You could overcome the problems in life by using your own skills rather than trying to find something from outside and you can use your own resources when you need."'

'I now realize that I was following a family tradition (cooking) and from now on cooking will have a meaning for me.'

'I think it is a really helpful awareness to know what helps us in life.'

'When we were generating the collective document, it was a time when we were in that moment, we didn't think about the pandemic, difficulties, anxiety, etc. We really enjoyed that period of time.'

'I am so surprised to receive responses from other people.'

'This project contributed both to our lives and to our therapeutic practices.'

EXAMPLES FROM CONTRIBUTIONS

I want to share one of my colleague's response to the collective document: 'When I looked at the collective documents, I felt like I was watching marbling art; all the documents are part of a unity, however, none of them interfere with others, like the colours in the marbling art.'

After sharing collective documents, precious contributions were received. Here are some examples from these contributions:

Contribution to the Collective Poem:
Someone wanted to add one more stanza to the poem:

Colour the life in your own way
Love everything in your heart
Give so generously that you can warm every soul on earth
Mingle the souls that no soul remains without love in the world

Contribution to the Formula:
All the difficulties/ordeals=0

Contribution to the Paragraphs:
'This document helped me see that the solutions in life are in ordinary things that we do here and now rather than sophisticated or outside.'

Contribution to the video:
'I thought that my own skills, values are so important.'

MY EXPERIENCE AS A THERAPIST

As a therapist, all the group processes were very exciting for me. At the beginning of the first session, there were only difficulties, problems, and feelings of hopelessness and desperation. But then I witnessed the discoveries of their responses to the pandemic. I usually have individual sessions, and when we discover double-stories with the people who consult for therapy, it really makes me feel excited. However, in group work, seeing the responses of and with more than one person added to my excitement.

In addition, the processes of generating collective documents were very creative, and I could see the evolution of the expressions from individual to collective. When the documents were prepared in a collective way, it was very different from the start. I felt like I was watching a riverbed to which the water flows in through different geographical areas.

On the other hand, because the students were being supervised by me, we knew each other. And after the group project, we felt warmth between us, and our relationship became closer. After the group project, some of the students did sessions with people who faced difficulties because of the pandemic, and they used the narrative ideas we had explored. I was supervising them, and I saw how good they were at narrative practices even though they did not have narrative therapy training. I could see that this project helped them both as individuals facing difficulties during the pandemic as well as therapists. The group project was very unique, creative, and constructive for all of us.

CONCLUSION

This group project began spontaneously in response to a need of the therapists who wanted to help people facing difficulties in the pandemic process. In group works, I preferred to see the pandemic as a liminal phase, where one has a sense of being lost. The trauma was also collective, being experienced by many people due to the effects of the coronavirus. Therefore, we tried to find *sustaining* skills rather than *solving* skills. As the feedback shows, the group members discovered their own skills, knowledge, and values in life. It was not coming from an 'expert' who told them what was 'healthy/unhealthy to do' in these days. The conversations in the group work encouraged them to look at their already-used skills and knowledge. They thus felt that they had already managed to survive under the pandemic, just as they had survived previous hardships in their lives. They also employed their creative skills in the process, whereby each group tended to choose the type of document that was related to their interests in life.

SOCIALIZED HEALTHCARE AND MEDICAL INTERNATIONALISM: CUBA AND THE CORONAVIRUS

Vinay Lal

Six months into the worldwide panic induced by SARS-CoV-2 and the calamitous consequences in its wake, a few countries are often mentioned in the world press as those that have been more successful in stemming the advance of the virus. These countries include South Korea, New Zealand, Taiwan, and Singapore. The supposition, it is very likely, is that countries which are still struggling to contain the virus may have something to learn from those which have (nearly) vanquished the virus, though countries, much like individuals, seem notoriously impervious to the idea that there are any 'lessons' to be drawn from history. Everyone likes to speak of the 'lessons of history', but the habit is ingrained enough in most that such lessons are deemed worthy of emulation by others though not by oneself. Moreover, that memorable adage which opens *Anna Karenina* comes to mind: 'All happy families are alike; each unhappy family is unhappy in its own way.'

One might complicate the narrative still more: barring New Zealand, the other three nations—and the sovereignty of Taiwan (formally, the Republic of China), let us recall, is disputed by the People's Republic of China—that I have mentioned fall within Southeast Asia, where, as many will argue, the historical memory of SARS (2003) played a role in preparing them for this iteration of the coronavirus' assault upon the human world. Some may, therefore, submit that the experience of these countries varies greatly from that of other nations. Similarly, barring South Korea, the other three nations are exceedingly small, and the containment of epidemic disease has almost always been a greater challenge for more populous countries. The experience of China would, of course, appear to belie this claim, but understandably, there are reasons to feel squeamish about putting forward China as a country that might be emulated in this connection. It is in China that the virus almost certainly originated, and there are substantial majorities in countries such as India, the United States, and Germany which, even as they may quietly marvel at China's success in squashing the virus after the first horrific scenes of its rampage through Wuhan had been flashed to the world, are clamouring to have China held responsible for the deep wounds that have been inflicted everywhere by COVID-19. Even those saner voices which rebel at the idea of holding one country accountable for a condition that has doubtless been precipitated by the reckless human advance upon reservoirs of nature are, nonetheless, constrained to admit that China almost certainly was dissimulating in withholding information about the virus, and the disease that it causes, from the rest of the world. Moreover, not every country is prepared, at least not yet, to follow the path of totalitarianism on which China seems set for the present.

It is in this connection that the near-omission of Cuba from the global narrative that has come into shape around the coronavirus is altogether striking. Cuba has been admirably successful in containing the virus, but there is comparatively little mention of it in the world press—certainly very little in comparison with the attention lavished upon the other aforementioned countries. While the United States exports arms, ammunition, and obesity-inducing diets to the rest of the world, Cuba has acquired a reputation the world over not just for its cigars but for its wholly unique corps of healthcare professionals. In the six decades since the revolution that overthrew the US-backed regime of Fulgencio Batista and brought Fidel Castro to power, and then turned Castro's comrade-at-arms, Che Guevara, into perhaps (besides Mohandas Gandhi) the world's most iconic figure of resistance to oppression, well over 400,000 Cuban doctors and healthcare workers have served abroad, rendered aid to countries at times of disaster and epidemics, and created what is unquestionably the most mobile force of medical professionals in history (Gorry 2019).

To be sure, not everything is hunky-dory in this island nation that lies around 100 miles to the south of Florida and has for the last 60 years resisted attempts by the gigantic hegemon to its north to bend it to its will. The US, by its own admission, has maintained a comprehensive economic embargo against Cuba since 1962 and has not hesitated to penalize and bully countries that have dared to violate or evade the sanctions that have to, varying degrees, been in place since the initial embargo was announced by President John F. Kennedy. A Central Intelligence Agency assessment in 1986 noted that the annual subsidy from the Soviet Union to Cuba, averaging in the first half of the 1980s to around \$4.5 billion, had shored up what was in every other respect a failing economy (US Central Intelligence Agency 2016). This subsidy took various forms, from the Soviet Union importing 80 per cent of all Cuban sugar to generous and favourable terms of trade extended to Cuba and heavy Soviet investments in the Cuban economy. The dissolution of the Soviet Union in December 1991 brought this period to an end and the withdrawal of Soviet aid, and the US has since taken various steps in attempts to throttle Cuba's economy, facilitate the country's collapse, and initiate what is called 'regime change'. To all these woes may be added the Communist Party's own stranglehold on power—manifested in a tight control on economic activity, the containment of political dissent, and adroitness in using a propaganda machine aimed at enlisting the power of the people to help resist 'Yankee imperialism'.

Interesting and germane as is the history of communist Cuba's survival as an independent nation in the face of unremitting hostility from the US, its enviable success in containing the threat of COVID-19 contrasts sharply with the chaos that has unfolded in the US. It is difficult in the US, even for a purportedly liberal and cosmopolitan newspaper such as the *New York Times* to admit as much, and the coverage of Cuba's experience with COVID-19 has been, as I have suggested, slight in the American media—an omission that appears all the more glaring when contrasted with the gushing admiration showered upon New Zealand and its young female prime minister. On 1 July 2020, Cuba had 2,348 cases and 86 deaths; this number had inched up to 2,608 cases and 87 deaths by the end of July. At the end of August, the tally stood at a little over 4,000 cases and 100 deaths. New Zealand, which has a population of 5 million in comparison to Cuba's 11.4 million, has done marginally better than Cuba. It had approximately half the number of cases and one-fourth the number of deaths. Both countries, after an initial spike, had been remarkably successful in holding the number of deaths constant: though in mid-August the number of cases in both countries began to rise once again, the virus was still remarkably under control and far from entering the community transmission stage.

But the comparison is also misleading in at least two respects: first, with a GDP per capita that is five times larger than that of Cuba, New Zealand has far greater resources at its command to tackle the threat; and, second, Cuba continues to remain under an economic blockade that has curtailed the supply of medicine, medical equipment, and other essential goods. A group of 'UN human rights experts', supported by independent experts and groups, was moved in late April to call upon the US to lift the blockade noting that 'the impact of the comprehensive embargo has imposed additional financial burden, increased cargo travel time due to an inability to procure supplies, reagents, medical equipment and medicines necessary for the diagnosis and treatment of COVID-19'. These UN special rapporteurs pointedly remarked that 'the lack of will of the US Government to suspend sanctions may lead to a higher risk of such suffering in Cuba and other countries targeted by its sanctions' (UN News 2020).

When the first case of COVID-19 in Cuba was detected on 11 March 2020, the country already had in place an elaborate plan to counter the threat of the virus; indeed, it may be said that Cuba has been well-prepared for such emergencies for decades, having shown the way to the rest of the world, not only through its consistent commitment to public healthcare expenditures but its expeditious if understandably controversial response to the AIDS crisis. Some commentators have argued that the country's commitment to public health can be seen from the outset of the revolution, in concerted efforts to improve literacy, nutrition, sanitation, and housing for the working class, and an article published in the socialist journal, *Monthly Review*, appears to offer what may justifiably seem to some as an idealized representation of the revolution's healthcare goals in suggesting that 'Che Guevara taught Cuba how to confront COVID-19' (Fritz 2020). The article points to Che's nine-month break from medical school in 1951–52 to gain, among other things, practical experience of leprosy that is chronicled in his *Motorcycle Diaries*, though he and his companion, Alberto Granado, were far from being the international leprosy experts for whom they were sometimes mistaken by villagers (Schell 2010, 71). If the halo around Che in some circles, and contrariwise the US-led efforts to cast his life as one of unmitigated and spectacular failure (US Central Intelligence Agency 1968), suggest that a nuanced assessment of Che's place in shaping the priorities of the revolution is entirely outside the scope of this brief essay, what seems to be relatively more indisputable is Cuba's success in having achieved milestones in healthcare that are not merely significant but a model to the rest of the developing world. In a densely compact report published in January 2016, the greatly respected *Lancet* noted the changes in the Cuban health system over the last several decades, registering shifts in emphasis in infectious diseases, community care, and chronic diseases, but suggesting that *throughout*, Cuba did not diverge from the objective of securing preventive care. The report states unequivocally that 'health became a major priority' since 'the regime came into power in the 1960s' and that the emphasis on preventive care has 'paid off' (Lowenberg 2016).

To gauge what circumstances have permitted Cuba to halt the advance of the coronavirus, it is also necessary to revisit the country's experience with infectious diseases. Cuba had set up a National AIDS Commission in 1983, well before AIDS arrived on the island in 1986, and all foreign-derived blood products were destroyed. As one scholarly study notes, 'although this action put a strain on the country's blood supply, it enabled Cuba to escape transmission of HIV to haemophiliacs and other blood recipients' (Hoffman 2004, 208–9). The government also instituted a system of mandatory isolation for persons suspected of suffering from a communicable disease, and sanatoriums were established, first in Havana and then extended to the rest of the country, for the forcible confinement of HIV-positive individuals. The sanatoria have been credited with helping control the epidemic; others have criticized them as prisons (Sananes 2016). By the early 1990s, Cuba had around 200 AIDS cases, while New York, which had roughly the same population, had 43,000 cases. In 1994, the system of compulsory confinement to a sanatorium was relaxed, but other stringent regulations have been retained. Pregnant women must undergo an HIV test; HIV-positive people are required to provide the names of all their sexual partners in the last six months, and each of those persons is required to take an HIV test; and patients released from a sanatorium must similarly continue to report to a physician at periodic intervals for education and counselling. Cuba developed its own HIV diagnostic test in 1987 and has since 2001 produced anti-retroviral drugs which are administered free to HIV-positive patients. It is not surprising, in view of these circumstances, that even as ethical concerns arise from the harshness of some of the country's regulations, including the forcible quarantining of HIV infected people, what impresses most is Cuba's success which has been virtually 'unmatched anywhere in the world'. Hoffman noted that, in Cuba, 'the collective community is protected by sacrifices made by the individual. Judging by statistics, there is little doubt that if other countries around the world had adopted Cuba's programme twenty years ago, it would have saved millions of lives' (Hoffman 2004, 208–9). The aforementioned 2016 report in *The Lancet* provided other startling figures—for example, there has been a decline in Cuba in infant mortality of 40 per cent since the 1960s, 'even as the basic economy remained flat... Today, Cuba's infant mortality rate is lower than that of the USA' (Lowenberg 2016).

Sometime in January 2020, the Cuban government, having taken the warning signs emanating from China seriously, put into place a 'prevention and control' plan, one also facilitated by the nearly unique system of community healthcare already prevalent in the country (Morris and Kelman 2020). Cuba has the highest number of doctors per capita in the world: 84.5 for every 10,000 inhabitants, while India, China, Brazil, the United States, the United Kingdom, and Sweden have 8.5, 20, 22, 26, 28, and 40, respectively (WHO 2018). These figures, unless parsed further, do not sufficiently reveal the immense gap between Cuba's investment in public healthcare and the appalling, indeed one should say criminal, neglect of it in many countries—especially a country such as India. There are no private medical practitioners in Cuba; in India, on the other hand, the state has increasingly withdrawn from critical social services, leaving most people to fend for themselves. The average of 8.5 doctors for every 10,000 inhabitants in India does not reflect the enormous and still-widening discrepancies in accessibility to healthcare between the poor and the affluent, and between those in rural areas and the urban-dwelling population; nor does it reflect the fact that accessibility is a function of both proximity and affordability.

Cuba similarly outstrips every other country in apportioning nearly 13 per cent of its GDP for healthcare. Each neighbourhood is assigned at least one general practitioner and one nurse, and medical personnel are almost always on intimate terms with their patients, living in the very neighbourhood, comprising generally of 150–200 families, that they serve. A little more than a week after the first case was reported on 11 March 2020, the government announced a ban on tourist arrivals—a much greater sacrifice than it may have been in other countries, since Cuba, operating under the chokehold that the US has applied for decades, is heavily dependent on tourism for revenue and its foreign exchange reserves.[1] Community health surveys are carried out periodically, and in this instance, as has happened previously during dengue outbreaks, teams were dispatched to carry out door-to-door surveys to identify those with greater vulnerability to the virus, identify and test those with symptoms, and place those proven or suspected to be positive under quarantine. 'The whole organization of their healthcare system,' a professor of government at an American university remarked, 'is to be in close touch with the population, identify health problems as they emerge, and deal with them immediately' (Augustin 2020). It is in this manner that Cuba was able to prevent the virus from entering the community transmission stage. A more critical assessment of Cuba's methods, while dwelling on the country's success in battling COVID-19, argues that what has been debated in some other countries—'whether you should wear masks, what that means for your freedom, whether people should be tested, or they should remain at home or be treated'—is in Cuba not debatable at all, and violation of the rule requiring the use of masks can lead to a fine and, after multiple offenses, a prison term (Hackel 2016). But requiring people to wear face masks is, or has been, mandatory in over 50 countries, including Austria, the Czech Republic, Israel, Argentina, Luxembourg, Germany, France, and Jamaica—none of these being countries that critics of Cuba would deign to characterize as 'fascist' or 'authoritarian' states.

In considering Cuba's success in keeping the virus at bay, a few simple facts merit mention or reiteration:

---

1. Cuba's reliance on tourism is underscored in a report filed by a Miami-based American journalist that betrays the flamboyance of the Yankee imperialist typically derided in Cuba. 'On official state media like "Gramma"', writes Tim Padgett, 'you *will* see headlines like: "Cuba has recovered and defeated the pandemic". The island has in fact reported fewer than 2,500 COVID-19 cases and fewer than 100 deaths. But whether or not Cuba has really subdued the new coronavirus, it's opening its doors again to foreign visitors.' The article is a sly attempt to question the official narrative stemming from Cuba, but its author might be better served critiquing the official narrative flowing out of the White House. See his 'Claiming "Recovery" From COVID-19, Cuba (Slightly) Opens The Door To Tourism', WLRN, 2 July 2020.

- First, healthcare in Cuba is universal and free, no mean accomplishment for any country in the world.
- Second, with its limited economic resources and comparative isolation, Cuba has displayed considerable wisdom in its investments in public health, literacy, and sanitation. Its achievement in containing the advance of the coronavirus is all the more admirable considering that the country faces a considerable housing shortage and that the system of queuing up for food and essential items at ration shops—a system known as *La Libreta*—means that the risk of infection increases just as it suggests that the enforcement of physical distancing poses difficulties that every country does not have to face (Deutsche Welle 2020).
- Third, the country has a history of showing a level of preparedness for public health emergencies from which most countries, and most particularly a behemoth such as the US which far from facilitating international cooperation has done everything possible to obstruct it, could take some cues.[2]
- Fourth, the system of community healthcare, which is at the same time interwoven into a national healthcare system that permits a rapid system of testing, tracing, treatment, and evacuation of the vulnerable, allows for a coherent system of response at every level.
- Fifth, and most critically, notwithstanding the fact that some Cubans are bound to experience the regulations that have been imposed in the wake of the pandemic as

---

2. *Granma*, the official voice of the Communist Party of Cuba, is forthright on this matter: 'United States officials are knowingly committing a crime, when in the midst of a pandemic they attack Cuba's international cooperation, seeking to deprive millions of people of the universal human right to healthcare services... No country should assume it is large enough, rich enough or powerful enough to defend itself, isolating itself and ignoring the efforts and needs of others.' See Ministry of Foreign Affairs statement, 'The COVID-19 pandemic makes clear the need to cooperate despite political differences', *Granma*, 16 April 2020.

> an imposition, the majority of the people feel invested in the healthcare system and have shown that the problems posed by the coronavirus can only be tackled if there is some synergy between the state and civil society.

A more exhaustive account of Cuba's healthcare system and its success in meeting the immense challenge posed by the threat of the pandemic would bring other considerations to the fore, two of which may be mentioned by way of a conclusion. Contrary to the prevalent orthodox wisdom which grants full and unquestionable sovereignty to allopathic medicine, Cuban medical education and practice have also been hospitable to homeopathy (Fitz 2010). Conventional physicians can do little more than express outrage or chuckle when they hear the word 'homeopathy', associating it with sugary pills, and the National Institutes of Health (NIH) in the US insists that 'there is little evidence to support homeopathy as an effective treatment for any specific health condition', just as the Federal Drug Administration (FDA) has not approved any homeopathic compound for medicinal use (Torres 2020). Considering the present state of the US, neither organization can be viewed as an undisputed fount of authority on such matters, and over 30 countries have sought to buy from Cuba supplies of PrevengHo-Vir, a homeopathic immunological booster used to help prevent viral infections. (The Cuban pharmaceutical industry has also developed an allopathic drug, Interferon alfa-2b, that has previously been used for the treatment of certain types of cancer, hepatitis, and AIDS, and has now been used in China to treat COVID-19 patients, but that is another story—though it is worth noting that Cuba 'has now received requests for the product from 45 countries' [Yaffe 2020].) It may well be that the treatment is not in the least efficacious; nor would it be surprising if PrevengHo-Vir, which Cuban authorities do not at all claim as a cure to COVID-19, should be dismissed by many as a form of quackery.

Some writers have argued that there is a record of Cuba having achieved some success in combating epidemics partly with the aid of homeopathy. One striking illustration of the homeoprophylactic approach, states a defender of Cuba's more ecumenical thinking on medical practice, is furnished by the greatly reduced incidence and control of leptospirosis, defined by the CDC as 'a bacterial disease that affects humans and animals caused by bacteria of the genus Leptospira', which struck Cuba in 2007 and was addressed in part by the administration of a homeopathic compound (Graham n.d.). Homeopathy is not a mere afterthought in Cuba, a remedy sought in desperation, or a form of treatment taken in a spirit of defiant rejection of allopathic or mainstream medicine. The point here is a more complex one, taking us to the heart of the politics of knowledge that is at stake here: where allopathy has insisted on its full and complete sovereignty, as the only form of medical intervention derived from the scientific method, the exponents of homeopathy—and of traditional Chinese medicine and Ayurveda—have a far more expansive and pluralistic view of what counts as science. In this respect, Cuba's integration of homeopathy into the curriculum of its renowned medical school, The Latin American School of Medicine, generally known by the acronym ELAM, is as far-reaching and radical as anything else that the country has done to secure the well-being of its people. What is also distinct to homeopathic practice, and aligns it more closely to the spirit embodied in the Cuban idea of healthcare revolving around neighbourhood doctors, is the kind of relationship it encourages between the doctor and the patient. As Paul Starr wrote in his magisterial work on the making of modern medicine, built on the edifice of a ruthless drive to weed out all competing systems, 'homeopathy stressed the need for sympathetic attention by the physician and individualized diagnosis and treatment of patients' (Starr 1992, 97).

This essay commenced with an invocation of Cuban medical internationalism and it is fitting that it should conclude on the same note. Cuban medical missions date back to 1960, when an earthquake struck Chile, and have since firmly established Cuba as a global health leader. The story has been told often of the 10,000 Cuban medical professionals who volunteered for a mission to West Africa during the Ebola outbreak, 260 of whom were selected to work, in the World Health Organization's own assessment, 'under very demanding conditions' (Yaffe 2020). Whatever one's view of the Obama administration, it had the decency to recognize the stellar work of the Cuban medical mission, which is credited with having worked effectively in Guinea, Sierra Leone, and Liberia to reduce the patients' mortality rate from 50 per cent to 20 per cent (Kornbluh 2020). The editorial board of the *New York Times*, no friend of Cuba, wrote at the time in grudgingly admiring terms that 'Cuba stands to play the most robust role among the nations seeking to contain the virus. Cuba's contribution is doubtlessly meant at least in part to bolster its beleaguered international standing. Nonetheless, it should be lauded and emulated'.[3]

What is insinuated here, namely that Cuba's medical internationalism is primarily a form of cultural capital sought by a largely or wholly discredited nation, which is also desperate for foreign exchange reserves, is given substantially more weight by critics who, apart from the general animosity harboured against the communist state, have taken the island nation to task for the violation of rights of patients and the labour rights of physicians. Cuban doctors, for instance, are only permitted to retain a small portion of the wages they earn overseas for themselves, having to transmit the rest to the state, but this criticism entirely overlooks the fact that their education is entirely subsidized by the state (Dantes 2018, 175–82). That is a far cry from the predatory practices of American medical schools where an MD degree would typically set a student back \$250,000—one reason among others why ELAM's graduates include Americans among other international students.[4] One could with good reason, similarly be just as critical of Cuba as

3. Quoted in *The Lancet* report 'Cuba's focus on preventive medicine pays off'.

4. One American student's report on the medical education he received in Cuba makes for instructive reading. See Warner (2016).

I have been of China in its draconian deployment of measures to contain the virus, but such criticisms must also show some awareness of the extraordinary resilience with which Cuba has faced the depredations of its neighbour *el norte*. In the present crisis, it has certainly done far more than the US in showing the way both to international cooperation and the way out of the pandemic—from its acceptance of a British ocean liner with 50 virus-stricken passengers and crew aboard that no other country was willing to allow to dock, to its dispatch of medical teams to nearly 40 countries, commencing with China and Italy, where COVID-19 patients were treated (see Yaffe 2020 and Kornbluh 2020). John Donne's poem, 'No man is an island', is familiar to nearly everyone; but Cuba, a small island nation, suggests a more apt modification: an island is not always just an island, and may yet even be a continent.

COVID-19: COLLECTIVE RESPONSES TO CHALLENGES IN HONG KONG

Ada Kot

INTRODUCTION

Hong Kong is located at the frontier of a battlefield fighting against the pandemic since the first outbreak in China and is still struggling with the third wave of COVID-19. When the world had no idea about the upcoming threat, the people of Hong Kong were aware of the news of a cluster of suspected pneumonia cases in the city of Wuhan in December 2019. From the beginning of the outbreak of COVID-19, in China, the people of Hong Kong responded calmly because of the lessons they learnt from the Severe Acute Respiratory Syndrome (SARS) epidemic in 2003. However, the COVID-19 pandemic lasted for more than half a year, precautionary measures were imposed and tightened up, which raised challenges for all sectors in society. With the practice of social distancing and limitations for public gatherings, education and in-person services including counselling are deeply affected. This opened up opportunities for helping professions to reconsider their modes of service, ethics in practice and self-care.

LESSONS LEARNT FROM THE SARS EPIDEMIC IN 2003 AND SOCIAL UNREST IN 2019

In November 2002, Guangdong, the nearby province in Mainland China geographically connected with Hong Kong, experienced an outbreak of the atypical pneumonia later termed SARS. It reached Hong Kong in March 2003 and caused a total of 1,750 cases, with 286 deaths from 11 March to 6 June 2003. People learnt the importance of adequate epidemiological information, risk of infection of medical and healthcare workers during the epidemic, and the need of improving the overall healthcare system in Hong Kong (Hung 2003). At the individual level, wearing a mask became a habit among people in Hong Kong (Ting 2020), not only as personal precaution but also for humility and for the community, in order to prevent the disease from spreading further.

This story repeated itself in December 2019. When there was an outbreak of cases in China, the Hong Kong community was alert. Precautionary measures were enhanced by individuals, such as wearing masks and washing hands. Prices of masks tripled in late January 2020. Mainland China netizens took to ridiculing the people of Hong Kong for buying masks, claiming it to be an overreaction, or just an excuse for continued social unrest. In fact, due to the pro-democracy protests, critical thinking, distrust towards the Hong Kong government, fact-checking, collective and mutual support actions grew among the people. Although the anti-mask law has been effective since early October 2019, during the social unrest, citizens tended to wear masks and ignore the law that prohibited the use of masks.

On 4 January, the Hong Kong government declared a 'serious response level' to the virus outbreak in Wuhan, while medical experts in Hong Kong urged mainland authorities to be more transparent in releasing Wuhan patient data for epidemiological study (Cheung 2020). People advocated the shutting of borders with China, in the community. Frontline medical workers launched a five-day strike in early February 2020 to urge for closing all borders, in order to relieve the pressure on the healthcare system. The Hong Kong government closed all but three border control points which remained open after the strike, and the demand made by the public was not answered completely. A huge increase of demand in disinfectant products such as alcohol and bleach, daily-use products including rice and toilet paper, and most importantly masks, led to an ongoing panic buying. Frontline medical workers were also under pressure due to shortage of protective gear, such as surgical masks. There was criticism levelled against the Hong

Kong government for being incompetent in fighting against the pandemic, in comparison with the Macau and Taiwan governments, which are located close to China and had also suffered from SARS.

The 2019 social unrest turned silent because of the pandemic. However, the knowledge and skills generated, which are rooted in the community, were promptly transferred to meet the challenges of the pandemic successfully within the community. In light of the situation wherein the people in Hong Kong strongly distrusted the Hong Kong government, fact-checking and speedy information circulation during the social unrest transformed into a website that worked as a hub for comprehensive information during the pandemic, including public places visited by patients and well-presented epidemiological relationships of cluster cases. Journalists urged the Hong Kong government to disclose details of cases in the daily press conferences held by officials with clues provided by netizens. In response to the panic shopping, community neighbours relied on Facebook groups to barter daily-use products, individuals supported the elderly and disabled people in the community proactively by checking in on their daily needs. Retailers, especially those who supported the social movements in 2019, mobilized resources to secure a supply of daily essentials with the purpose of protecting people and ensuring their safety and health especially of the most vulnerable in the community. Many retailers donated surgical masks for frontline medical workers in the healthcare system. Netizens designed an online 'Mask calculator' for people to estimate the need of masks based on the number of household members and working days, and encouraged people not to stock up and share extra masks with the underprivileged. Proactive collaboration in the community, together with a high level of self-discipline and social distancing, helped the city flatten the confirmed cases curve in the first wave imported from China in January 2020, and in the second wave imported from people infected overseas in March 2020.

THE THIRD WAVE OF COVID-19 IN HONG KONG

Unfortunately, collective practices could not save Hong Kong from COVID-19. The city experienced a third wave in July and August 2020. The daily new confirmed COVID-19 cases reached as high as 149 on 30 July, the city had 4,692 confirmed cases and 77 deaths as of 24 August 2020. Sadly, the death toll increased sharply during the third wave and the elderly, or the infected in elderly care homes, accounted for most of these cases. The Hong Kong government not only refused to close all the borders with the Mainland to reduce the risk of the virus entering Hong Kong, but also ignored medical experts' advice. Experts pointed out the extent of home quarantining where there ought to have been mandatory quarantine camps for returnees from overseas. The government exempted testing and quarantine for people like seamen, aircrew and executives of listed companies, which allowed around 200,000 people to enter Hong Kong with no medical inspection which proved to be one of the loopholes in the system (HKU 2020).

Since the second wave, the government had implemented precautionary measures such as limiting public gatherings, temporary closures of public and entertainment premises such as gyms, cinemas, libraries, suspension of public services, restricting 'dine-ins'. All these measures were tightened during the third wave. In late July, the Hong Kong government did not allow dining in restaurants, other than hospital and police canteens, which forced blue-collar workers such as cleaners, street promoters and construction workers to eat on the dusty streets in heavy rain and heat. The community demonstrated solidarity again in response to the inhumane measures implemented by the government; churches, small shops, including hair salons and clothing shops welcomed people to eat inside their premises with social distancing measures in place. The government agreed to open community halls for people to eat inside but suspended this facility after two days. Sentiments of anger, frustration and complaints against the government increased, but the government refused to apologize and hold itself to account for the third wave that led to a sharp increase in the death toll, or the inhumane rule of prohibiting eating in restaurants. Furthermore, it is said that the precautionary measures and financial support in response to the downward slide of the economy were to protect the corporate consortia with no consideration for grassroots causes. Moreover, the Hong Kong Police is being criticized for implementing precautionary measures to control protests. With the implementation of the National Security Law and the postponing of legislative council elections, the sentiments of hopelessness and helplessness grew among the public over the summer of 2020.

IMPACT ON HELPING PROFESSIONS

The education sector has been deeply affected. Schools, including kindergarten, primary schools, secondary schools, special education schools, and universities were suspended since January 2020. Although face-to-face classes resumed since late May, the third wave took away the memorable event of the graduation ceremony for a lot of students and smashed their hopes of resuming face-to-face classes in the new academic year starting from September 2020. Teachers faced huge challenges in conducting online classes; parents in dual-income households were tired of balancing taking care of children and working at home; students with special education needs lacked face-to-face services. Kindergartens are at risk of closing as parents have tended to assume that face-to-face classes cannot be substituted by online classes for young students. They thus stopped paying tuition fees. This was particularly seen in families facing financial difficulties due to COVID-19. Educators are not only facing challenges and risks in their careers, but are also tired of answering to the demands from parents and the Education Bureau, when most of the school arrangements in response to COVID-19 are delegated to the school authorities for the final decision of implementation. In addition, schools are expected to cooperate with the government under the National Anthem Law and the National Security Law that have come into effect recently. Schools are facing a dilemma with pressure from the Education Bureau to cater to the pressing need of caring for students' mental well-being due to the social movements in 2019 and COVID-19. Due to the social movements, and the implementation of the National Security Law, not only students, but also educators are concerned with issues of trust and privacy, which hinder their ability to seek help and advice for the mental well-being of students.

The social welfare sector is also affected by COVID-19, especially those serving foreign domestic helpers. On top of the entry restriction due to COVID-19, language barriers, lack of information regarding COVID-19, compulsory quarantine, poor living environments in hostels and employment issues during the pandemic, the workload of workers supporting foreign domestic helpers has increased, especially with a cluster of Indonesian domestic helpers with confirmed cases during the third wave. In order to maintain social distancing, work from home arrangements in various agencies also multiplied the workload of this group of helping professionals. Efficiency in work among the people of Hong Kong is well known, and work from home arrangements implied that people would extend working hours as there are now no clear boundaries between work and personal life. While there is a concern and support for the needs of the underprivileged population during the COVID-19 pandemic, there is a lack of concern regarding psychological support for the helping professions.

With increasing frustration, concerns about mental well-being were raised. However, counsellors and therapists in Hong Kong are challenged by restrictions during the pandemic as their traditional training and modes of service are largely in-person. Different from the scenario overseas, despite high accessibility in the city, the services of online counselling are underdeveloped. There is a lack of training, ethical concerns such as confidentiality, knowledge of supportive devices and interface, etc. Only a few agencies are offering counselling services for suicide prevention, AIDS prevention and youth engagement, etc. To a certain extent, maintaining social distancing meant suspension of much of the psychotherapy and counselling services in Hong Kong during the outbreak of COVID-19. The urge to change and adopt technologically-assisted modes of service induces pressure on psychotherapists and counsellors, whether they work in the public or the private sector.

APPLICATION OF NARRATIVE PRACTICE UNDER COVID-19

Text counselling is an alternative way to offer support when social distancing needs to be maintained, and people are living in small, crowded flats that do not ensure privacy. Online video counselling needs a person to have a physical place ensuring privacy, where their conversation may not be heard by others, along with a password-secured stable internet. It has also been difficult for families in Hong Kong to avail such services if all members stay at home, simultaneously sharing Wi-Fi to access the internet. Text counselling is an alternative way for people to share their worries, concerns, and stories, with real-time or delayed responses from their counsellor via apps or email. With the integration of narrative practices, a postmodern approach based on the meaning of the language used in which people understand their lives and narrate their life stories, text counselling could be a mode of therapeutic documentation for people. In narrative practices, documentation is used in multiple and creative ways (Dulwich Centre 2020). Although it is applied during in-person meetings, 'rescuing the said from the saying of it', the mindful principles and practices are good reminders in text counselling. According to Newman (2008), it is important to double-check with people for the words or phrases they use when writing documentations. Through the process, preferred actions and values of the person might also be explored. The counsellor is the audience of the person, connecting with the person through a sharing of resonance. It also serves as a 'responsive diary' for the person that encourages the person to spend time on self-care and can have them reflect on their life under the seamless daily routine of working from home. In the safe space of text counselling, people do not need to show their face to ensure privacy, especially when it has become a great concern in Hong Kong now. Both the person and counsellor have the obligation to ensure security of the device and internet used, by using VPN, and changing and not disclosing passwords to third-parties. Furthermore, although people are separated due to social distancing, through careful and anonymous circulation of documents with the consent of the person, local knowledge and skills in tackling challenges generated from the individuals will be a contribution to the wider community that may connect with other people in a similar situation, but may not be willing to speak up due to privacy concerns.

SUPPORT FOR HELPING PROFESSIONS

There is a huge demand for training in transforming services online for helping professions, including teachers and counsellors. When people were getting used to Zoom, there was a privacy concern, which induced additional pressure on them. Teachers were facing the pressure of not being able to ensure students' attendance and attention, as online pedagogies were not widely applied before COVID-19. For counsellors, especially those in private practice, business dropped sharply as they were forced to avoid in-person contact, which caused financial pressure on them. In addition, there was a lack of guidelines in tele-health and online counselling as well. Although training and review of guidelines on ethical issues for online counselling are offered by training and professional bodies, the need of support for the mental well-being of helping professions has been forgotten. Ongoing supervision is not a requirement for a registered counsellor in Hong Kong. Without support for personal growth and guidance in professional development, caring for the self needs awareness and initiative from the counsellors themselves. Under the COVID-19 pandemic, counsellors need to be well-prepared psychologically—before the economic downfall sets in heavily on the city—to serve people with a healthy mental state. It is an ethical issue if the counsellor is under financial pressure, and is thus providing promotions or offering services in ways that put a strain on the needs of providing mental healthcare.

SUMMARY

In conclusion, people of Hong Kong must be proud of their collaboration in fighting against the COVID-19 pandemic, and not being beaten by the third wave. COVID-19 brings challenges and crises for helping professions, but it also creates opportunities for educators to equip themselves with more updated pedagogies, and it is a time for students and society to understand the importance of school life. For counsellors, it provides a break to review ethics issues in providing services, expand and transform modes of service, and most importantly, to make time for self-care.

RESILIENCY AND ABUNDANCE: FINDING OUR PATH TO WELLNESS DURING COVID-19

Yvonne Sandoval

In the morning, I open my window and smell the fresh air. The smell of rain from the previous night fills my nose. It reminds me to be grateful for the precious gift of the rivers, the oceans, and the waters that live inside of me. I can see the subtle new growth in the garden as the sunflowers smile back at me. I say a prayer of gratitude for all that is growing, ask for abundance to multiply so others may have the sustenance they need as well.

With each passing day, as more people are impacted by COVID-19, this prayer is being amplified. COVID-19 has become a teacher for both wanted and unsolicited life lessons.

COVID-19 has taken its toll on human beings across the globe. People of colour and poor people are being impacted at alarming rates. Choices made by political leaders based in greed and corruption have furthered the damage to the point of a global economic collapse. Fracking and poisoning our earth's waters are happening every day. While healthcare workers and teachers fight to afford their lives, billionaires' profits increase.

In the US alone, millions of people have filed for unemployment, a safety net that is not available in most countries around the world and are on the verge of eviction. Businesses are closing at alarming rates, many people are on the brink of hunger if they were not already there. This is the result of not valuing the sacredness of our land, water, children and elders.

The average income in the US is $52,000 a year. In the valley I call home it is only $14,000. COVID-19 has dropped incomes significantly. Many people are out of work doing their best to make ends meet, as the cost of food skyrockets. Panic and hopelessness grows daily. There is a global perspective that the US is wealthy. Not everyone here has that luxury. A large wealth gap exists. Those most vulnerable are people of colour and people with already low incomes. There are many families that will go to bed hungry this evening. COVID-19 is widening the disparities. Our culture of individualism is coming to haunt us. Those who wear a mask and those who do not is practically split down party lines. More conservative individuals are making it more difficult to control COVID-19 numbers in their refusal to maintain their 'rights'.

Consideration for elders and immunocompromised people are at the mercy of this individualistic freedom seeking mentality. As I write this, six million people in the US have been infected with COVID-19.

In my practice as a therapist, parents tell me they are down to their last bag of beans: 'We don't have enough to pay the rent. How will we survive without a job?' one client asks.

My teenage clients talk about their bleak futures and broken dreams as they enter the world of online schooling. The challenges for people continue to mount. I have a hard time keeping up with the number of referrals of people seeking help. My connection with clients is now through a computer screen on Zoom. Thoughts about my own stability creep inside my mind while I am in session. It takes more work these days to redirect my thoughts and to stay in the present. How does one stay calm in the midst of a pandemic and mounting tensions?

Eight years ago, I was invited to a join a group of women to talk about the challenges of living in our rural area of northern New Mexico. One month prior, I had moved from a big city to the valley affectionately known as El Valle. The valley has about 2,500 people, it is one hour from any grocery store. Many people questioned my decision to move to such a rural area as a single parent with a one-year-old daughter.

Women gathered in the front room. Plates filled with delicious food we all brought were on our laps and we began to share our stories. The women shared their joys and struggles of living in the valley. They spoke about the isolation, of not being able to see friends while appreciating the beauty rural life in the high desert brings. Feelings of concern were shared about access to healthcare. The valley is located one hour from any store or hospital. Many of the women had health concerns and were unsure of what might happen in an emergency. Several of the women had concerns about how to make a living with so few jobs in the surrounding area. The conversation lasted for hours, filled with laughter and tears. As the women brainstormed their ideas, they were placed on the wall on a paper. Dreams of communal farming, harvesting herbs for health and starting a thrift store was placed on paper and then into action. We began to call ourselves the El Valle Women's Collaborative.

Less than 30 days from our meeting, the group began renting an old house, bringing unwanted wares from home to start a thrift store. The first day of organizing the thrift store was momentous. We saw what is possible when people come together for the common cause of humanity. Like the lesson mycelium teaches us, our reliance on one another began to grow and our network began to spread. With each passing week the thrift store continued to expand. More donations continued to come in locally and from the city one hour away. However, we were beginning to struggle with pricing the wares. Many women wanted to price the used items to make it accessible to the community. Others felt that if we priced the items higher, we would draw in more people from the city and the money could be used for other emerging projects. Everyone had good reasons for their pricing. There was just no consensus.

I began reflecting on how healers would make a living many years ago. Many people valued the healers in their community and brought items to support their families' needs.

There was no need to charge money because they were supported by the community.

My friend and I began reading articles about sacred economics and the gift economy. These seemingly new ideas were not new at all. They were in fact how many earth-based people around the globe have operated outside of the modern currency system. After all, our currency is only a couple of hundred years old. After multiple discussions and challenges with pricing, we decided as a group to try a policy of 'pay what you want'.

In the beginning our neighbours were confused. 'You mean I can take these clothes and pay anything I want?' 'Yes, that is exactly what we are saying.' Some neighbours would come in and clear out a section of the store and pay a nominal fee. But that slowly started to change. Neighbours started to see it as a means to share with others. The donated items increased and people started to pay more to offset the cost of those who did not have the same financial resources. One woman who had very little resources came in and gave me her necklace. The necklace was a family heirloom. 'I wanted you to have this. You gave me clothing and blankets when I could not afford them.' Her generous spirit deepened my understanding of what true abundance is. Abundance is not finite. It is an energy that comes from a source ready for us to tap into.

I see those same lessons of abundance highlighted on my farm. Our farm called Bueno Para Todos is a project of the El Valle Women's Collaborative. A few months after starting the thrift store a group of women including myself discussed the importance of growing food together. We began dreaming of creating a beautiful garden where we could feed our neighbours and ourselves alongside the thrift store. The dreams began to unfold and we soon had a community garden. The garden only lasted two growing seasons before we decided to close the thrift store. We attempted to negotiate a better price on the building and land but we were unable to do so. Just two years later, we closed the store and had to look for another place to farm. One season, we planted at a neighbour's house. The travel to a less central location and growing tensions with other renters on the land made it less favourable than before.

At the time I was debating whether to return to the city. My contract as an adjunct professor ended. I had no money living in a small town, with a sick 13-year-old dog and struggling to hide my tears from my daughter. I did not want her to see me cry from being stressed out. I surrendered and began praying. 'Creator if I am meant to be here in this valley provide me with a safe house for my daughter and give me land and give me water to work the land with... Help me understand my purpose.' I had nothing left to give but my prayer. Three and a half months later I received a call from some dear friends. 'There's a place on the other side of the valley we think you'd like.' How was I going to pay rent? I had no real income. I just left teaching at the university. In all honesty, I went to see the property out of a false sense of obligation. As I got out of my car I could hear the sound of the birds chirping. The first step on the land and I knew I was home. The property was 10 acres with a brand-new home and water rights. A perfect place for a community farm. Was this really happening? This was my prayer manifested. Within two weeks my friends negotiated a minimal rent and my daughter and I were in our new home with plenty of space to plant.

Today Bueno Para Todos ('Good for all') is a shared partnership with neighbours. It has become a mutual-aid for COVID-19 as many people lose their jobs and employment becomes scarce. Each one of us takes turns watering and weeding. On the weekends, we mask up and practice social distancing to do farm projects together to build camaraderie and grow food together. Native indigenous practices, sometimes called permaculture, have been used to build up healthy soil and increase production. We plant with intention.

All of our planting practices begin with an offering of traditional medicines of our people such as blue corn and tobacco. Our relationship to the plants is important. We treat them with respect as living beings by using pronouns or their names to address them. As Robin Wall Kimmerer writes in her book *Braiding Sweetgrass*, 'In some native languages the term for plants are those who take care of us.' This type of synergistic mutualism is all over the natural world. A strong case for the antithesis of free-market capitalism.

Before COVID-19, I was driving 12–16 hours a week to go to my office in the city, sometimes weeks would go by without going outside. Today, seeing clients online comes as a welcome blessing. These days, after my prayers and morning meditation,

I walk outside to the farm. It is my place of grounding before seeing clients online. Sometimes, my daughter Yolotzin will join me in the morning if she's not too tired. I treasure these moments when she joins me. Looking around I see the explosion of colours. The bees and ladybugs hard at work, pollinating and caring for their plant friends. Sometimes I am in awe thinking about how each of these full-size plants grew from tiny seeds. These plants are now my friends offering nutrition and a full spectrum of medicine. All they ask of me is to water them and pick them. On one hand the relationship with them is simple, I water and pick and they grow. Over the years I have learned that I can deepen this relationship by connecting with the plants. This can be done through offerings of blue corn, tobacco or a song. They like when I spend time with them watching them grow.

The garden will always give if I am intentional with the relationship. When I commune with her the abundance is even greater.

Bueno Para Todos has become a symbol of hope. Students from the United World College, an international high school have partnered with us over the last three years to build a large hoop house, craft raised beds, and start an edible food forest. The hands and minds of these young people have laid the foundation for the farm's success. Students join us monthly for a weekend to work on the farm and learn about healing the mind, body and spirit. We get the honour of engaging with them for two years. It is difficult to see them off when they graduate. The students become family. The mending of my heart comes when they call or message to say they are interning or taking a job to support Mother Earth. I feel like a proud mama whose child has returned home for a visit. Just last week, one of our students from Germany launched a fundraiser to support refugees and the environment. Another student from Greece told me she is helping protect bats as pollinators. Meanwhile, one of our other students is taking a gap for a year to work on a farm inspired by the work she did with BPT. My daughter is gaining a broader perspective of the world through the students without having to step outside the land. These precious students have been a blessing, a welcome blessing.

Along with the offerings of tobacco and blue corn that go into the earth when planting, so do these stories. When someone comes to gather vegetables, they are taking in the goodness at a cellular level. Students from the United World College come from all over the globe. I can recall a day when we had over 60 people at the farm raising the hoop house. That day we had six continents represented, 13 countries, 11 languages, and seven religions present. A friend leaned over and said, 'Do you know how amazing this is? Jews, Muslims and Christians are here on Passover working together.'

I have always held high hopes for humanity. In that moment I knew that a new world was possible. The earth is our common ground and here we were caring for her together.

In trying to stay present and looking towards the future I remind myself to remember the past. The high desert lands that I stand upon were once home to the Pecos Native American Tribe. The Pecos people were one of the largest Tewa Pueblos (villages) at one time. Tewa territory, which consists of multiple pueblos, covers a large part of the state of New Mexico. Three years ago, in a fit of frustration and feeling my body overheat, I sat down in my chair and asked why I was even here.

'I am from the city.'

'I am not a typical farmer.'

'Why, Creator, do you have me here?'

I was suddenly prompted to look at my computer. I was being guided to look at different webpages and found the history of the territory. During the Spanish conquest most of the Pueblo people were killed. The remaining 17 Pecos natives fled to be with their kin in Jemez Pueblo. I had recently learned at a family reunion that we were Jemez Pueblo people. My great grandparents had even been in the boarding schools. I heard a voice, 'You have come full circle.' I understood in that moment I was exactly where I needed to be. My work was to honour those who have passed by paying respects to the land.

Learning to regenerate land has been a steep learning curve

for me. The pretty pictures they show in magazines or a Google search takes a lot of work. Very rarely are we given a real perspective on what it takes to regenerate the land. On the same note we are rarely shown the gifts Mother Earth gives to us. These gifts are not quantified the way we might count a tomato or an apple. No. These gems come in the form of my daughter getting excited after trying a home-grown strawberry for the first time. She looks at it with such joy and realizes the taste is different from store-bought strawberries. When I can make herbal tea for a friend who is feeling anxious, or when you start to learn the healing properties of herbs, and where you once saw weeds, now you see food and medicine, the moment when you can hear your plant allies speak to you, you realize you are not alone in this world. In fact, you are surrounded by immense support and beauty.

The lessons plants teach us are the laws of the natural world. We are interconnected and we are blessed when we have the courage to be in the right relationship with the living world around us. Like most healthy relationships, land regeneration takes time.

Learning to honour the ancestors' land we are upon, hearing the plants and water speak and learning how to defend the sacred is a process. Each layer of wounding we shed opens up space for these lessons to be learned. COVID-19 has given us the opportunity to be in the right relationship with one another and all other living beings on this planet. If we take these lessons forward in this uncharted territory of civil unrest and COVID we may have a chance to recalibrate the heart of Mother Earth and open up a pathway for the next seven generations to come. Every day will be a test of our strength and our courage moving forward.

DISCOVERING THE JOY OF LIVING IN TIMES OF CRISIS, INSPIRATION FOR GROWTH

Ruxandra Anghel

TWO BIG QUESTIONS

The real joy of living is found in the most unusual circumstances. For many, this might be a difficult truth to digest, and yet a truly relevant truth in the current times of a pandemic. Existential philosophers and those who have been through great challenges would argue that true happiness can only be found through challenge. The worldwide existential crisis of 2020 seems to have generated a phenomenon of rebirth for existential philosophy. Issues such as crisis, meaning, death, anguish, and the joy of living have come to the fore in the collective consciousness as the world experiences a significant shift of paradigm and great uncertainty.

Confined in lockdown, many people all over the world turned to philosophy to try to find an explanation and possibly a way out of this unusual crisis. Albert Camus and Victor Frankl regained mass popularity with a spike in the sales of their books *The Plague* (Camus 1947) and *Man's Search for Meaning* (Frankl 1949). Even Nietzsche, otherwise controversial and among the most challenging thinkers to comprehend, is being cited during casual conversations between friends. What if Nietzsche was right? Perhaps there is no God and it is up to us to make meaning of our frightening and uncertain existence on Earth? The existentialist perspective of the pandemic is complemented by popular culture, medical science, and personal prophecies. Many new theories of the world circle our social networks, and yet there are two big questions still in search for an answer, the same ones as ever:

What is the meaning of what is happening to us?
When will we get any certainty?

THE EXISTENTIAL ACADEMY IN LONDON

I joined the New School of Psychotherapy and Counselling at the Existential Academy in London in 2017. For some years, I had been looking for the right postgraduate course to complement my career in psychology and become a psychotherapist and an academic. What I was looking for was a framework to match my personal view of the world and my values. In a casual conversation with a work colleague, I found out about the NSPC and their existential framework. They have a variety of postgraduate courses in the helping professions that are based on the principles of existentialism, including existential coaching and pastoral care. Having studied philosophy in the past and having heard of the emergence of existential psychotherapy, which truly appealed to me, I was delighted to find out about the possibility of getting a doctorate in this field. I applied within a month, and soon after, I received my offer letter. There I was, becoming an existentialist.

I find the experience of being part of this world of existentialism truly inspirational, particularly at the Existential Academy. It showed me the importance of knowing myself and my personal values in facing life challenges and making life choices. It helped me understand who I was, who I was not, how I see the world, and what kind of life I would like to create for myself. It is not just about *the who* and *the what*, but also about the *with whom*. It is about the courage to make the most appropriate life choices for yourself. Probably the greatest gift of my experience with the NSPC is having this sense of belonging to a framework that I resonate with and being surrounded by others like me, people with whom I share important principles, valuing human liberties, and supporting meaning based living. Yet, of all the meaningful gifts of existentialism, the most important one is that of finding meaning in the most challenging of life circumstances.

EXISTENTIAL SUPPORT INITIATIVES

Considering this year's pandemic, which we could look at as a pan-existential crisis, adhering to the principles of existentialism has meant that I was able to try to transform this period into an opportunity for personal growth, for myself and for others. With inspiration from my supervisors and all my existential experiences, I have managed to make the lockdown one of the most fruitful moments of my life. Two existential principles stood behind the initiatives we took to help ourselves through the lockdown. The first one was about accepting that life is a series of paradoxes happening simultaneously. We cannot avoid them, but we can embrace them and choose to face them with courage and grow from them. The spring of the pandemic brought with it the paradoxes of loss and the opportunity for personal growth, the paradox of physical isolation and spiritual connection, of fear of death and hope for rebirth, the despair, and the excitement in the face of a new world paradigm. The other existential principle that proved to be of help in the lockdown is that of activating one of the most important aspects of human existence, our wiring for belonging and connection. Despite the challenge of not being able to meet in person, but having more time for virtual meetings, we were able to connect and reconnect with friends and family from all over the world. In some cases, the lockdown created the context for new solid connections.

Emmy van Deurzen, the principal of the Existential Academy and one of the most prominent figures in establishing existential psychotherapy as a discipline, used the online to connect with the world. She shares her wisdom through short videos on her Emmy van Deurzen YouTube channel. Emmy posts frequently and often uses personal examples from her own existential dilemmas and her personal ways of facing this world crisis.

Joel Vos, one of the directors at the Existential Academy and the founder of Meaning Online, organized a weekly online support group to create connection through the lockdown. He also organized a full day of talks online at the International Meaning Conference London (www.meaning.org.uk), where people from all parts of the world united for one day in July in the search for meaning in times of coronavirus. The conference videos are available on the website to purchase post-conference, and they are accessible for people from all walks of life, not just psychology professionals.

In 2021, both Vos and van Deurzen published books about rising from existential crises and navigating the COVID-19 pandemic using the tools offered by existential philosophy and meaning focused techniques. Emmy van Deurzen offers a rich perspective on the meaning of crisis in her new book *Rising from Existential Crisis* (2021), helping our understanding on why and how existential crises are a given of existence. She encourages her readers to search within for vital courage and strength that are to be found in all of us human beings. To arrive to a place of courage and vitality, it is necessary to challenge our own mindset about crisis, survival, responsibility, and mental health. Vos in *The Psychology of Covid-19: Building Resilience for Future Pandemics* (2021) invites us to apply critical thinking to explore the meaning of the pandemic, by evaluating its social, political and health dimensions. Vos suggests that by opening our minds to see beyond the uncertainty, by questioning the status quo, and actively participating in social change we can create a more resilient world.

Inspired by all these wonderful acts of support, as well of those of many Londoners who volunteered to pass on their expertise to help others, I decided to launch a Facebook group, Project Gladness, with resources and monthly online meet-ups that promote the joy of living as a philosophy of life, especially in times of challenge.

MANAGING PARADOX AND CHOICE

From an existential perspective, life experiences are shaped by the way we make meaning of and engage with the paradoxes of living, the paradoxes between knowing and not knowing, of being independent and needing to belong, of the absurdity of life and the passion for living (van Deurzen 2015).

This existential perspective is one way of looking at the

world during the pandemic and generally in any circumstance of life. The paradox perspective might at first leave us with the impression that life itself is rather harsh, even unbearable. In fact, seeing and accepting the paradoxes helps us embrace life as a whole, with its ups and downs, and the never-ending stream of existential dilemmas. After all, as Irvin Yalom (2011) said, life is a very long exam with no right answers. Here is where freedom of choice comes into play. Existential paradoxes might restrict our living, but the freedom of choice of perspective belongs to us. It is what Frankl encouraged in his work on the pursuit of meaning. We can look at crises as moments of reaching a crossroad where the two options forward are the road to catastrophe and the road to meaning. If one chooses to see meaning in all that comes their way, adverse situations have a chance of becoming more valuable to one's existence. A crisis, such as the pandemic, could make us better, stronger people. Despite the fear and the sorrow, the world has also experienced great altruism in the past months.

Perhaps another choice could be what Nietzsche suggested in *The Gay Science* (1910)—to stop taking life so seriously. Of course, the pandemic is a profoundly serious situation. However, allowing ourselves to have moments of laissez faire (French for 'let it be') could help us be more resilient in the end. When taking a situation too seriously, the mind could easily slip into overthinking, catastrophizing, and hence, paradoxically closing itself from finding useful solutions to overcome the challenge.

THE GIFT OF SELF-REFLECTION

Irvin Yalom, one of the most appreciated existential humanistic psychotherapists, wrote in his autobiography that life is a permanent process of becoming (Yalom 2017). The key to existential therapy is the process of exploring one's own identity through self-reflection. For the novice mind in self-reflection, the process can feel intimidating, just like navigating an agitated sea in the dark without a compass. Yet, once we get the courage to start the adventure of reflexivity, we discover that it is the most accurate navigator. Practitioners and practicants of reflexivity promoted it wholeheartedly during the time of lockdown. In the sometimes extremely busy times of recent years, people often complained they did not have any time to themselves. The lockdown brought the opportunity for exactly that, developing our own headspace. That was indeed a rare opportunity that crises do not usually offer and to some that led to great revelations about the most important aspects of their lives, their families, their careers, their relationships, and their health.

BELONGING

Belonging is a fundamental human feature. Much of the advice given during the pandemic stressed upon the importance of staying connected even if through technological means. Despite being physically isolated, many of us have connected like never before. Togetherness is crucial in both good and troubled times. Celebrating life's victories alone is meaningless, whilst suffering life's tragedies alone is unbearable. Meaningful relationships are the key for a purposeful life. In times of global crisis, the spirit of community can make that difference between growth and despair in managing the existential paradox. A great gift of the initiatives inspired by the Existential Academy is the creation of different meaningful communities, both online and offline. The community of the International Meaning Conference (IMEC) is a good example of harmony in action and positivity. Finding meaning as part of a relational process is an invaluable resource for growth, whether it is a professional therapeutic relationship, a friendship or a romantic partnership (Vos 2018).

If we were to draw a helpful conclusion from the framework of the Existential Academy in London, it would be that in order to survive life's existential crises it is essential to build our own emotional Noah's ark. On the ark, we can invite our community of likeminded people, and together, navigate the storms and the calm seas, accepting that the joy of living is not about clear waters but about the courage to navigate together in the unknown.

Learning Narratives

EARLY LEARNING ROADMAP IN RESPONSE TO COVID-19: KEEPING YOUNG CHILDREN SAFE, LOVED AND LEARNING

Sara Dang

The pandemic threatens young children's development in unparalleled ways. Before the COVID-19 pandemic, an estimated 250 million children (43%) younger than five years were at risk of not reaching their developmental potential (Black 2017) and millions of children were facing a global learning crisis, where even after several years of school, they could not read, write or do basic math (World Bank 2018). Global surveys studying the impact of the pandemic have shown that over 1.5 billion children have missed out on school and 10 million may never return, especially girls who are now being forced into early marriage (Save the Children n.d.). Moreover, a third of households experienced domestic violence, 82% of poorer households reported a loss of income, and 89% had difficulties accessing healthcare and medicine due to the pandemic (Edwards 2020).

Effects of prior pandemics confirm the risk of both immediate and long-term adverse consequences for children, with particular risks faced during early childhood, when brain architecture is still rapidly developing and highly sensitive to environmental adversity (Shankoff 2012). When children grow up deprived of stimulation, with low interaction with adults, and ongoing, persistent stress, their young minds fail to build or maintain important brain connections. This ongoing 'toxic' stress causes visible changes in brain structure and can have damaging effects on children's learning, development, behaviour, and health across the lifespan (National Scientific Council on the Developing Child 2014). Yoshikawa et al. (2020) claim that follow-up studies of individuals in utero during pandemics, natural disasters and famines show the potential for life-long negative consequences of such shocks (Almond 2006). Save the Children must ensure that early learning and well-being is an essential part of the COVID-19 response.

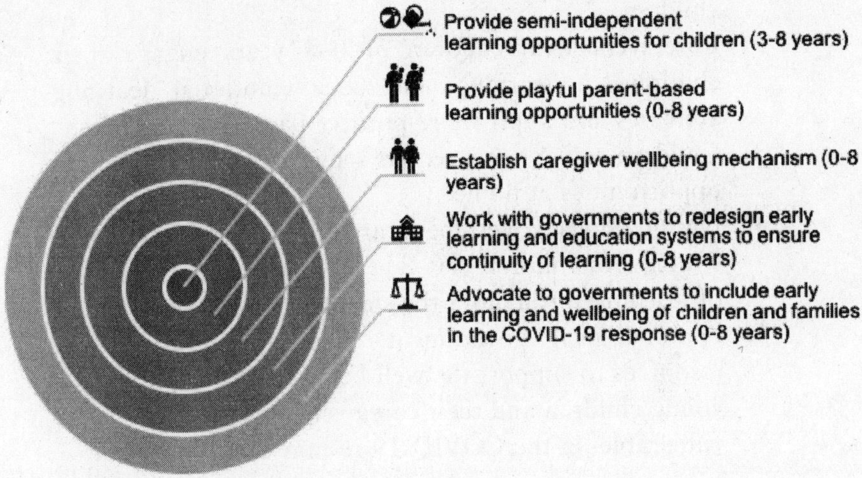

This roadmap to ECCD programming in the context of COVID-19 aims to support countries to implement, monitor, and evaluate experiences throughout the stages of a crisis and to enable governments and other ECCD actors to advocate for and operationalize caregiver well-being, parenting and semi-independent learning. It focuses on establishing a caregiver well-being mechanism to set the foundations for early learning and development, strengthening the capacity of the caregiver to support young children's learning, providing semi-independent learning opportunities, working with governments to ensure the continuity of learning throughout the stages of the pandemic, and advocating with key actors to include ECCD in response efforts. The roadmap draws from country experiences to demonstrate how to create an environment for homes, in partnership with supportive caregivers, as well as how to ensure that young children receive quality semi-independent experiences through other channels. The roadmap aims to foster a shift in thinking around how enabling homes can protect childhoods and mitigate learning loss in emergency contexts. The expected results are that:

1) Caregivers with children of 0–8 years have knowledge of stress management strategies for themselves and their children.
2) Caregivers with children of 0–8 years engage their children in learning and socio-emotional learning activities and apply more positive parenting practices.
3) Children of 3–8 years receive semi-independent learning opportunities at home.
4) National/local governments are implementing a learning strategy for children of 0–8 years that ensures continuity of learning throughout the stages of the pandemic.
5) National/local governments plan for and allocate resources to support the well-being and development of young children and their caregivers, especially the most vulnerable, in the COVID-19 response.

Objective 1. Establish a Caregiver Well-Being Mechanism (0–8 Years)

In times of crisis, caregivers are more prone to stress, anxiety and depression, which reduces their ability to engage with their children (Yoshikawa et al. 2020). Therefore, caregiver well-being, which encompasses mental health and psychosocial support and the ability to identify and manage stress, is a prerequisite for positive parenting. Families can be enrolled in a programme as members of a small, supportive network (virtual or phone-based), with a group facilitator. Through these networks, families can learn essential skills to recognize their own stress and how this can affect young children's behaviour (more crying, more defiance, regression, etc.). Messages and prompts can encourage caregivers to manage stress, practice self-care and respond appropriately and equally to girls' and boys' behaviour and needs. The messages can cover psychosocial education, socio-emotional learning activities that can be done at home, self-care, connecting with existing family violence services and referral pathways, how children experience stress and positive parenting. This programme can be coordinated with a MHPSS programme to provide phone consultations with professional counsellors as needed and support referrals of identified cases. The group facilitators can be trained in psychosocial first aid and basic emotional support. The 'Dissemination Strategy' section describes how the programme can be delivered. Through this component, caregivers can receive the support they need to unlock their potential to engage their children in experiences.

Objective 2. Provide Caregiver-Based Learning Opportunities (0–8 Years)

Save the Children can empower both male and female caregivers with the capability, knowhow, and confidence to integrate early stimulation and responsive care into everyday activities, promoting all developmental domains, and help to provide children with a safe, loving, and nurturing home environment. These learning activities can be disseminated through a parents' audio and SMS programme, the radio, mobile phones and any other available communication channels. The programme can convey both caregiver well-being and positive parenting practices, as well as simple ways to turn routine tasks into enjoyable learning activities. Household materials can stimulate joyful interactions that promote brain development, parental self-confidence, the bond between caregivers and children, and the child's sense of security. They can also address gender stereotypes that restrict young girls' and boys' ability to play with materials of their choice. Specific adjustments can be made for more disadvantaged communities and families, including children with disabilities and caregivers with disabilities.

Objective 3. Provide Semi-independent Learning Opportunities (3–8 Years)

In addition to strengthening parenting practices at home, early learning programmes can offer a learning programme that children can engage in semi-independently. This children's programme can be delivered through mass media, mobile phones, videos, radio, television and social media. Gender-transformative role models can be highlighted and encourage thinking, exploration and learning outside of stereotypical social norms. Programming can include songs and stories, and the distribution of a home learning kit for the most disadvantaged communities and families, following government safety guidelines. The home learning kit may include construction toys, playing cards, counters, self-learning materials, story books, dolls, balls, paper and drawing materials, a calendar of activities portraying girls and boys engaging in non-stereotypical activities, and a guide for parents to create their own home play area with safe materials for semi-independent learning (e.g. unbreakable plates, cups, spoons, cloths, shakers). The children's programme can include games, songs and stories appropriate for children under five years.

Objective 4. Work With Government to Redesign Early Learning Models, Education Systems for Young Children to Ensure Continuity of Learning for All (0–8 Years)

Save the Children will need to redesign early learning models and education systems for young children, including children with disabilities, by devising creative and effective solutions to address disparities. We can ensure continuity of learning by offering flexible in-person and remote options that can be administered individually and in small groups (see figure). We can strengthen the culture of innovation within country offices by encouraging the design of creative non-centre-based early learning programmes, drawing on our many years of programming experience in this area. We can also introduce platforms for collaborative reflection that encourage country offices to study issues, apply creative and relevant solutions, use rapid assessments to evaluate their effectiveness, and then either refine promising approaches, or try out new ones. Monitoring and documenting our experiences will be pivotal to informing the government on good practices for implementing ECCD during COVID-19. Participating in an inter-departmental early learning task force could be a forum to share field experiences and support scale-up by the government. Closely working with the government to review ECCD COVID response action plans, back-to-school strategies, coordinating the delivery of training and sharing best practices are examples of ways to engage with the government to ensure delivery of quality early learning.

Objective 5. Advocate to National and Local Governments and Donors to Include Early Learning and Well-Being of Young Children and Their Families in the COVID-19 Response (0–8 Years)

The final objective of the roadmap focuses on advocacy to include early learning and development from birth within the COVID-19 response, especially for the most disadvantaged girls and boys. The early years are much more formative than many realize, and the impact of the pandemic on young children's lifelong learning and success could be very serious without intervention. Caregivers from more disadvantaged groups are less likely to have the skills and confidence to engage their children at home, and require more intensive, practical and coordinated programmes. Save the Children's impact evaluations have shown that simple and low-cost home learning programmes can significantly improve early learning and development scores and reduce inequity. Save the Children can work in partnership with the government. We can support the creation and implementation of policies that plan for, fund, pilot and scale up effective early learning and well-being programmes, especially for the most vulnerable communities. These home-based programmes must be delivered not only to children who are not able to access ECCD centres due to the pandemic but also children who were never enrolled in the first place.

COVID has forced us to rethink ECCD programmes for the future, and it has become clear to us: We have a choice to make. If we invest only in older children, young children facing adversity, whose parents cannot engage them and cannot meet their basic needs for safety, food, shelter and well-being, will be at a significant disadvantage that will continue to deepen. But if we work with government systems to design flexible, innovative and effective early learning programmes that extend beyond the school walls, with home-engagement and cross-sectoral caregiver well-being components, we have the potential to mitigate this learning loss and ensure that even more children have the early learning foundations they need to succeed in life.

LESSONS FROM COVID-19

Aarti Ramaswami

2020 has been an incredible year for everyone. Our families, teams, schools, workplaces, communities, and governments—across countries, industries, and age groups—have undergone tremendous disruption requiring new ways of thinking, being, living, learning, educating, travelling, and working. That said, COVID-19 can be thought of as only symptomatic of challenging situations, crises, and disruption. What have been the lessons from the past months?

The changing nature of education, the varying appetite for anything digital (education, marketing, operations and supply chains, leadership, and so on), the varying preparedness of various internal task forces and the resources at hand, have forced us to reimagine our present educational and business models, reflect on what from the past would still be relevant, and have greater preparedness for the future.

In this article I will share with you a few actions we put in place as part of our preparedness—preparedness for questions from stakeholders (be they parents, students, staff, faculty, alumni, corporate partners), preparedness for better teaching and learning, and preparedness for managing in the new normal.

PREPAREDNESS

2020 has been a challenging year for us across campuses and across programmes. The silver lining is the continued positive retention of students, successful launch of digital initiatives, and a renewed work style—online—with our employees. While we are separated by distance we are connected by a sense of community.

Our preparedness took into account short-term and mid to long-term actions involving various task forces to understand needs and ensure organizational capability. We had task forces each for recruitment and business development, programme experience, career and professional development, faculty pedagogy, executive education, infrastructure and facilities, employee well-being, and managing stakeholders.

While many of our activities under lockdown moved online (the Talent Day Career Fair, open house, webinars and master classes, staff meetings, and teaching of course) we observed higher participation and engagement online.

We also conducted across campuses surveys of online learning. We found that there are some challenges and opportunities that online teaching presents: for example, the IT equipment at home or at school, the dynamics of the classroom (participation, mood, preparedness of students for courses, time zones they are in), multi-tasking faculty, adjustment to grading and assignments and of course the time that faculty have to prepare for such a situation.

The challenges also bring opportunities that we have seen based on surveys done among various stakeholders. For example, we observed that students who would normally not raise their hands were comfortable typing their questions in the chat box. Online learning also opens up strategic opportunities for the future—how shall we continue to deliver our pedagogy? Technical opportunities come about through research and provision of better infrastructure, learning of new tools. There are also practical benefits such as saving commute time.

In order to prepare for the next normal, we also offered pedagogical resources to students and faculty, such as resource websites and tutorials dedicated to online and hybrid teaching, online communities and forums to share experiences in classrooms, upgrades to all classrooms into video-conferencing mode, with more screens, speakers, and recording facilities.

Before arriving on campus, common concerns among students and participants across all programmes included travel restrictions, visa process, quality of online learning, perceived limitation in interaction with faculty and other students, accommodation and post-arrival adjustment, the fees and perceptions on ROI. Continuous communication with the students and participants on experiences of others, the transition period, and so on were helpful.

After arriving on campus, the student experience task force concerned itself with arrivals, quarantine requirements, team building under online conditions, induction into the programme, assessing various formats of learning, social distancing in the classroom, libraries, cafeteria, and other gathering places for our various communities. Campus social life and company projects were also affected, given the social distancing requirements and travel restrictions. Professional development is another area that needed adjustments to online delivery of coaching, training, workshops, alumni and industry talks, virtual field visits, meetings, and so on.

The physical and psychological safety of our communities remains the first priority. In terms of student or employee well-being, to help deal with burnout, social and physical isolation, anxiety over the uncertainty of the situation, professional counselling has been offered.

THE LEADERSHIP CHALLENGE

The pandemic has brought to fore the need for a special kind of leadership that embodies empathy, communication, connection, ultimately for a sense of community and hope. I believe there are no 'new' lessons—this is indeed not the first, only, or last time the world has gone through upheaval. But rather, there are reminders of what matters most in such situations. Here's what COVID-19 reminded me.

THE IMPORTANCE OF MINDSET

I want to state upfront my biases: I embrace change, and don't mind for the most part to shake up the status quo. The lens through which I view the COVID-19 situation shows me a picture of opportunity in chaos. As much as the dark clouds have hovered above us for months and will continue to, I want to see how this situation will help me answer the new 'what ifs' and the new 'what else'. This is not always easy or natural for everyone.

Someone with another lens is likely to see the situation quite differently. That said, the mindset a leader brings to the situation influences the mood of meetings, the conversations, and the possibilities one sees in the situation for future action. Can we bring a more present and future oriented mindset? Can we bring a learning, playful mindset? Can we encourage ourselves and each other to have a growth mindset? What new conversations are we then able to have? What new actions can we then bring about?

LEADING WITH EMPATHY

Speaking of lenses through which we see the situation, success in our leadership comes from recognizing that the 'other' is not like 'me' and understanding what lenses they use to see the situation. We are very aware that each of our colleagues and friends have different personal circumstances, different levels of support and resources at home, different learning and/or working styles. Perhaps they now have extra costs and inconveniences to work from home, deal with dependent children and relatives, not to mention a demand on already strained psychological resources. Leading with empathy requires us to understand and accept every personal situation, communicate that understanding, and relate to the emotion they are experiencing—be it pain, fear, anxiety, frustration, boredom, relief, or joy. Leading with empathy requires us to remain flexible in order to get the work done through our teams.

Our stakeholders (managers, colleagues, customers, suppliers, clients, and so on) continue to have expectations from us. How can we enable our teams to deliver despite the disruption?

EFFECTIVELY COMMUNICATING EXPECTATIONS

Working from home, and especially under such unprecedented circumstances requires trusting, and building trust remotely. One could not have a limit on honest, frequent communication. We need to communicate expectations from each other (your colleagues or family, for example), set boundaries (with colleagues and family). These might be some new conversations that our colleagues, friends, and family members will need to have but this is the time to do so. When in doubt, talk it out. Asking our managers, colleagues, or family members for clarification or support, as the situation demands or allows, opens the possibility for new and critical conversations to not be missed.

STAYING CONNECTED

When physical contact and the ease of walking across to your colleague's desk are taken away from us, the 'out of sight out, of mind syndrome' may be heightened. During such times, there may be a need to over-communicate and over-connect and be over-available at least initially, so that a routine may be established for connecting online. This also helps to resolve any misperceptions or misunderstandings about commitment, accountability, and so on. It is imperative we take the initiative to work it out with relevant colleagues the frequency and mode of connecting per day/week individually or as a team.

STAYING AGILE AND DISCOVERING HIDDEN OPPORTUNITIES

Agility is not just about speed, agility is mobilizing the team for responsiveness. Recognition of the urgency of the situation, the volatility and uncertainty of the crisis leaves no room for denial—our stakeholders are waiting for action and help to deal with ground realities. Clear guidance, access to resources, creatively innovating new solutions despite lack of resources, pivoting to new ways when the data direct us, using digitalization to improve personal lives and work-lives—the nature of the challenge will demand a range of responses and the goal is not to find the quickest response. Yes, in a way it is, but the higher goal is to find an optimal response that aligns with our values and one that the team can buy into, engage with, and implement. The need to be agile may open up conversations about opportunities to reimagine the 'old ways'.

BUILDING TRUST AND ACCOUNTABILITY

Such crises also lead to discoveries about team members: Who can handle uncertainty and ambiguity? Who can be accountable? Who are the catalysts for change? Who are the keepers of the culture? Situations like COVID-19 amplify the existing dynamic within teams and shed light on challenging pathways in the organization. If a team has trust and works well, a crisis situation can amplify that trust and synergy. For a team that is already challenged by its dynamic, a crisis situation can amplify those challenges, making trust among team members diminish, with members assuming bad intent. Whether a team falls apart or comes together in periods of strain is very much anchored in the initial mood and dynamics. It is of particular importance to enable the smooth coordination of teams that are more likely to struggle in crisis, working and building back the trust remotely.

TAKING CARE OF ONESELF

We all react to change differently. Be patient with yourself and your colleagues, and assume good intent before any judgements are made (of yourself or others). Beyond work hours, taking the opportunity of the situation to step back, disconnect and reflect, or reconnect with loved ones, our hobbies, or activities that energize us—whatever the need of the situation, these have held me and my team members in good stead.

RE-AUTHORING CONFINEMENT: ENDURING COVID-19 AND CREATING A COLLABORATORY

Peggy Sax

> We found on Re-authoring Teaching a common house, a watering hole where everyone can come to drink and quench their thirst for discussion and exchange.
>
> —message from Pierre Blanc-Sahnoun, Bordeaux, France, on behalf of the Galactic Federation of Narrative Planets (2020)[1]

Around the world, we face the COVID-19 crisis. While not in the same boat, we are in the same storm as each community—local and global—striving to come together to harness its unique skills, knowledge, and experiences. This paper explores how Re-authoring Teaching—a global learning community of narrative therapy practitioners, teachers, and enthusiasts—is drawing from experiences as narrative practitioners in the digital age to create a watering hole congruent with the sensibilities, ethics and practices that guide a narrative approach. We explore communal practices that create audiences, link lives and reclaim the community out of catastrophe, as expressed through our online Re-authoring Confinement project. We hope these endeavours illustrate our shared commitment to embody the spirit of collaboration and community by being such a community.

---

1. See 'Together Enduring COVID-19: Events and Resources', Re-authoring Teaching website (https://reauthoringteaching.com/resources/together-enduring-covid-19-events-and-resources/)

WHY NARRATIVE THERAPY?

For over 25 years, the ideas, practices, and ethics of narrative therapy have highly influenced my practices as a family therapist and teacher. Narrative therapy pays attention to how people make sense of their experiences and assists in changing their relationship with problems affecting their lives, focusing not only on a given problem but also on what stands outside of the problem. Co-founders David Epston and Michael White characterize this approach with particular philosophical foundations, interviewing practices, and a range of playful possibilities (White and Epston 1990). In addition to guiding counselling conversations, these principles and ways of working offer tremendous possibilities in community, organizational, and coaching contexts. For this reason, the term 'narrative practice' is sometimes used instead of 'narrative therapy'.

Rather than thinking of human difficulties as manifestations of deep or underlying structures, narrative therapy seeks to separate the person from the problem and explores how stories shape people's identities and the development of a storyline. Narrative practitioners are always double listening—listening to the problem and to accounts of what lies outside the problem. Through our questions, we invite people to notice and explore initiatives or events, otherwise known as 'sparkling moments' or unique outcomes, that would not be predicted by problematic stories and thereby offer different meanings and possibilities for people's lives (Carey and Russell 2003). In recent years, David Epston and his close colleagues are identifying specific practices that contribute to the art of counter-storying (Ingamells 2016).

Built on folk psychology traditions, narrative practice privileges experience-knowledge over expert vocabularies. Significant care is taken to ensure that language conveys people's actual experiences rather than others' 'interpretations of these experiences' (White 2004). In narrative practice, 'co-research' refers to the process by which people inquire together to create original research about insider knowledge—to learn from people's direct experiences about what is most meaningful to them from life situations and relationships (Epston 1999).

Several important ethical considerations inform narrative conceptions and practices. Envisioning training as collaborative research, Michael White often reflected on the ethic of collaboration and of de-centred practice as assisting practitioners to break from despair and reinvigorate their work and lives (White 1997a). An ethic of hospitality refers to the consideration and practices of meeting with families as though they are 'guests' in the practitioner's 'home' (Hancock and Epston 2005). Often, this approach attracts people intrigued by Foucault's notion of 'modern power' and committed to social justice (Combs and Freedman 2012).

CREATING AUDIENCES, LINKING LIVES, AND RECLAIMING COMMUNITY OUT OF CATASTROPHE

> If you want to go fast, go alone. If you want to go far, go together.
>
> —African Proverb

As a postmodern therapy, narrative practice rests on the belief that our identities are socially constructed. This signifies a shift from centring individuals and their actions to centring processes of relating, and from 'aboutness' thinking to 'withness' (Hoffman 2007). In addition to impacting our ethical considerations, this difference in approach influences how we envision contexts for healing practice (McNamee 2007) and legitimizes communal practices as an alternative to traditional clinical practice (Hoffman 2011). A growing literature on resiliency and post-traumatic growth explores alternative accounts of surviving traumatic events such as solidarity, joy, friendship, love, generosity, spontaneous acts of courage, resourcefulness, and resiliency (Solnit 2009).

Rather than centring individuals and their actions, narrative approaches views strengthening webs of connection, and community supports as an integral part of the therapeutic work.

Often, narrative practitioners seek to incorporate audiences in efforts such as letter-writing campaigns, outsider witness practices, reflecting teamwork, Tree of Life gatherings, 'reclaiming community', and other community rituals. In an article entitled 'Reclaiming Community Out of Personal Catastrophe: Communal Practices That Build on Naturally Sustaining Webs', I explore ideas, practices, and teaching stories that support the deep healing and satisfaction that can come from ally to ally relationships, getting involved with local/community resources, giving back to others and making meaningful contributions to others' lives (Sax 2013).

NARRATIVE THERAPY IN THE DIGITAL AGE

Having embraced postmodern pedagogy, I have been exploring since 2000 how similar principles can guide narrative pedagogy in the classroom, trainings, and online. Over the past decade, these interests in teaching narrative therapy online have focused on building the Re-authoring Teaching virtual community. How can we apply similar practices to help us as individuals and communities as we endure the current pandemic in the digital age?

Teaching Narrative Therapy Online

I first experienced the possibilities and limitations of distance learning narrative therapy while teaching graduate students 20 years ago in the rural state of Vermont, USA. In those days, teacher and students travelled to various local computer labs to meet up at specific times. Akin to reserving the room-sized calculator for statistical analysis as a graduate student in the 1970s, big technical machines dominated distance learning labs. It was both awesome and overwhelming to gather in high-tech rooms, facing the challenge of overcoming the prevailing bankers' approach to adult education (Freire 1970), positioning the teacher as the epistemological authority, and students to receive, file, and store deposits of knowledge.

Since then, online education has developed a number

of technological tools conducive to collaboration, rich conversation, and co-sparking ideas around shared materials. While asynchronous tools allow people to exchange from a 'different time-different place' mode at each person's own convenience and own schedule, synchronous methods offer opportunities to meet up in real time through Zoom, Skype, Google Hangouts, Microsoft Teams, and/or other synchronous methods. It is now possible for a non-geek to construct one's own website using Wordpress and other open source website creation platforms.

Re-Authoring Teaching: Creating a Collaboratory

In 2008, I wrote a book titled *Re-authoring Teaching: Creating a Collaboratory*, based on nearly a decade of experiences using the online medium to supplement teaching narrative approaches to graduate and undergraduate students (Sax 2008). The term 'Re-authoring Teaching' is a play on the term 'Re-authoring Conversations' that Michael White and David Epston coined in their original description of narrative therapy. I was compelled to write this book having experienced vast online possibilities for students and teachers meeting across geographic distances, to interact between classes, and to learn not from the teacher but from each other and guest visitors. The book wove together my voice alongside students' reflections, shifting the position of teacher as an expert to more of a reciprocal two-way process, congruent with the focus and values of narrative therapy (White 1997). Having carefully constructed a central meeting place with discussion forums, I became the facilitator for exchanges of ideas with students participating at their own convenience and own schedule from the asynchronous 'different time-different place' mode.

Michael White died unexpectedly in 2008 at the age of 59. Shortly after his death, I started the digital version of Re-authoring Teaching as an online study group to share the commitment to honour Michael's legacy. Bonded by our grief over losing such an important mentor, we co-created an island of belonging where people drawn to narrative practice and other collaborative approaches could continue our narrative studies together across geographic distance. Over the next decade, we rebuilt the Re-authoring Teaching website through several reiterations to become the hub for a range of narrative therapy offerings and resources.

Having become a non-profit organization, our board shares the commitment to building a global learning community—both synchronous and asynchronous—that transcends geography, professional status, and other differences. As a collaborative venture, our mission is to share expertise through training opportunities and online learning resources designed for practice, reflection, replenishment, and community-building. Throughout all our endeavours, we seek to embody that spirit of collaboration and community by being such a community, and invite our participants to join us in preserving, developing, and extending the legacy of narrative therapy.

GUIDING LEARNING PRINCIPLES

Five learning principles guide Re-authoring Teaching's growth as a learning community where participants can, at times, meet in person and otherwise use computing and communication technologies to connect and co-spark online.

Collaboratory. It blends the two words collaboration and laboratory to convey an environment without walls where participants use computing and communication technologies to connect with a sense of discovery over a shared project. All of our online features—The Collab Salon, Online courses, and webinars—build on this principle.

Tewhakaakona. This New Zealand M ori word includes the concepts of teaching and learning which, traditionally, in Western ways of thinking, are viewed as different processes involving different positions for the participants (Lewis and Cheshire 2009).

Making space for multiple voices. Our participants come from different parts of the world, from different cultural and racial identities, professional backgrounds, levels of experience, and access to resources. We strive to be aware of structural inequalities and to act according to our belief in social justice and human kindness.

Flipping the Classroom. We deliver content through various forms such as sharing online videos, PowerPoint slides, and readings. Whenever possible, we deliver content outside of the real-time meetings, thereby preserving time to engage each other to explore topics in greater depth and to facilitate meaningful exchanges. We encourage our facilitators and faculty to guide and support rather than didactically 'teach' and encourage peer-to-peer interaction and learning.

Build dialogue, create bridges. Our narrative training aims to create a space where people can meet under the banner of curiosity and collaboration to learn from each other, build bridges, and engage in conversations about how we, as practitioners, can be most effective in the work that we do. As practitioners, we all come from different theoretical, geographical, and ideological backgrounds. These backgrounds define where we come from as professionals but do not limit where we are going. In the work that we do, we believe it is hugely important that we remain curious and open to learning from others both within and outside our theoretical framework(s).

BUILDING A HUB FOR NARRATIVE THERAPY TRAINING AND RESOURCES

Re-authoring Teaching Inc. strives to bring together the best of teaching experiences and everyday practices from narrative practitioners around the world, with a focus on skill-building and application in a range of contexts. As an introductory online course, 'Narrative Therapy: Foundations & Key Concepts'[2] identified three key ideas influencing narrative therapy:

2. On the Re-authoring Teaching website (https://reauthoringteaching.com/narrative-training/ce-courses/courses/foundations-and-key-concepts/).

1) narrative inquiry guided by poststructuralist philosophy; 2) the narrative metaphor and how stories are shaping identity; and 3) intentional understandings of identity that connect us with our values and commitments. Since then, we have been developing additional online courses as well as the monthly Collab Salon, Faculty Consultation Groups, Workshops and materials for Higher Education.

In addition to narrative training opportunities, we continually update resources on the Re-authoring Teaching website. Drawing from our sensibilities and skill set as narrative practitioners as well as belief in multimedia, we created a YouTube channel where we continually add new free videos, organized in playlists. Each video gives glimpses of rich online content from Narrative Camp, workshops, glimpses into our online courses, and presentations recorded by our partners.

Most recently, we created Twelve Hot Topics for The New Decade. Each theme brings together a range of multi-media materials and is curated by a small group and coordinator: 1) Building on Michael White's Legacy; 2) David Epston: Innovations & Collaborations; 3) Emerging Voices Across Narrative Generations; 4) The Affective Turn; 5) Cultivating Diversity & Accountability; 6) Narrative Skill Development; 7) Narrative Practices around the World; 8) Sustaining our spirit in the work; 9) Earth's Environmental Crisis and Opportunity; 10) Narrative Applications; 11) Teaching & Supervision; 12) Using Technology Constructively. At the bottom of each topic, we encourage our readers to contribute materials of their own.

DOUBLE-LISTENING TO THE PANDEMIC

> Do not get lost in a sea of despair. Do not become bitter or hostile. Be hopeful, be optimistic. Never, ever be afraid to make some noise and get in good trouble, necessary trouble. We will find a way to make a way out of no way.
>
> —John Lewis

COVID-19 is fraught with very real challenges in everyday life. Facing the unimaginable, many of us are dealing with worrisome, terrifying, and heart-breaking crises or worrying about the future for ourselves and our loved ones. As narrative practitioners, we are also drawn to initiatives and events that might not be predicted by the problematic stories generated by the pandemic. What are we discovering as we endure this pandemic together? What are some of the sparkling moments where the dominance of the pandemic problem disappears?

Dickerson (2020) describes a post-structural approach of responding to the pandemic by flipping the usual ways of responding. Rather than getting captured by the current problem, we look for openings or gaps that build on what already works. In her article 'The "Flip"—Sustaining Complexity and Multiplicity Post-Quarantine', she highlights Re-authoring Teaching as one of three programmes that employs a practice of 'disciplined improvisation' to flip more traditional ways of responding.

> Each programme has a built-in structure that depends on technology to make it work; each has a disciplined approach that allows the helpers to improvise to meet the needs of the receivers. It is this 'flip', this way of thinking, that can sustain us and our work in times of great complexity and multiplicity. (Dickerson 2020)

The remainder of this paper will explore how we are now building on our mission, guiding learning principles, themes and resources. Re-authoring Teaching is crafting online responses to the pandemic. Regularly updating our website, we created two community pages: 1) Together Enduring COVID-19: Resources and Events; 2) Re-authoring Confinement: Inspirational moments in everyday life. Throughout, we aspired to create a central place for remembering our commitment to walk the talk of collaboration and community.

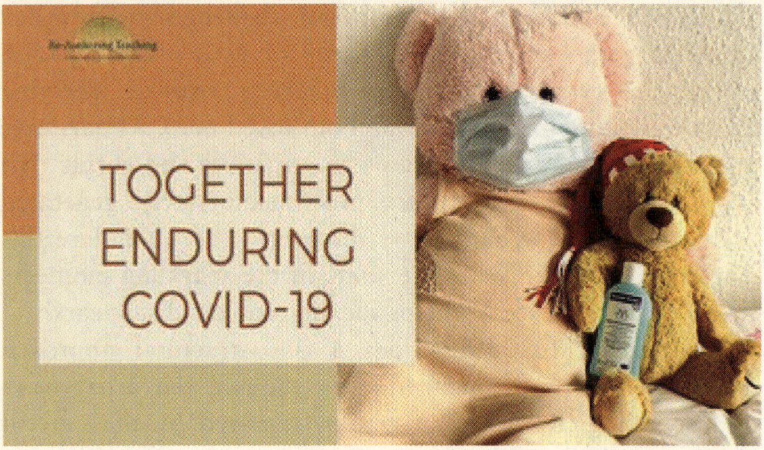

PLANETARY PROBLEM, GALACTIC SOLIDARITY

> Today, in the face of an unprecedented, traumatic situation, we wish to welcome all our colleagues who love narrative ideas in this undertaking of common construction of meaning and connection. We welcome you to share your ideas, your feelings, your indignations, your unique outcomes, your magic spells, your moments of poetry, your wonderfulnesses...and everything that is important to you in this very particular—and tragic but not only—moment of our lives.
>
> —message from Pierre Blanc-Sahnoun, on behalf of the Galactic Federation of Narrative Planets

Wherever in the world, our members face real effects of the pandemic on their lives, relationships and work. With help from our 'Narrative Practices Around the World' team, we constructed the 'Together Enduring COVID-19: Events and Resources'[3] page for people to share their favourite resources as well as to serve as a discussion forum. As COVID-19 impacted some of us sooner, we did our best throughout to highlight 'voices from the future' to give tips learned along the way. In addition, we reviewed our monthly Collab Salon to highlight

3. On the Re-authoring Teaching website.

the effects of the pandemic on their particular topic. First, we offered a special Enduring COVID Collab, which we made freely available to everyone, regardless of Collab membership. We also conversed with presenters to think together how best to bring forward this theme into their upcoming presentations.

RE-AUTHORING CONFINEMENT: INSPIRATIONAL SPARKLING MOMENTS IN EVERYDAY LIFE[4]

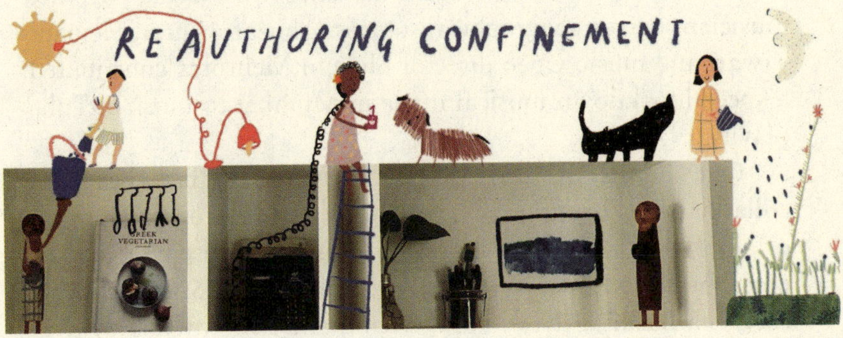

Illustration by Ananya Broker Parekh

Our Re-authoring Confinement resource brings together contributions from members of our community: a YouTube playlist with video reflections from around the world, COVID inspired music, fundraisers, communities collecting wisdoms, children and family projects, animal companions, arts & crafts, gardens & nature, performances, poetry & prose and a discussion forum. By making it easy for people to send in contributions from around the world, we are together aspiring to 'create a collaboratory' together. We chose the following illustrations: 1) Making music; 2) Communities Collecting Wisdoms; 3) Poetry.

4. See also 'Re-authoring Confinement: Inspirational sparkling moments in everyday life', Re-authoring Teaching website.

Making Music

> Thank you for encouraging people to be their preferred and amazing selves!
>
> —message from Elena Baskina

During home confinement, many people are not only making music but creating original songs. Current collaborations take advantage of technological advances that bring together musicians across geographic distances. Abuzar Akhtar, Hemant Tiwari and music video director Shamin Mehrotra contributed a special lockdown musical made in Mumbai to our YouTube playlist.

Our audio musical playlist brings together beautiful collaborations from across the world: 'My Forecast' is an original song with lyrics by Maria Tiunova (Moscow, Russia), music by Dean Lobovits (El Cerrito, California, USA) and vocals by Elena Baskina (New York, Miami and Moscow). 'Covid' is an original song by Pierre Blanc-Sahnoun (France), sung by Charlie Crettenand (Sion, Switzerland) and produced by Dean Lobovits (Berkeley, California). 'Stephen' by Will Sherwin (Michael Castelli on slide guitar, Gene Combs on guitar) is another cherished contribution. Michael Castelli (Middlebury, Vermont) contributed 'Redrocks' along with his friend Tim Joy who laid down the piano and organ tracks; having played this song at live gigs, he started recording it about a year ago: 'It only took a global pandemic for me to finish it.'

Communities Collecting Wisdoms

> Over conversations, reflections and silences, the participants located hope in its little-big acts of resistance, in metaphors of nature and in acts of solidarity, in picture-books and poetry verses, in music and acts of care. These conversations of hope were coming alive in parallel, through illustrations and each of them sought to weave in their hope into the collective. The collective document is a testimony to people's acts of response

and resistance to the current distress, their acts of collective care and continuing to access hope for the coming days.

—message from Narrative Practices India[5] and the Mental Health Team, Ummeed Child Development Centre, Mumbai[6]

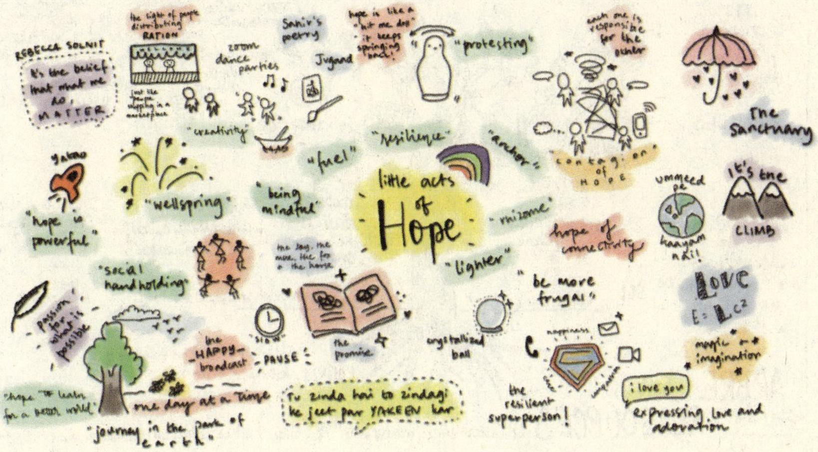

A number of communities have been getting together for special lockdown gatherings to share their wisdoms and create collective documents with each other. France, Turkey, India each adapted The Tree of Life in a Community Context[7] to support each other, create collective documents and generate hope. The Narrative Group Project: Exploring Different Responses to COVID-19 from Turkey—as further featured in this journal—explores skills, 'knowledges' and values that help endure such effects as uncertainty of the future, anxiety of losing loved ones and feelings of loneliness with links to enduring values, hopes, dreams, skills and knowledges. By posting their project on our Re-authoring Teaching page, they hope to inspire others to respond to their questions, by sharing their own ideas and feelings.

5. See https://www.narrativepracticesindia.com/.

6. See https://ummeed.org/people/.

7. See 'The "Tree of Life" in a Community Context', available online (https://dulwichcentre.com.au/wp-content/uploads/2014/01/tree-of-life-community-context.pdf, last accessed 9 November 2021).

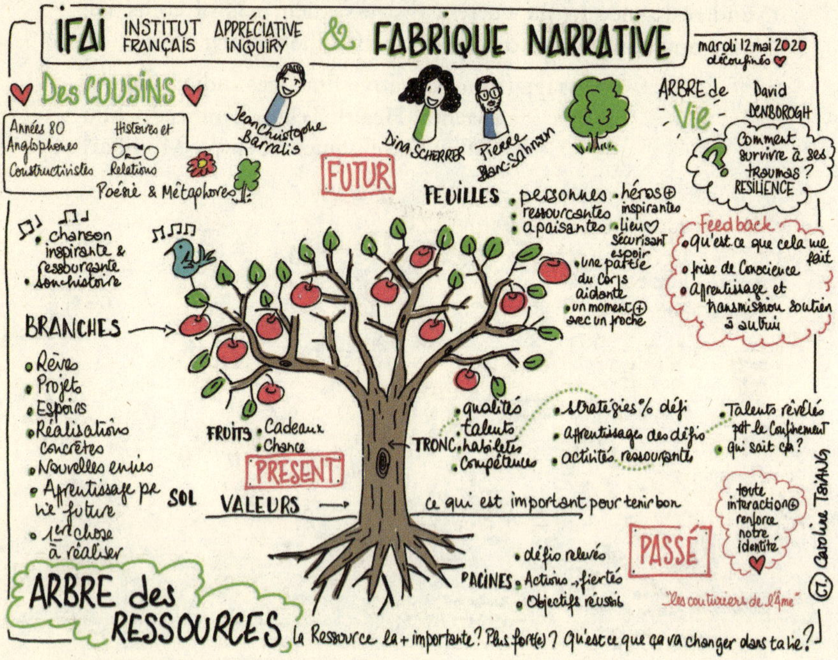

This sketch noting graphic by Caroline Tsiang[8] (Ville d'Avray, France) illustrates a special Lockdown Tree of Life for children and family collected by narrative practitioner Dina Scherrer (Paris, France) for people who live and/or work with children and teenagers.

Poetry

For some of us, sheltering at home can offer contemplative writing time. Pam Burr Smith (Maine, USA) shared this poem:

Poem from the Early Pandemic

All of a sudden
all of us have been tossed
with exquisite aim
into a new world.

Busyness which has demanded
such loyalty in our recent lives
lies useless in empty streets.

8. See https://www.pensee-visuelle.fr/.

And quiet at home,
we face a simple truth
that we need each other.
We need each other
like the teenage boy and his mother

who stand at sundown on a small balcony
and raise trumpet and violin
in the soft fog of a night that grows.

Together they begin Beethoven's Ninth.

Soon through the mist, distant piano joins
then vivid, close, a neighbour's cello.

The hesitance of beginning
drops away
replaced by the wakened air of music.

Windows open to the surprising joy
of gorgeous sound.
A new song of hope flows into motion
and fills the world anew.

CONCLUSION

> Whatever emerges on the other side of our current mega-crisis, community will be key in turning it towards the good.
>
> —Gene Combs, Evanston Family Therapy Center

This pandemic will have a beginning, middle, and end. While sheltering at home, there are enormous differences in contexts and privileges. As we face challenges in enduring COVID-19, Re-authoring Teaching hopes our initiatives will strengthen a global learning community reflective of our values, commitments, and preferences.

INTERNATIONAL EDUCATION AS A RESPONSE TO COVID-19: AN INDIAN PERSPECTIVE

Arundhati Sharma

The International Education sector has created multiple job opportunities for teachers from around the world. ISC Research, a market research company that collects data on international schools, places the privately-owned international schools in China at about 850 (Atack 2019). China's relaxed policies towards international education and its attempts at refurbishing its reputation in education to become the international education destination has seen an increase in the number of foreign nationals taking up teaching positions in several international schools and universities (Huang 2003). An increasing number of wealthy Chinese nationals are driven by the need for their children to pursue higher education in universities abroad and are vigorously seeking international education. This coupled with the need for higher exposure to English, have been the reasons for the increase in international schools in China. Returning Chinese, whose children now hold international passports, want the same level of education as abroad, and therefore seek to enrol them in international schools. Thus, the number of students in private international schools have increased around 64% in the past five years to about 245,000 (Atack 2019). Such schools offer Cambridge International AS and A levels and the International Baccalaureate curriculums. Most of these international schools pride themselves in hiring native English-speaking nationals from countries such as UK, Canada, America, and New Zealand. Apart from those hired for teaching curriculum subjects, international teachers take up positions for teaching English to Chinese students. As per 2017 statistics, there were an estimated 400,000 foreign teachers in China (Cadell 2019), with higher numbers until 2020.

In a majority of such schools, COVID-19 presented a unique situation for the internationally employed teaching staff. The first news of the COVID-19 outbreak was published in China on 31 December 2019. The World Health Organization (WHO) confirmed cases of COVID-19 on 5 January 2020 in a published news article. Having confirmed the first few deaths from the novel coronavirus in China around 19 January, its impact on international teachers was still unanticipated. China was preoccupied with its New Year celebrations in the latter part of January 2020, where all schools and educational institutions closed for a period of two weeks. The majority of foreign teachers employed in China often travel to parts of Southeast Asia during this time, while others travel to their home countries in the United States and Europe. Thus, when COVID-19 was at its peak in China lots of teachers were outside of China. In the fear of catching the coronavirus, many teachers extended their stay in places where they were stationed during the holidays. Teachers stranded abroad experienced tremendous anxiety and stress due to the uncertainty of returning home to China, since many have married Chinese locals and now call China their homeland.

INTERNATIONAL TEACHERS, COVID-19 AND ONLINE LEARNING

Schools set to open in the first week of February, saw a transformation of learning overnight. Teaching changed from face-to-face instruction to online learning. However, teaching students who have very little English-language capabilities, along with teachers who have little Chinese-language capabilities adds an interesting set of challenges in an online environment. Students in China follow the 'Confucian value system' in education. Kennedy (2002) describes the very nature of Confucian educational value system which includes respect for the teacher's authority, with an utmost reluctance to question the teacher. The teacher is always the 'one with the right answer' (Carless 2011) and any individual opinion regarding any matter is discouraged and considered selfish. In order to save 'face' or *mein-tzu*—which translates to maintaining status in front of others, student interaction is minimalistic, and student responses to teachers' questions are often met with silence and blank stares (Carless 2011; Kennedy 2002). The perception of teachers is compared in relation to how well the teacher prepares students for the test, and thus, the teaching and learning methodologies should be test-focused. Hence, international schools that cater to the pure Chinese population of students, often struggle with incorporating an engagement-based student learning culture. However, despite lack of engagement, a face-to-face class provided physical cues to the teacher about a student's level of learning, but the use of online learning methods during COVID-19 eliminated the input of these physical cues. Therefore, along with the limited English capabilities of students, cultural perspectives, lack of physical cues and no class engagement created multiple challenges in effective lesson delivery, classroom management including student attendance, feedback, assessments and student learning. Along with these, the limited online teaching experience of many teachers, as well as their limitations in using online teaching technology effectively, such as Google Classroom, Microsoft Teams, and Zoom led to stressful days for many teachers.

Along with classroom preparation, using new technological tools and preparing for a completely new way of teaching and learning overnight, teachers outside of the country also taught online classes at odd hours in the night due to time differences of up to 12 hours. Additionally, education bureaus in different provinces in China provided different directives to educational institutions regarding next steps, and this created panic and confusion, along with misinformation to foreign staff in China. However, despite challenges, teachers were able to adapt to this methodology. Restrictions in the effective use of online teaching and learning were for a few specific subjects. Physical education lost its meaning of being physical, as students could not indulge in any activities outside of their house. Many schools focused on the theory of physical education, as physical education in its truest sense was impossible. Other subjects such as art and chemistry that required the use of school facilities were limited in their learning, as facilities were inaccessible, and students had no access to these at home. Although the first few months of online education were riddled with confusion, uncertainty, and anxiety, it has paved a new way of learning.

EDUCATIONAL LEADERSHIP DURING COVID-19

COVID-19 was at its peak in China during the latter part of February 2020 and there were no signs of schools opening any time soon. Schools changed dates frequently for re-opening, and there was uncertainty about the next course of action, especially for those teachers stranded in other parts of the world, not necessarily their home countries. They faced huge monetary losses to sustain in another country. If leadership was important, then this was its time. Arnold Glasgow, an American businessman's quote summarizes what educational leadership needed during the COVID-19 pandemic: 'One of the tests of leadership is the ability to recognize a problem before it becomes an emergency' (Daskal 2015). If one thing was certain, it was the fact that nothing was certain. Decision-making was divided in terms of those who valued their employees and those who saw this as an opportunity to cut staff. Some leading international schools in Beijing and Shanghai realized the emergency and provided clarity, informing teachers about their possible return dates. Other schools provided an opportunity for teachers to decide their own course of action, whilst others were quick to make staff redundant. Provinces in the southern part of China were not as prompt in evaluating the situation to be an emergency like schools in Beijing and Shanghai, as they depended on the education departments in these provinces to provide a directive. Therefore, many teachers in these parts found themselves stranded within China during the peak of the outbreak.

Leadership in international schools was stuck in a catch-22

situation, effectively engaging their stakeholders—with immense pressure from parents and students to provide quality teaching, and at the same time, to support its teachers who had little to no training or experience with online teaching. Along with these, new policies and procedures were crucial to be developed, those that were never thought of before the COVID-19 era. Technological support in terms of improved internet connections were provided to the teachers, new platforms such as Zoom were tested for online delivery. Student protection in the wake of online learning, the nature of online classroom discipline, and assessments were just some of the crucial points to be considered by educational leadership. This time also saw parents getting involved in their children's learning, as taking assessments online required supervision, and it was up to the parents to monitor their child's learning and assessment environments. Teachers were directed to discuss topics about sincerity, discipline and truthfulness in work and action as part of learning online.

Authorities tried to support their foreign teachers by providing the necessities, such as food and masks. They worked on changing schedules, and reducing class time to range from 30 min to 45 min. However, the biggest challenges faced by authorities was to ensure continuous quality learning despite COVID-19, convincing parents of the value of education online in comparison to the cost of international education, and ensuring that online schools would provide the necessary preparation for the upcoming exams in the month of May and June 2020.

In response to the parents' concerns, schools had to let the Chinese authorities medically test their foreign teaching staff for the virus. During the peak time of COVID-19, the majority of teaching staff were asked by their schools to comply with health checks by the local authorities. Foreigners during this time were monitored closely as fear of contamination from foreign nationals was high, due to the increasing number of infected cases being reported from other parts of the world. Although the schools had to support government directives for the testing of their foreign teachers, these were also questioned by the schools as many foreign teachers were tested multiple times despite results being negative. However, the majority of schools supported their teachers, ensuring that any stress caused due to the testing was reduced. Necessities such as transportation to and from the hospital, or ensuring that food was delivered to the teachers, were taken care of.

STUDENTS AND LEARNING DURING COVID-19

The student experience of online learning was driven by anxiety in terms of exam preparation and subsequent performance. The overall time frame that students went through online learning was from February to May 2020, after which the majority of schools in China went back to face-to-face teaching. Many younger students faced linguistic and technological challenges in understanding instructions and following the lessons. China's internet restrictions further raised concerns with accessing online content on YouTube and other websites, unless a virtual private network (VPN) is used. Most schools access the VPN through their internet provider; however, since students were in their own homes, many parents did not have access to a VPN and hence student learning on many occasions was limited. The learning experience was overwhelming, to say the least, as students were forced to engage with it under a rising sense of panic, chaos and anxiety due to the virus and the uncertainty of performance in the exams. Further, university placements added to their woes. Along with these, fulfilling parents' expectations and to 'save face' added to the feeling of grief and doom for many students. The breakdown of internet services due to the overwhelming scale of internet consumption also limited access to learning resources. Students therefore suffered mentally and emotionally.

However, students' resilience was also observed during this time as they did cope well with the change in the mode of content delivery. Thus, students were able to cope with the overall anxiety and adapt to the changes quickly.

TEACHING AND LEARNING POST THE CLOSING OF INTERNATIONAL BORDERS IN CHINA

China issued a directive to close it borders to international visitors by the end of March 2020. This has continued of 23 August 2020. This was done largely in order to curb a second wave of infection from individuals coming in from countries such as the US or the UK. The closing of the borders has created a massive shortage of teachers available to take face-to-face classes in China. Those schools whose teachers were directed to return by mid-March, before the closing of the borders and who failed to do so, lost their jobs. Other schools asked their teachers not to return. The current scarcity of teachers caused by the closing of borders has created many job opportunities for foreign teachers within China who are willing to relocate. Amidst this chaos, the rampant racism within the international education industry came to light and the international teacher recruitment practice was questioned. Governing bodies such as the Council of International Schools (CIS) and leading international teacher recruitment firms have pledged to fight structural racism in the international education sector. Therefore, COVID-19 has challenged the very fabric of what international education stands for—*global citizenship*, the unbiased and un-prejudiced recruiting of its teaching faculty across international schools, based simply on merit.

Most schools in China have resumed face-to-face teaching since May 2020, however, teacher workloads have extended beyond normal, as schools are struggling with hiring teachers who are subject specialists. The closing of borders has made it difficult for teachers to come back to China, thus putting pressure on existing staff to deliver the same quality of teaching despite shortages. This has called into question existing policies and practices of teaching and learning and flexible work-time possibilities. Many schools have decided to hire local staff to cover classes, thereby raising doubts about the capabilities of local staff to bring in the same diversity most crucial for an international experience of learning. To counter this shortage, many teachers stranded abroad continue to take classes online to support their students in every way possible.

CONCLUSION

COVID-19 has demonstrated that humans are resilient beings and will evolve and adapt to circumstances that were completely unfathomable before the pandemic. Education, therefore, is in a phase of evolution, as it seeks to answer the question: 'Does the current education system develop people for a new world?'

COVID-19 has brought some additional questions into focus for the education industry:

1) How must the nature of education and assessment evolve for the future?
2) How can leadership evolve to support high-quality learning remotely?
3) How can policies evolve to support higher work-life balance within education?

It remains to be seen how individuals will direct teaching and learning post COVID-19. Until then, all teachers across the globe continue adapting, and innovating to develop a new generation of well-informed, learned men and women to guide the world to a better future.

RECONNECTING IN A POST-PANDEMIC WORLD

Elena Baskina and Masha Tiunova

Even before the pandemic, human connections have been challenged in many ways. New forms of relationships have emerged, confronting people with more options. Those options often, as Peggy Orenstein put it, provoked us into 'a constant state of negotiation, trying to live out more modern ideas yet unwilling or unable to let go of the old ones'. New technologies providing joyful and novel ways of connection have also been bringing painful forms of disconnection. Work environments have often equated our identities to work objectives and goals—which we then apply to ourselves, our partners, and our relationships.

The COVID-19 pandemic has only made this harder, as humans attempt to connect from larger distances, behind masks, and amid high pressure and stress. More and more conflicting expectations of what should be done brought new, painful frontiers of loneliness.

As a result, people have more things to figure out and reflect upon. There are even more discourses that affect them. A whole new language emerged out of the pandemic.

Some of the practices that emerged throughout the pandemic were discovered through desk research, and others through interviews and talks we conducted with people from different countries (sample: 25 people). Please note that these practices are not the only ones. This paper can, in fact, be an open call for more relational practices that we would like to further explore.

BECOMING AUTHORS OF THE NEW REALITY

1) There is a saying attributed to philosophers such as Wittgenstein that is quoted by the founder of the narrative

approach, Michael White—'words create worlds'. Social constructionism brings forward the idea that our realities are co-constructed through verbal exchange. *The Economist* published an article on the effects of the pandemic on language ('Pandating', 2020), bringing forward such words as:

ドライブスルーお見合い *(doraibusurū o miai)*. Drive-through matchmaking (noun). Singles in Japan flirt with one another from their cars, in the empty car parks of wedding halls, arranged by matchmaking agencies.

Coronalingus. To get down to it (virtually) during lockdown (verb). Refers to dirtier sexting.

Cuomosexual. A devotee of Andrew Cuomo (noun). Andrew Cuomo is the governor of New York.

Zumping. The act of ending a relationship during a Zoom call (noun).

Coronavirus and Chill. To watch (virtually) a film or TV show with your quarantined partner (verb).

Quarantinderen. To use Tinder while in quarantine (verb).

Covidivorce. A COVID-induced break-up (noun).

冷静期 *(lěngjìngqī)*.
a) Cooling-off period (noun).
b) A 30-day wait to get a divorce in China (noun).

From the narrative standpoint, creating new words to describe the experiences is a powerful way to reclaim the authorship that was taken away by the events we seemingly do not have power over (the pandemic, the lockdown, the limitations in communication, government handling of the crises). It's interesting that the new word formations, so easily available in contemporary American English, are not at all a norm in some other languages like Russian. Having looked for the post-pandemic words that appeared throughout the quarantine (carantine), we really can't name a few. This topic should thus be further explored to find out how it relates to the overall feeling of authorship among primarily Russian-speaking people.

2) There is a great sense of urgency that people mention in our conversations. There is clearly a group of people who realize that now is the time to explore, experiment, try things out.

First of all, this relates to their connection with themselves. People started sewing, playing the piano, moving apartments, travelling, taking vocal lessons, and considering changing jobs and countries of living. Many started trying out new spiritual practices—like new meditation formats and attending new personal development programmes. All of this came out of the desire to better connect with themselves, their 'true and authentic' selves. One of our respondents said: 'You can only discover yourself through living. And I haven't really allowed myself to live.'

There are people who decided to open up relationships, to end or start relationships, to come up with new relationship formats. For some, those were thought-through decisions; others decided to go for new practices because 'it's better to regret the things done rather than the things not done'. Practices that were previously regarded as fantasies, something that 'would be nice to try out' started being regarded as opportunities now. For instance, young men and women in Russia and the US reported exploring their potential polysexuality through dating apps—which was not relevant for them before. They knew of polysexuality but identified as heterosexuals. Yet, the pandemic invited them to try out different versions of their sexual identities.

3) Some people in Russia and the US started living in communities. Obviously, communal ways of living existed previously. However, throughout the pandemic, this tendency was intensified as people's response to the lockdown was to go out of the city with a group of friends. After the lockdown was over, they chose to stay with the same group of people and make it their new standard rather than a time-bound practice. This response is also related to the loss of trust in governments

and institutions and the desire to create a sustainable 'state' around themselves. Renting houses together, doing group meditations and reflections, sharing meals became an option not just for 'hippie-type' intellectuals, but for broader circles of people. Communal living for them now stood for security, belonging, and being able to share joy and pain and manage the otherwise difficult-to-manage reality. In San Francisco, we met people living in friendly communes, visiting each other's houses and attending events. Being disappointed with governments and how they arrange our lives, they created a network of communities around themselves that has a potential to grow into an alternative system with shared values.

4) Following the previous topic, it is important to mention protests which became stronger in 2020. While there is a lot of awareness about the Black Lives Matter protests, and obviously there will be papers devoted to this very important movement reshaping the face and soul of American society, we would like to talk briefly about the protests in Belarus. After the current president Lukashenko falsified the election results, the people of Belarus started peaceful protests that were met with extreme violence from the government police and military forces. The people of Belarus, however, kept the protests entirely peaceful, not breaking even one window glass or attacking police. The images of women dressed in white giving flowers to the police, singing songs invited a wave of solidarity among people with Post-Soviet roots all over the world. The call of US-based Belarusian entrepreneur Mikita Mikado to those in military forces and police to refuse to fight the peaceful population received numerous applications. Having been fascinated by the beauty and peacefulness of the protests on top of the government violence, people all over the world stood in solidarity with the people of Belarus.

5) A very different and large topic is remote relationships. The lockdown brought about both the extreme helpfulness of and extreme disappointment with the remote. Having been first excited to jump on Zoom, people shortly developed Zoom-out and started returning to voice messaging, calls, and even

email. Of course, one of the answers to the lockdown and socializing limitations became the post-lockdown euphoria (to be described later). However, some people did form new relationships and started using online formats they hadn't tried before (and this is not about Zoom or Miro used for personal, besides professional, communication).

One of the formats that we discovered was voice messaging among friends or remote roommates. For people living separately, away from families and communities, this has become a great way to be in close, casual, practical relations and not have to move in with people they don't want to live with. Everyday casual exchanges on a variety of topics starting from what one had for breakfast or what they are putting on helped people create closeness on a very deep level.

Another format that became more acceptable for adults was sexting. While previously sexting was seen as a dangerous occupation of young people, during the pandemic, it became a way to create intimacy and sustain closeness for adults as well. Sexting provided to our respondents a magic circle where they could be safe and welcome, opening a door to creativity and improvisation. While still not talked much about, we are wondering whether practices like this will contribute to sex positivity.

6) Post-lockdown euphoria: Seeing crowds on the streets of Moscow after the lockdown was over, and crowds on the beach of San Diego, we talked to people at both places about how this corresponds with pre-lockdown behaviour. It appears that limitations for people were so difficult and the lack of interaction with the world and people so painful that their post-lockdown response was to connect in all possible ways. Of course, this was mostly true for younger people. While some of the people are still quarantining, and large cities like New York are showing a lot of COVID-19 cautious behaviour, some places are celebrating the end of being socially distant and disconnected by going into the beaches and streets.

7) Of course, there are a lot of practices, responses which still have to be discovered. If previously closing one's face with

a burqa was regarded as causing doubt and undermining trust, for many people now, an uncovered face is causing exactly the same responses. People reported that they acquired an automatic behaviour of leaving the room with a mask which stayed with them even when they were going out of their bedroom into the living room. Though masks of all colours and fabrics became available, so people can express themselves, they still don't leave a lot of space for facial expressions. The question is which practices become a response to closed faces. Except for the obvious protesting-to-wear-masks behaviours.

8) Business and politics require a lot of immediate attention, amidst the need for 'getting back to normal' fast. While talking to Anne Liese, Guerin-LeTendre (UK), and Aurelie Glorieux (France) at a discussion group on this topic (that actually provoked part of the thinking behind this article), we concluded it would be helpful to give some space to recognizing that this has been a tough experience, to give space to grief and sorrow, to understanding what's emerging for people and between people. Many people reported a sense of being lost, and lacking connection with themselves first of all.

Anne Liese expressed a particular concern about caregivers, who have significant influence over people and haven't been receiving enough care and recognition (especially in countries like Russia with high numbers of doctors' deaths).

9) Not being able to touch/hug people led to the growing interest in bodily practices, next to the desire to explore sensuality and be more around people. While new gestures have emerged (like saying hi by touching elbows), the lack of physical contact is continuing to provoke responses that also have to be further explored.

Further research has to be done on how shifts in practice and their impact on contact during the pandemic have altered communication between human beings.

Coping Strategies

GLIMPSES OF SERVANT LEADERSHIP IN MAURITIUS: A BOLD AND EFFECTIVE RESPONSE TO COVID-19

Basantsingh Deerpaul

INTRODUCTION

As soon as the WHO characterized COVID-19 as a global pandemic (WHO 2020), various continents have braced themselves in different ways to face this unprecedented and unexpected challenge. Consequently, responses have been varied both within and across continents. Some countries responded to the COVID-19 outbreak with draconian, mandatory social distancing policies whilst others have reacted more timidly, either by deliberate choice or due to implementation constraints, leaving individuals to choose for themselves an appropriate degree of self-isolation. Others still have opted for a relatively permissive approach based on institutional and cultural underpinnings.

China implemented extraordinary public health measures at great socioeconomic cost, moving swiftly and decisively to ensure early identification of cases, prompt laboratory testing, facility-based isolation of all cases, contact tracing, and quarantine. In the community, mobility was at a near standstill, with social distancing implemented at a grand scale. China's massive transmission rates called for extreme measures, and the measures were successful. Remarkably, South Korea lost control and regained it with no lockdown and simply strong application of the above principles, enhanced by using novel digital technologies for contact tracing (Fisher et al. 2020). Kerala was the first Indian state to encounter the virus and had kept deaths down to three initially. It had largely curbed COVID-19 but later on was dealing with nearly 200 cases, all people arriving from other parts of India. Senegal from the

African continent seemed to be quite innovative in its approach, having devised a cheap test for the virus and using 3D printing to produce ventilators at a fraction of the going price. China, South Korea, India and Senegal had one common feature and that is, preceding experience in dealing with coronaviruses and other viral outbreaks.

The Republic of Mauritius, located off the southeast coast of Africa, shining as a democracy with roughly 1.3 million inhabitants on its three main islands: Mauritius, Rodrigues, and Agalega, with no prior experience in dealing with an outbreak of such declared magnitude and cost, had a unique response to the COVID-19 test.

To a parliamentary question (Mauritius National Assembly 2020) addressed to the Honourable Prime Minister, Pravind Kumar Jugnauth, the Minister of Defence, Home Affairs and External Communications, Minister for Rodrigues, Outer Islands and Territorial Integrity in regard to the opening of the Republic's borders amid the COVID-19 Pandemic, stating which actions will be taken to ensure the safety of the population against the second wave of COVID-19, replied as follows:

> The World Health Organization had estimated that Mauritius had the highest risk of exposure in Africa, and would have the second-highest rate of infections in a report dated 11 March 2020 amidst the new pandemic:
>
> Number of mild infections: 87424
> Number of severe infections: more than 1000
> Hospital admissions: more than 22000
> Deaths: 837. ('Due to extreme urgency', 2020)

The projection from the WHO seemed to cast apprehensions, for the majority of Mauritians, as to whether the government would be able to handle the looming crisis. Not only did the island have extensive links with hotspots in Europe and Asia—tourism is the foundation of its economy—but it is also the tenth most densely populated country in the world. These were fertile conditions for the spread of the new coronavirus.

The infection rates of COVID-19 as from March 2020 in Mauritius offer a startling distinction though. This paper attempts to explore how Mauritius responded strategically in terms of prevention, outbreak management and communication to the COVID-19 challenge through the 'Servant Leadership' philosophy of the Prime Minister and how the latter institutionalized this value to his government, the heads of ministries, frontliners and NGOs when the COVID-19 pandemic beckoned ominously.

One of the core tenets of servant leadership theory is that servant leaders instil in followers a desire to serve others. Research in this field has convincingly argued that servant leaders are uniquely effective in developing and nurturing service values among followers. More specifically, it is thought that servant leaders represent strong role models that influence followers via learning processes and vicarious experiences and, thus, eventually imbue the importance of service within their teams (Liden et al. 2014).

Greenleaf (1977) who coined the term servant leadership gave a broad definition and stated how to best measure the phenomenon:

> The difference manifests itself in the care taken by the servant—first to make sure that other people's highest priority needs are being served. The best test, and difficult to administer, is: Do those served grow as persons? Do they, while being served, become healthier, wiser, freer, more autonomous, more likely themselves to become servants? And, what is the effect on the least privileged in society; will they benefit, or, at least, not be further deprived?

Many find it hard to accept the phenomenon of servant leadership because they do not understand how a servant can be a leader and how a leader can be a servant; that is, it seems to be an oxymoron. Graham (1991) identified humility, relational power, autonomy, moral development of followers, and emulation of leaders' service orientation as characteristics of servant leadership. De Pree (1992) listed 12 characteristics of leadership in which he included integrity; vulnerability; discernment; awareness of the human spirit; courage in relationships; a sense of humour; intellectual energy and curiosity; respect of the future, regard for the present, understanding of the past; predictability; breadth; comfort with ambiguity; and presence. Spears (1995) published a list of 10 critical characteristics of servant leadership based on Greenleaf's writings which included listening, empathy, healing, persuasion, awareness, foresight, conceptualizing, commitment to growth, stewardship, and community. Spears's list remains to this day the most respected and referred to list of servant leadership characteristics (Focht and Ponton 2015). The above list is by no means exhaustive but open to considerable interpretation as well as value judgements; therefore, an attempt is made to utilize the foresight, stewardship, conceptualizing, listening, healing, awareness, and commitment to the growth of people characteristics to analyse the Mauritian response to the COVID-19 challenge.

FORESIGHT

Chinese authorities had started containment measures on 1 January 2020 and blocked all public transportation links between Wuhan and the rest of the world on 23 January. Meanwhile, cases were identified across other Asian countries. The Government of Mauritius willingly started screening people on arrival at its airport from 22 January, introducing fever measurements and separation of at-risk passengers on 29 January. Based on the increasing number of COVID-19 cases worldwide, the Ministry of Health and Wellness issued several communiqués regarding travel restrictions from high-risk countries. On 16 March 2020, Mauritius extended travel restrictions for a period of two weeks on foreign passengers coming from or having transited during the last 14 days in countries of the European Union, including the United Kingdom, Switzerland and also from Reunion Island. As for Mauritians coming from these countries, they were automatically placed in quarantine for a period of two weeks (Jeeneea and Sukon 2020).

Still, COVID-19 arrived anyway. Official press briefings by

the spokesperson of the National Communication Committee on COVID-19 later revealed that before 18 March 2020, 28 infected persons had already entered the island despite checks at air and seaports (press briefings, May 2020).

Foresight is a characteristic that enables the servant leader to understand the lessons from the past, the realities of the present, and the likely consequence of a decision for the future. It is also deeply rooted within the intuitive mind. Foresight remains a largely unexplored area in leadership studies, but one most deserving of careful attention. Based on the exploration of Greenleaf's foresight in his analysis, Wong (2014) suggests that this characteristic can in fact play a significant role in shaping strategies to mitigate risks, eliminate danger, and harvest growth in an organization or agency.

Rather than studying foresight in an organizational context, Slaughter (1995) examined the concept in a broader framework of future study. He argued that the future could not be predicted precisely, nor were there any 'iron laws' or 'blueprints' governing 'the process of human or cultural development' that might contribute to shaping the future. Slaughter further postulated that instead of being an ability to view the future for what it precisely is, foresight is a 'human attribute that allows us to weigh up pros and cons, to evaluate different courses of action and to invest possible futures on every level with enough reality and meaning to use them as decision-making aids' (ibid.).

STEWARDSHIP

On 18 March, the first three cases were confirmed. Prime Minister Jugnauth set up a high-level ministerial coronavirus committee. This was the driving force behind the country's response and included the ministers of health, finance, tourism, infrastructure and commerce. It was chaired personally by the Prime Minister. The committee met every day, including weekends, and sometimes meetings would go on for three hours. Initially, the meetings were face-to-face—later, when one of the committee members became infected, they started meeting online.

'Having a Prime Minister meeting and chairing the meeting every day, it's a commitment that I have never seen in any other country,' said Dr Laurent Musango, who sat on the committee. Musango, a Rwandan physician with extensive public health experience, is the WHO's representative in Mauritius. He played a key role in advising the Mauritian Prime Minister. Almost every day, the Prime Minister would call him or send him WhatsApp messages, asking for WHO guidelines on specific issues (Allison and Brima 2020).

Robert Greenleaf's view of institutions was one in which CEOs, staff, and trustees all played significant roles in holding their institutions in trust for the greater good of society. Servant leadership, like stewardship, assumes first and foremost a commitment to serving the needs of others. It also emphasizes the use of openness and persuasion rather than control.

Reinke (2004) explores the relationship between perceptions of leadership and the level of trust between employees and supervisors. More specifically, her article seeks to begin a theoretical discussion of a particular leadership approach—that is servant leadership—and introduces an instrument for measuring servant leadership. The results show that one component of servant leadership, stewardship, is a determinant of trust level, indicating that 'service before self' is not just a slogan, but a powerful reality that builds trust between employees and supervisors (ibid.).

CONCEPTUALIZATION

Upon the declaration of the first three confirmed cases of COVID-19 in Mauritius on Wednesday, 18 March 2020 (Outbreak Day 1), Mauritius closed its international borders to all foreigners and even its citizens the following day (Day 2). Closure of all educational institutions also became effective the same day. The prevention strategy also consisted of community confinement. A national lockdown was implemented as from 20 March 2020 (Day 3) which was enforced into a curfew order on 23 March 2020 (Day 6). It is to be noted that the curfew order was extended thrice on 30 March, 10 April and 1 May and was valid until 30 May 2020 midnight (Sun and Wah 2020).

The ability to look at a problem or an organization from a conceptualizing perspective means that one must think beyond day-to-day realities. For many leaders, this is a characteristic that requires discipline and practice. The traditional leader is consumed by the need to achieve short-term operational goals. The leader who wishes to also be a servant leader must stretch his or her thinking to encompass broader-based conceptual thinking. Servant leaders are called to seek a delicate balance between conceptual thinking and a day-to-day operational approach.

LISTENING

Listening is described as the active acceptance of employees' opinions, ideas, and suggestions (Spears 1995). Johnson and Bechler (1998) found strong positive relationships between listening skills and leadership emergence. Kramer (1997) tested interpersonal skills and found relationships between listening and transformational leadership effectiveness. Bechler and Johnson (1995) reported a relationship between listening skills and leadership effectiveness. These studies document the importance of listening skills for leadership effectiveness (Barbuto and Wheeler 2006).

The strategy adopted by the Mauritian authorities for outbreak management followed WHO recommendations (WHO 2020). All confirmed COVID-19 cases were immediately transferred for isolation in dedicated treatment facilities. As highlighted by the WHO Scientific and Technical Advisory Group for Infectious Hazards (STAG-IH), working with the WHO secretariat (Heymann and Shindo 2020), close monitoring of the number of confirmed and suspected cases were undertaken in Mauritius. Acknowledgement is provided to the valuable contact tracing which was undertaken in a diligent manner by teams of health professionals for rapid isolation of cases. Laboratory testing of suspected cases by PCR (polymerase chain reaction) started on 3 February 2020 in Mauritius and has been crucial in the diagnosis of the COVID-19 cases during the outbreak. Mass screening of frontline staff by rapid diagnostic testing started on 27 April 2020. As of 15 May 2020, 24,608 PCR tests and 60,867 rapid diagnostic tests had been carried out (Sun and Wah 2020).

Leaders have traditionally been valued for their communication and decision-making skills. While these are also important skills for the servant leader, they need to be reinforced by a deep commitment to listening intently to others. The servant leader seeks to identify the will of a group and helps clarify that will. She or he seeks to listen receptively to what is being said. Listening, coupled with regular periods of reflection, is essential to the growth of the servant leader.

HEALING

A servant leader—with reported behaviour characteristics such as empathy, compassion, and altruistic calling and healing—builds not only a mentally and emotionally healthy workforce but also inculcates a sense of cohesiveness, collaboration, and sustainable relationships among the followers by understanding and addressing their feelings and emotions. The servant leaders, with characteristics of empathy and compassion, are oriented towards the followers' suffering. This leads to empathic concern and compassion that trigger in them an urge to take action to relieve the followers' suffering. This action, also termed as compassionate responding, manifests itself in a three-step behaviour: 1) patient listening and discussion; 2) empathetic handling that includes comforting and calming as well as guiding and counselling the suffering employee; and 3) taking personal responsibility and providing support (emotional, social, financial, and administrative) (Jit et al. 2017).

The next stage of escalation of COVID-19 infections came on 24 March, when the number of detected infections had climbed to forty-two and people were still overcrowding supermarkets. The Prime Minister announced that the country would be under complete lockdown until 31 March 2020 with only essential services being operational. A total 'sanitary curfew' was instituted. Supermarkets, bakeries, and shops were no longer allowed to operate, with immediate effect. Evidently, the most vulnerable of the society would be affected by such draconian measures. The government decided to undertake the following measures:

At the start of the lockdown, the government announced the immediate distribution of 35,000 food packs to families in poverty (as per the Social Register of Mauritius), to the disabled and to at-home residents. All labour contracts set to expire this year were extended through to December 2020. Wage and income support measures to employers were introduced, ranging from US$125 to $315 for workers with salaries below $625 (on a 15 days' salary basis) per month to $315 for those in the $625–1,300 range (through the Government Wage Assistance Scheme). Workers earning over $1,300 received no support. Self-employed individuals, as well as trade persons in both the formal and the informal sector, received financial support of U$130 (equivalent to half of the monthly national minimum wage) through the Self-Employed Assistance Scheme (SEAC). These measures were extended until 31 May. The government also announced about 1.6% of GDP increase in spending along with extra tax deductions for SMEs (de Melo et al. 2020).

One of the great strengths of servant leadership is the potential for healing one's self and others. Many people have broken spirits and have suffered from a variety of emotional hurts. Although this is part of being human, servant leaders recognize that they also have an opportunity to 'help make whole' those with whom they come in contact.

AWARENESS

Servant leaders lead through awareness and healing. A person with relation-awareness and situation-awareness is able to identify situational, historical, religious, cultural, and social elements in a complex situation (Song 2018).

The data communicated on a daily basis by the National Communication Committee on COVID-19 was used to examine the effectiveness of the measures being undertaken to contain the COVID-19 outbreak. The daily communication of that information was considered an effective means of sensitizing the population to control the outbreak. From Outbreak Day 1 (18 March 2020) to Day 24 (10 April 2020), the number of confirmed cases increased daily from 3 to 318. That number started to stabilize and reached 332 on Day 40 (26 April 2020). On 15 May 2020, as the first phase of easing curfew restrictions began, no new COVID-19 case had been reported for 19 consecutive days. On Day 20 (6 April 2020) the first four recoveries were reported, and the number of recovered patients kept increasing since that day. The number of active cases peaked at 286 on Day 24 (10 April 2020) with nine deaths. There was subsequently a steady decline, though there was an additional death on Day 41 (27 April 2020). Day 55 (11 May 2020) was an important date as there were zero active COVID-19 cases in Mauritius (Sun and Wah 2020).

General awareness, and especially self-awareness, strengthens the servant leader. Awareness also aids one in understanding issues involving ethics and values. It lends itself to being able to view most situations from a more integrated, holistic position.

COMMITMENT TO THE GROWTH OF PEOPLE

Servant leaders believe that people have an intrinsic value beyond their tangible contributions as workers. As a result, the servant leader is deeply committed to the growth of each and every individual within the institution. The servant leader recognizes the tremendous responsibility of doing everything possible to nurture the growth of employees.

The COVID-19 pandemic is testing the limits of societies and economies across the world, and African countries are likely to be hit particularly hard. All possible resources are being rallied to help countries meet people's immediate health and survival needs while also safeguarding livelihoods and jobs in the longer term—including calling for a standstill on official bilateral debt service payments which would free up funds for strengthening health systems to deal with COVID-19 and save lives, social safety nets to save livelihoods and help workers who lose jobs, support to small and medium enterprises, and food security. Growth in Sub-Saharan Africa has been significantly impacted by the ongoing coronavirus outbreak and is forecast to fall sharply from 2.4% in 2019 to -2.1 to -5.1% in 2020, the first recession in the region over the past 25 years (World Bank 2020).

Despite this bleak situation, the Government of Mauritius promptly committed around 12 billion rupees ($300 million) to support its businesses and workers, even as the effect of COVID-19 is likely to be felt well into 2021 and beyond (Jeeneea and Sukon 2020).

CONCLUSION

For the Republic of Mauritius which had never handled a pandemic before, the response seemed effective. When human, political, economic, social and health stakes are high, servant leadership, as this study highlights, is not a 'soft' philosophy. The Prime Minister, through the COVID-19 challenge, was able to institutionalize servant leadership across key stakeholders at a crisis time. It is evident that:

1) People's highest priority needs had been served. The government's prevention strategy to curb the pandemic curve worked. A major health disaster had been averted.
2) Those served grew as persons. Mauritians, while being served had become healthier, wiser, freer, more autonomous and aware of the handling of an epidemic. The age-old adage 'Health is Wealth' never perhaps rung so true. The sanitary curfew along with the 'early

hard lockdown' was an illuminating experience for many on the island.

3) The authorities and public, after having garnered experience, went out and helped underprivileged countrymen and thus became servants in turn.
4) The different financial assistance schemes provided will affect the country's reserves. Yet a choice was made between health and wealth. The former won this time.

COLLECTIVE DOCUMENTATION OF LIVES DURING COVID-19 IN KATHMANDU

Raji Manjari Pokhrel and Prathama Raghavan[1]

INTRODUCTION

Collective documents are an archive of a community's knowledge, wisdom, skills, hopes, and dreams for a future world. Collective documentation is a practice informed by narrative practices that take the form of poems, books, collections of pictures, interviews, lists, illustrations, drawings, letters, etc. 'Narrative practice is a term that is replacing "narrative therapy". Many practitioners work in public sector settings such as early child care and education, social services, and community mental health where "therapy" does not adequately describe their roles. Applications of narrative practices in community circumstances also demonstrate the limitations of speaking about therapy' (Narrative Practices Adelaide 2015).

Michael White (2003) and David Denborough (2008) have introduced several examples of collective narrative documents. Denborough described collective narrative documentation as involving the process of collaboration in constructing ways to archive and 'describe the skills and knowledge that people are engaging with to deal with hard times' (2008, 28).

Collective documentation can also record a moment in time, the responses of communities to a moment, and stand as an alternative to the dominant narratives generated by the mainstream ways of documentation. Myerhoff (2007) called them acts of 'cultural creativity'. They can represent the past, the current moment in time, and possibilities and imaginations for the future. The hope of sharing these documents is for the

1. With contributions from Rihana, Uma Bista, Safal Lama, Tripty, Pranika Koyu. Photographs by Uma Bista.

audience to stand as witness to these preferred ways of being and living of communities. Sharing increases the visibility of these often-marginalized experiences and brings with it the possibility of nurturing diverse narratives of people and communities.

In the case of this article, they are an archive of the responses of a few people with diverse life experiences, living in Kathmandu, Nepal, during the COVID-19 pandemic. Here we have chosen the form of a document of responses to some key questions determined by the authors. We have woven together a tapestry of diverse responses that each stand out in their uniqueness and together resonate in their shared values and principles.

PEOPLE WE INTERVIEWED

Safal Lama: 21 years old.

Tripty: 25 years old, a photographer on her way to becoming a professional house sitter. She loves cooking, gardening, and petting other pets.

Rihana: Activist and ex-drug user, working at the intersection of transgender rights and addiction. Currently co-managing a women's drug rehab centre on the north side of Kathmandu.

Pranika: Poet and activist, living with her son P and his father Prajwal. To read her writings, go to *Setopati*.[2]

Uma: A photographer, a visual storyteller who has been working as a photojournalist for almost a decade. To see her work related to the pandemic, go to her Instagram page: uma.bista

What has been the experience of living during COVID-19?

Safal: I am an outgoing person, so it was really difficult for me. COVID made me stuck in one place; it made me suffer from stress. I was lonely, bored, and tired. I used to feel sleepy all the time. In the beginning, I felt like there is nothing in the future.

2. See https://www.setopati.com/author/892.

I got alopecia, which also got me worried. In the beginning, not only me, but my friends were also suffering from financial difficulties without any support from their parents. Now we are adapting to the situation.

Tripty: In the beginning, after the lockdown was imposed, I was really scared. My family is in Jhapa, and they called me and asked me to come home. I thought I am just going to stay here; it would be safer. I might get infected going home. We had started a COVID-19 response campaign at work. We would put out information around COVID-19. We were working 8–10 hours, which kept me busy and not thinking about this situation. I was living alone. I would only talk to friends and family on the phone. Having something to do was good for me.

I have been house sitting for some people. I also started working on relief distribution and documenting the work. I have moved from house to house. It has been constant change—personal space as well as the situation outside. This has been confusing sometimes, but I am trying to work it out.

Rihana: Before the first lockdown in March, I had started working at the women's drug rehab centre north side of Kathmandu. The centre was started by female drug users. We currently have six residents and three caretakers, and I am one of them. I am a transgender woman and an ex-drug user, and now I find an overlap in my work, something I want to do, so that was good. Personally, at the beginning, it was a bit monotonous. And the noise and news all around was too much. I stopped listening to the news at one point and focused on providing day-to-day structure for residents.

Pranika: I like the side of Kathmandu I live in because it is quieter, fresher. I live in a big space which feels like a lot to work on daily. I think an apartment would have been better for us. I live with Prajwal and our son P and we co-parent together. There is not much difference, in a sense, because prior to lockdown too I wouldn't go out much; the lockdown has also been the same mobility-wise. Before lockdown, I would get invited to so many discussions, including speaking engagements but couldn't go to all these places, but now it's all virtual, so now I can actually participate in more. Sometimes, from 11 am to 6 pm, there are marathon webinars. This situation has made it possible, due to internet access. People who have access can listen to me talk all over Nepal on violence during conflict, caste issues, citizenship, women's rights issues, the books I am reading or have read, and I have reached a new audience I think. This has all happened because of this lockdown. However, how it will translate into my future work is still in limbo. I don't know whether people are serious about following it; it isn't clear whether this online engagement will continue and be sustainable or not. So these days I am again refraining from speaking. How effective is it? Could it be just a show?

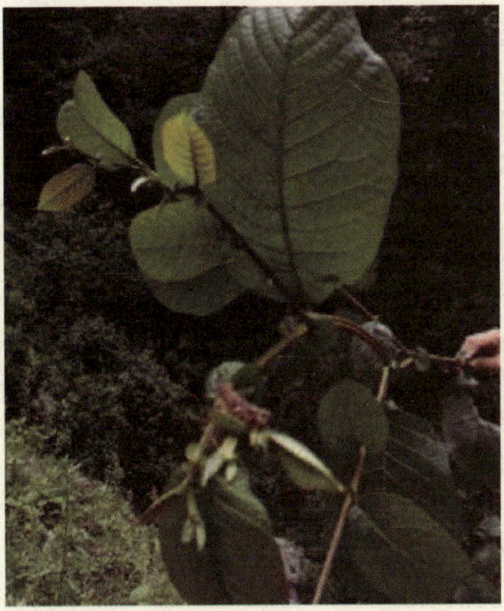

Uma: Once I came to Kathmandu, I didn't think it would be so bad. I went to work and on the lift I saw notices about social distancing and mask-wearing. The notices were everywhere. People were panicking and I felt the panic too while going to the office every day. Then it was decided we wouldn't have to go to work regularly but would have to work during the lockdown anyway. Our team of four decided to work alternate days to be safe. One of my co-workers would work every day to help out. The joy I felt was to see the city feel clean as I went out to work as an essential worker. I was afraid but seeing the changing face of the city I felt *ananda*, calm.

Along with office work, I also took pictures for myself and showcased them which became a way to engage myself, console myself about the fear. Earlier, I used to watch a lot of news, but I decreased the frequency, which helped reduce my state of panic. At home everyone was normal, acting like nothing will happen, but I would panic and was told not to think too much.

Who has made it possible for you to get on with your day-to-day life?

Safal: At first, I didn't talk to anybody; I was so worried. After I got alopecia, I started talking with someone at the organization where I intern. I shared with her my feelings, my insecurities about beauty and the hair fall. Then I started talking to some friends that I trust. Talking to them I realized that others were also suffering in a manner similar to mine. They helped me by talking to me every day.

Tripty: Friends and people around me have been trying to help me. I know I will be okay because of this. Even when I have to leave the house I am in currently, I know I won't be on the street because of these friends. Even though the first two months I was living alone, over phone calls I could talk to people if I needed to. One surprising thing during COVID was how you made the effort to talk to people over video calls. I also realized that it was the same for so many of my friends—having reunion calls with high school friends—people were making the effort to wake up in different time zones to talk to each other. We didn't do that before Corona. After I started doing relief distribution work, I would see people thrice a week—being in the same space with other people, eating the same food—I missed that. One of the people doing relief work was my neighbour. During the lockdown phase, we bonded, we cooked for each other, went for runs and cycling together. This neighbour in particular helped me. One of my friends sent me flowers when I told her I was not feeling so well.

Rihana: My sisters who have been doing this work on addiction for a long time have been a huge support for me. And now being able to work here, helping women struggling with addiction has given me a sense of purpose. It has brought us together. Also the NA (Narcotics Anonymous) groups I am part of and the international NA groups for LGBTIQ folks have been a huge source of support. Nature, surprisingly plays a big role in helping me get through my day, and I never thought I would ever say such a thing! Seeing the vegetable garden grow, the scenery around here, it is such a wonderful experience.

Pranika: Time-wise, even before the lockdown, we had a schedule and I would be able to find time to do my work. We cook. I don't like to order food anyway. Before, I would eat out a lot; now we eat more at home. My grand-aunt was living with us for a while. Prajwal and she, both of them liked cooking—so that was sorted for me. And the food that I cook or prepare is what P chooses to eat! I got some fleeting thoughts of picking up a hobby. And now, gardening, which I have begun to learn, has become a hobby all of a sudden. And it's been nice, though I do so little.

Uma: My fellowship class for photography, narrative diploma class, the community of women photographers working on the pandemic on Instagram, these are some areas where I have been able to contribute. Collaborating and getting to know photographers and international networks have helped me a lot. I live with my family. Since the age of 19, I have been away doing this work and I am unaware of what goes on at home. I haven't been aware of the changing of seasons—wheat fields followed by paddy fields. The timetable followed during the day at home. New noises and distractions and having to play with the children at home; they would call me to interact with them, play with them. My home is a bit far away from the centre of the town so we have the advantage of a more open environment and it feels good to spend time with family. There is a forest a walk away. My mom cooks and we eat together and it's a new experience. *Dai chiura khane din Asaar ma*: June is the time to eat curd and beaten rice; it had been eight years or more since I sat during the day leisurely observing small moments with my family.

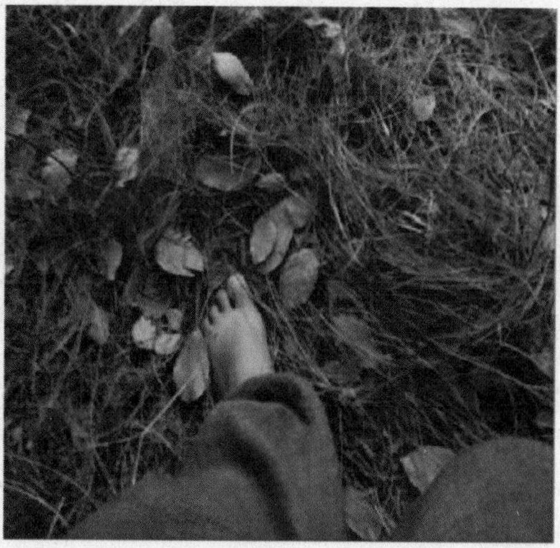

What have you made possible for others around you in their day-to-day life, that with you being there, their lives have felt safer, etc.?

Safal: I was talking to disabled queer persons—they were distressed that their parents will find out they are queer. Their parents are queerphobic and being disabled, being queer and not being accepted in their family was very hard for them. Some of my friends are HIV+; they were worried that their parents will find out. Since I know their parents too, I would talk to them and deliver their medication to their houses. We got to understand each other's worlds. We made groups to talk about and share experiences, memes, funny moments of queer people during this COVID-19 situation. I have talked to many unknown people in this lockdown. We can share positive energy even without knowing people.

Tripty: For my neighbour, I did for him what he did for me as friend, as family. We were there for each other for food, for exercise. I went for relief distribution for a few days and to take photos and interview people. After I interviewed people who were receiving relief, it hit me how bad the situation was. I was safe, I was in a bubble. I realized how people were struggling after the lockdown; the reality struck me. I was very sad for weeks after that. I felt so helpless, the relief we were distributing helped people but their problems were so much more than that.

Rihana: For the residents here I provide a structure in their day-to-day life. I provide dance classes and yoga. I have always been vocal about my own struggles with addiction. Last year I was having a really difficult time in my life and even while facing difficulties, I did not stop going to meetings. I stayed connected with the ex-drug users' community and stayed sober. I think that was possible for me because they are such a big part of my life.

Pranika: For Prajwal to have a break during the day, I schedule everything in the morning. When I have calls in the afternoon, I can turn off the video and be with P as well and that works out. Doing online engagements has made it possible for me to be with P. In the past I would travel for work without P and it didn't work at all. I have been told that I make a fuss about having a child and I have to explain that P is not like other children. If I were to take P to a public event and he would get upset and cry, people would look at me like I wanted attention.

Uma: In the home front I tell my family members to be cautious, I provide information. I help with doing the groceries. I interact with family members and I am around during the day, which wasn't possible before.

What is something you learnt about yourself that surprised you?

Safal: Firstly, I always felt that I am a useless person. I had never thought I will do this or that in the future. I usually think of the past. But in this COVID-19 situation, I thought I could be a sex therapist, which helped me a lot. I was researching about sex therapists and sex cultures, especially queer sex cultures. I find it easy to talk to my parents, family, brothers and sisters about sex cultures. I also find that I can easily connect with people, people listen to me. I do not feel negative about the alopecia I am suffering from. I feel beauty never stops, everything is beautiful. In Nepalese society being disabled, having alopecia, being a queer person is a problem. I read, I explored myself, I accepted myself—so I can help other people accept themselves. I am confident nowadays about myself. I feel unique. I talk openly about any subject on different platforms. I talk about sex openly—I shared articles about sex on Facebook. I asked sex therapists in Nepal if they knew about sex cultures, and they said they didn't. This makes me feel I need to be a sex therapist in Nepal. Now I have a goal, I need to do this.

Tripty: I am the kind of person who makes plans; I get upset if things don't happen the way I planned them. But now, I am trying not to do that in larger plans involving my living space. I still get upset when plans change with friends, etc., but with this living situation I am surprising myself.

Rihana: I have always been a complete unbeliever, *naastik*, when it comes to things like yoga and meditation. But due to the lockdown, I met this new Rihana who has started meditating and doing yoga. There is faith and self-love in me, I realized that about myself. There is special growth and I am amazed at myself! I am coming face to face with this real me at this moment! Where I am these days, there is a forest and a hill nearby and a river beside it. And I go on walks. Dance has been a big passion of mine and one of the ways I spend time is creating dance classes for people with different needs—that's been the profit of the COVID-19 lockdown time for me!

Pranika: I would think I would be way more anxious right now but I am not. I don't know if this is acceptance or denial! I am not taking a lot of work even though I should pay my loans, but I am so relaxed. I have been financially independent since I was 19 and I would only get comfort with a certain amount of savings in the bank. Right now I am using my savings. So I do look for work and apply but it doesn't seem so urgent to be working to earn. I am not feeling the heat! And this is definitely not ME, you know. I have LOANS. Looking at my son, I do feel desperate. Maybe there is calm because of what is going on. Now it's all the world that is helpless: could this be why I am calmer as opposed to other times? Everyone is arrested in time, bound by time right now. Before, the world was on the move and I would feel so helpless. And it would trigger me. There was the consolation that it's not just you, but it felt like an excuse to try to pacify myself. But now it's actually that.

Talking about what's surprising—I am surprised how I can live with this anger and resentment I have against the government. Writing abstract poems (Koyu 2020), warning our present regime that they better not let there be an uprising because then they won't have a place to hide…I wrote that and many people read it and I felt happy about it.

Uma: Wouldn't call it surprising. But I get the sense that I know myself better. I realized I sleep when I am upset or angry! As for my job, I wasn't satisfied at work for a long time and I would tell myself to quit but would then keep going. But now I have a sense of clarity. I didn't gain much and there is no space to showcase what I know. *Jyan vanda thoolo jaagir hoina*: a job is never more precious than life. I spent a lot of time in my 20s investing in the organization so I feel sad. And I now realize that there is no use committing myself wholeheartedly. I can look for other work. I used to think I have to work hard, but if there is no space, no open communication…it isn't worth it. This issue had already been here but came to the fore now. As a photographer I am surprised by how even without a camera with a regular screen I can capture moments through screenshots; there are portraits that I have taken like that.

Exhibitions aren't possible in physical spaces. Now to meet or network with a veteran I don't need to go somewhere, it can happen online—that possibility has grown.

What has this moment got you thinking about? What would you like to be different in the world? What would you like to keep and what would you like to change in the world?

Safal: Caste, cultural discrimination, race discrimination has been increasing in the world during COVID. We should never judge people by their circumstances. This is a situation where we should be together. We need to support each other, we need each other without caste, discrimination, without any conflict. We can help each other. We can explore what we want to be, with access to the internet in our homes. We can make parents understand our experiences, since we have time during this lockdown—showing them interesting videos, materials, online tools. Everything happens if we are together and we help each other without any judgement, without any discrimination. Identity doesn't matter—what I feel, how I identify—if we help each other with a pure heart, a pure soul and share positive energy. People are bullying each other but there are also people helping each other without any fear, being strong themselves. We never know who is helping us—like we don't know who is distributing relief, but we are taking it and therefore accepting help from people we don't know.

Tripty: Difficult times like the pandemic affect different people differently. I would like that to change. It is so unfair. People should have access to the basic things. I interviewed someone who said that you are giving relief and that's great, but we don't have gas to cook the ration you are giving us with. Everyone should have access to free healthcare and basic supplies to live a simple life and not have to struggle so much just to eat and live.

A lot of people came together to do so many things—relief distribution. People were doing things for others for free. I wish this would continue and not just be a thing that happens when something bad like the pandemic is going on. At the photo circle where I work, we were doing reading sessions for the photographers' community. People came not only for reading but to talk to each other and do something meaningful and to stay productive and connect to people they like. People were trying to be there for each other in different ways, being thoughtful.

Rihana: *Nature risayera malai nai time deu vaneko jastai chha*: nature is angry and is saying, 'Give me all your time!' Nature is so important. It has been a very new realization for me and I would like to keep nature safe. Also, this system we are forced to live within, I have always been against this system, it has ruined everything. It is not the fault of the individual and my desire is to change the system. I know at present so many transgender individuals must be struggling with substance abuse. I am an ex-drug user and a transgender woman and there is no representation for us at all. While doing this work, in the beginning I felt proud, but now that pride has been replaced by a sharper focus on the motive of the work. And now I feel there's a greater possibility of opening up and using my own experience.

Pranika: Online participation is economic, environment friendly, and it's less time consuming (saves time spent on travel, which can get hectic and tiresome in Kathmandu's traffic). Let's hope this continues. Earlier, I would feel I couldn't do anything online. But the other day a dear friend said I am very present in online discussions and she said you can do it! I give importance to being physically present but that has changed. Also, I wish we were more of risk takers. I wish we were bound by different things. If I didn't have P, I would be out in the street for sure. The State wants the citizens to do things on their own: PCR, do it on your own; 26 lakh for a ventilator, pay it yourself. Social injustice is rampant and it's propagated by the State which is apathetic, corrupt. They don't do it directly but the refusal to take measures for health, denying even dignity in these badly put up shelters is killing Dalits, aiding in trafficking of women and other individuals. All this proves that they don't care whether we live or die. So why are we silent? Social media activism is a safe resort at this time and it feels like it has minimal impact. It's as good as not using it and staying at home and accepting the situation for our own survival. We have been reduced to this. I wish I could work on that, changing the mindset of people. We don't have to be passive recipients. To what extent can I write if no one is influenced by it to act? In the US, people coming out against the lockdown...that could be silly, but they are expressing their individual needs. Here in Nepal, we say social, communal needs are more important than an individual's need. So how come we don't come out to protest together, because it is crippling all of us? There are people who are doing it of course but we need to have a ripple effect. Taking P out would make it look like I am seeking attention. If he could walk then it wouldn't have been a problem. Unless they have a child like him, they will not understand. And this is not only in times like this. The situation for families of people with disabilities has always been the same in Nepal—the absence of a comfortable and healthy atmosphere (both mental as well as physical) that allows you to take a child like P out has been absent. The onus is on us to the extent that it is burdensome and discouraging.

Uma: Being at home and eating home-cooked food, my health has become better, so I would want to keep it that way. We need to get rid of Corona! We can't go back to normal now and it's affecting everything. Personally, for me, the assignments that I get might need me to travel. Since I do need to work to make a living, I can't refuse and insist that I will only work from home. This is a crisis and people need to work together. Also, as photojournalists, our work needs to be appreciated by the institutions we work for.

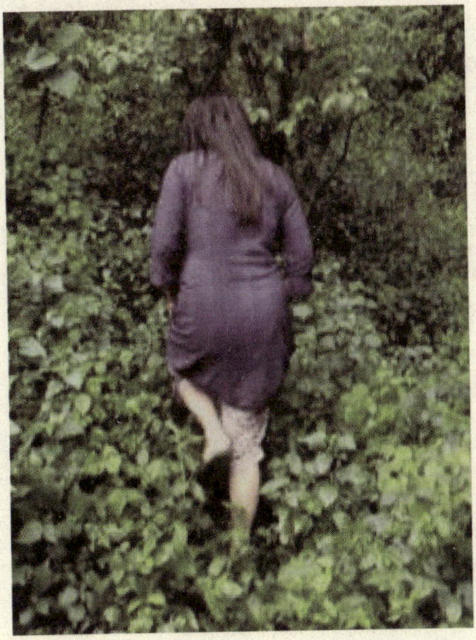

COMMON THREADS IN THIS DIVERSE TAPESTRY; CARE FOR OURSELVES AND OTHERS

Care for others and how it is intricately linked to caring for ourselves is something many of our interviewees spoke about. Making new connections and talking to people we would not have done in 'normal' life circumstances is also visible in many of the above narratives. Helping unknown people and accepting help from unknown people resonates through many of the shared experiences. This is further highlighted in how nature comes up in the conversation and the feeling that it has nurtured us and that we have the responsibility to nurture it in return.

EXPLORING NEW TERRITORIES OF IDENTITY

Whether it is learning to adapt to changing circumstances and embracing them or exploring new interests and discovering ways in which we would like to take our lives forward, this time has allowed, amid the chaos and distress, to anchor ourselves in newer ways of being.

Connecting more deeply with various facets of one's own identities, being surprised and amused at those discoveries has also been spoken about and resonates throughout all the conversations.

But people also speak about learning to live with the sadness that this moment brings due to the gaping disparities in society, or the helplessness and inability to do everything we would like to, and the constraints our lives and society put on us.

Reflections on Inclusiveness

'TAKING CURRENT STRAIN AND FEELING PAST PAIN, AGAIN': A REFLECTION ON BLACK SOUTH AFRICAN WOMXN'S[1] EXPERIENCE WITHIN THE CONTEXT OF COVID-19

Jude Clark

> We are, each one of us, locations where the stories of our place and time become partially tellable.
>
> —Miller Mair

This brief commentary provides a gendered reflection on this critical moment in a time that is characterized by the global pandemic of COVID-19 and looks specifically at the South African context. It draws on my identity and experience as an African feminist, a Black cis womxn, a mother, a partner in a heterosexual partnership and a clinical psychologist journeying with other Black womxn in therapeutic processes. It takes as its premise three points:

1) that a gendered lens is invariably an intersectional analysis, acknowledging the simultaneous multiplicity of social identity as a kind of prism through which multifaceted power is experienced (Crenshaw 2017). This commentary, therefore, does not aim to be and cannot be representative of all Black South African womxn's experiences under COVID-19, given that we are not a homogenous group, but differently interpolated in the social geometry of identity and power.
2) that the 'the personal is political'. This feminist slogan

1. The term 'womxn' represents an explicit inclusion of a broader intersectionality of gendered identification that includes trans, Black, and variously othered womxn.

and truism is alluded to in the opening quotation of Mair—that the story of my everyday lived experience is also a telling of the socio-political and historical context within which I live and the systems of power that act upon me and that I internalize as well as resist.

3) that how we understand/research/make meaning of COVID-19 has considerable implications not only for the ways in which we come to 'know' and represent womxn's experiences within the pandemic, but the ways in which we come to know and represent the broader historical, cultural and political systems of power that position these womxn in specific ways during crises.

~

It has been 26 years since South Africa's transition to democratic governance. In post-apartheid South Africa, the interwoven constructions of 'memory' and 'trauma' continue to be played out in discourses that traverse both private and public domains. The COVID-19 contextual phenomenon can be seen as a significant conduit for historical and personal memory of the effects of gendered power upon the daily lived experience of individual womxn, Black womxn in particular.

Particular moments such as the current COVID-19 moment we are living through remind us that the past is always alive in the present. These moments create a rupture in our investment in the discourse of 'putting the past behind us'. This pandemic, like other moments of crises and disasters, brings to the foreground the deep social divisions and inequalities of the past created by the legacy of colonial systems and other interlinked ideologies of dominance that persist and are perpetuated along the fault lines of our racialized and gendered everyday experiences. We carry this painful past with us, in our (gendered) bodies, in our (gendered) social relations—our behaviours, our conscious and unconscious biases—in our (gendered) systems and ideologies. So, there is a strange 'déjà vu' to the phenomenon of COVID-19, historicity to the shape and texture of 2020 that seems to reverberate through our individual psyches and the collective national imagination. One reason that the trauma of the South African past is never very far from the surface of our consciousness is that violence is the main historical continuity between 'then' and 'now'. For Black womxn in particular the main continuity through colonialism, apartheid and democracy, enacted in our social relations has been gender-based violence. For Black womxn, in a manner of speaking, the more things change the more they stay the same. While our Constitution has been lauded for the progressive nature of its gender policies and legislation, it co-exists with our reality of having among the highest rates of gender-based violence in the world. And so, in both embodied material ways and in symbolic ways, this period of COVID-19 is traumatic for Black womxn. COVID-19 brought with it a familiar militarization, reports of police brutality and 'heavy-handed' enforcement of curfew and prohibition laws, heightening the ever-present threat of violence.

For the Black womxn with whom I have formally engaged in therapeutic processes and informally connected within feminist circles, this period of COVID-19 has been a time which many have described as having 'pushed them to the edge'. Past violations and traumas have re-emerged in symptoms of anxiety, depression and burnout that are rooted in dynamics of disempowerment, fragmentation and loss of autonomy and agency. These central experiences of trauma, disempowerment and disconnection from others (Herman 2015) are being relived in the current moment as womxn remember in a visceral way under the 'lockdown' and physical and social distancing and isolation, the sense of having their sense of power and control over their lives taken away. They remember the contexts and feelings of volatility and uncertainty, of the surveillance and regulation of their bodies and their mobility. It is critical that, in any efforts and intentions of supporting Black South African womxn's psychosocial well-being during these times, we take seriously the ways in which the COVID-19 context triggers our individual and collective history of trauma, so as not to pathologize the various ways in which Black womxn are responding to COVID-19 stressors. The personal is political. We need to be cognizant of the ways in which the feminized burden of care significantly compromises the mental well-being of womxn, Black womxn in particular. Womxn who are formally employed (and have not lost their jobs) are having to cope with the already heavy workload of their paid employment, in addition to the expectation of assuming and resuming the duties of the domestic domain: domestic chores, child care, care for parents and extended family members—the unpaid and 'invisibilized' labour that comes with being physically present in the domestic space during 'office hours'. At the centre of this crossover between private and public labour is the deployment of notions of femininity that draw heavily on the naturalized and normalized effective role of womxn as nurturers and carers. These normalized discourses function coercively, mobilizing notions of cultural authenticity to reinforce patriarchal agendas that perpetuate the servitude of women (Lewis 2003). It is, therefore, important to interrogate the notions and discourses of 'caring', 'coping' and being the 'strong African woman'.

In my personal and professional experience, many womxn have sought psychological support asking for tools that could help them cope better with the increased workload and heightened stress of the COVID context. There was also a tangible self-blame and shame that many womxn named regarding 'not being able to cope as normal' with the 'COVID load'. The gendered expectation of patriarchy (which colludes with a cultural expectation of the role of womxn within African patriarchy) is to 'keep going' and successfully juggle increasing responsibilities, expectations and demands. There is very little social permission for Black womxn to admit that we are taking strain, we are not okay, that we are just barely coping. We do not give ourselves that permission either, so deeply entrenched is the messaging that 'care' is in the service of others, external to ourselves. Admitting that we need support or care is accompanied by shame and guilt that precludes us from sourcing and resourcing the support and care we need.

This dynamic exists even within the feminist movement where we intellectually understand and profess the importance of self-care and collective care as a necessary politics of self-preservation:

> We are wary and weary of the trope of the strong African woman, ever-willing and able to sacrifice, to subsume her well-being in service of others, to carry an ever-increasing burden with humility and a tacit pride in being able to do so. These discursive representations obscure the reality of our systemic oppressions as gendered oppressions and set us up to blame ourselves when we feel powerless, helpless, overburdened or generally overwhelmed. These tropes do not offer us a way out or through our racialized and gendered internalized oppression and we are critical of the ideological imperatives in response to which the Black African womxn is constructed. (Clark et al. 2019, 3)

So, many of us are 'coping' with COVID in ways that do not take us any closer to our well-being and perpetuate the patterns and structures of power that are at the root of the problem in the first place. As we extend and over-extend ourselves under these COVID-19 conditions, it is important to remember that we cannot be well until the structure of the institution of the family as a patriarchal, classist, heteronormative site of inequity shifts. We cannot be well until the feminized burden of care is completely overturned. This commentary hopefully alerts us to the ways in which the strain and pain of Black womxn under COVID-19 in 2020 is inextricably linked to the multifaceted legacies of our past and challenges us to do something about it—today.

TIME FOR A PARADIGM SHIFT: ENGAGING WITH DISABILITY IN THE AFTERMATH OF COVID-19

Lata Dyaram

> The only disability is when people cannot see human potential.
>
> —Debra Ruh

While the world went into lockdown trying to contain the outbreak of COVID-19, economies came to a standstill. Several companies are suggesting an uncertain business climate. Millions are losing their jobs. All of these paint a bleak picture of the future. Yet, one segment within India's population of 1.3 billion is still hopeful and optimistic. People with disabilities see the demand for flexible workspaces rising as companies embrace work from home as part of their work culture with aplomb. Some companies may be open to exploring the 'work near home' policy, whereas many other companies may consider leasing smaller spaces at different locations in tier II/tier III cities. These and other related trends will immensely benefit people with disabilities as employers are in the best position to cater to flexibility demands.

While the nation has been developing or reforming social protection programmes and schemes to provide better support to persons with disabilities and their families, the majority remains unprotected and unsupported. Such a situation limits the capacity to provide effective relief in the current crisis. Often, these policies are too generic and pay scant attention to the specific situations faced by disabled people, the apparent assumption being that the interventions targeted will accrue equally across all social groups. However, there are strong social gradients across the life course in the prevalence of disability. There is abundant evidence that people with disabilities are disadvantaged with regard to factors that promote social mobility such as education, employment, and labour market experiences, social and cultural capital, health and well-being. While the disabled have significantly reduced employment opportunities, those in employment are less likely to be employed in high-status positions/occupations and are employed with significant pay disparities in relation to their non-disabled counterparts. Further, the onset of disability while in employment can increase the risk of subsequent unemployment. Hence, while the nation has shown remarkable resilience reorienting itself to the crisis demonstrating its underlying strength and innovative thinking, can industries and organizations in India take a 'leading role' in the post-COVID times not only in the building of the post-pandemic economy but also in promoting social mobility and social fluidity?

Undoubtedly, industry will deliver major productivity benefits for the economy and businesses through science and technology. It is important to note that industry is 'uniquely positioned' to alchemize society and harness social/human capital. Industry can enable fundamental changes in the occupational structure aiding greater social mobility/fluidity with opportunities for the disabled for elevation and progression within the social hierarchy. One positive consequence of such mobility can be a better use of the disability community's talent, potential, and aptitude. This can enable the achievement of social and economic equality.

COVID-19 AND PEOPLE WITH DISABILITIES (PwD)

While we continue to face the ravages of the COVID-19 pandemic and one of the *most* dreadful economic recessions in recent memory, studies show that this recession has not been felt evenly across the labour force. Systematically marginalized communities—such as the disabled, women, and others—have experienced higher unemployment than average, and job seekers with disabilities are among the groups that have been hit the hardest. The global pandemic crisis has posed a greater threat to lives and livelihoods for people with disabilities who have been facing pre-existing marginalization in social, economic, and health terms with limited access to education, employment, healthcare, and community participation. This is so because despite the government's several welfare/special schemes for the disabled to integrate PwD into the mainstream in terms of tax exemptions, scholarships in professional courses, low-interest rates for loans, etc., there are huge disparities between the disabled and non-disabled population when it comes to jobs.

A brief review of recent literature on disability and COVID-19 indicates that there are several sources of distress that disproportionately impacted people with disabilities and more so when disability intersected with other marginalized identities such as gender, age, and income stratum. A study by the National Centre for Promotion of Employment of Disabled Persons (NCPEDP) highlights the issues and challenges confronting PwD in India during the COVID-19 crisis. Disability helplines have witnessed overwhelming responses with issues ranging from the inaccessibility of medical care/essentials to dire financial challenges. More than 2.6 crore persons with disabilities in India are at greater risk of COVID-19 and are unevenly impacted as varied social, infrastructural and economic barriers limit or prevent people with disabilities to access public health/hygiene services and other resources. These barriers are known to heighten their need to rely on support personnel, which could pose different challenges amid the pandemic norms of social distancing. The diverse nature of disabilities and pre-health conditions/comorbidities are noted to pose risks of serious illness/fatalities with COVID-19. There is overwhelming evidence originating from varied quarters on how persons with disabilities are facing increased social isolation and loneliness, discrimination from support personnel in medical facilities, denial of support services including sign language and tactile interpretation, violence, abuse and other extreme vulnerabilities emanating from socially intersecting factors such as gender and age. Hence, while the impact of COVID is felt across all sections of the society, attitudinal, environmental, and institutional barriers have magnified for people with disabilities, increasing their marginalization.

Whatever literature evidence as it stands, warrants attention to people with disabilities in the face of difficulties compounded by COVID-19. Actions taken now can promote unity and solidarity towards upholding not only public health but also human rights and human development. Considering these lived experiences of PwD, several recent publications have highlighted how this could put them at increased risk from COVID-19 and have called for a disability-inclusive pandemic response. However, not much is attended on several underlying factors that preclude movement towards addressing inequities. For instance, much of the information/data on the impact of COVID-19 on people with disabilities remains unknown especially with varying estimates of the prevalence of disability and its intersection with other factors of inequity including age, gender and income. In the case of people with disabilities, such systematic inquiry has been limited both before and during the pandemic. Much of the current documentation on disability risks and status comes primarily from caretakers and assisted living facilities which cater to only a fraction of the population with disabilities. These gaps in COVID-19 investigation can actually miss high-risk individuals among not just PwD but also other vulnerable groups. Inaccurate and unreliable estimates can misguide public policy-making and can lead to inappropriate allocation of limited resources. While there are many ideas on disability-inclusive COVID-19 responses, without proper records and statistics, not much can move forward with mere good intentions and anecdotal evidence as who gets reported cannot determine who gets included. Further, this presents a unique opportunity to create a more evidence-based approach to address inequities as most government policy-making is data-driven. Failure to consider this would deprive us of a full comprehension of the magnitude of the outbreak's impact and undervalue the life experiences and contributions of PwD to society, limiting the possibilities of equitable services to them. Unintended discrimination and social injustice can also contribute to such exclusion of people with disabilities from mainstream discussion and policy. Collecting disability data with evidence-driven steps can help create an inclusive response under the pandemic and lay the foundation for equitable public policy planning. This necessitates a systematic review of the pandemic response to characterize current shortcomings and identify areas for improvement. Further, addressing disparities by age, gender and other factors allows researchers and officials to provide an accurate evidence of disparities, and form the basis for a data-driven pandemic response. Such systematic investigation can become a fundamental pillar of social and public policy.

Therefore, including persons with disabilities and perhaps their families in prevention, treatment and recovery from COVID-19 will contribute not only to the fight against the pandemic but also in tapping the unique talent people with disabilities possess. Mere acknowledgement that COVID-19 is a global pandemic requiring national and international cooperation to save lives and livelihoods is not enough unless we aid the support needed to include and integrate PwD into the mainstream. It is thus important to call on various stakeholders: government, industries, employers, financial institutions, international cooperation agencies and private donors to be inclusive of persons with disabilities in their response to COVID-19 and help protect, support and nurture their talent at both the individual and systemic levels. Despite the disabled constituting more than three per cent of the population of India, their inclusion and meaningful employment needs remain unmet as only one lakh persons with disabilities in India have been employed in industries. There are myriad additional struggles for women with disabilities and people with intellectual and developmental disabilities. For jobseekers with a disability, the safety threat posed by the coronavirus—coupled with pre-existing barriers to employment and a now struggling national economy—creates compounding barriers that make finding a job extremely difficult. Given this, one of the most critical enablers for harnessing this marginalized talent are employers and their proactive intervention. What are the proactive steps that various firms, organizations and managers can initiate to ensure equal opportunities, greater representation, inclusion and integration, providing a level playing field for the disabled at all levels of the organizations?

EMPLOYERS AND SOCIAL MOBILITY/FLUIDITY

While everyday examples showed the ways in which the disabled are left behind in our pandemic response, the industry has adapted to a new normal by creating more innovative roadmaps, game plans and strategies towards building and sustaining their competitive advantage. In these flexible times is the opportunity to tap the needed talent from diverse quarters which are shackled by social structures and hierarchies. Given that it is important to understand and address issues related to the inclusion of PwD at all levels of society from a different lens, some of the key perspectives from the point of view of employers or organizations become pertinent. Industries and businesses have long been instrumental in driving social change—like successful initiatives towards addressing the challenges of diversity and inclusion, for instance, resulting in several modern progressive organizations that can be seen as having the fundamental attribute of being inclusive. Despite such concerted efforts to address disparities in gender and age, disability continues to remain neglected. For instance, although there were tax incentives from the government for private firms and the legal requirement for PwD to be hired by PSUs rose to four per cent, integration of PwD into the labour market remains low—not even one-fourth of their overall population are employed.

Despite experts in the disability arena having raised concerns about the effective implementation of the Rights of Persons with Disabilities Act (RPWD), 2016, India has become one of the countries with a robust legislative framework addressing the rights of PwD. As the Act addresses the employment rights of PwD, organizations and employers can be seen as important stakeholders in the implementation of the Act. How can organizations, employers, disability services agencies and

PwD work together in creating solutions towards inclusion and workplace equity? Needless to say, there could be several support structures that organizations might need to put in place ranging from infrastructure readiness to work culture attitudinal changes before they explore recruiting/recalling talented people with disabilities. This support and effort on the part of organizations towards embracing a multifaceted workforce have not only known positive impact on the overall business in terms of goodwill, a positive brand image, a motivated/talented employee base, low attrition/absenteeism rates, tax incentives from the government and so on, but also in creating a more equitable and healthier society. To this end, let us explore how organizations can continue to promote and sustain workplace inclusion of PwD in the aftermath of COVID-19. With governments imposing quarantines and companies imposing travel bans, the human and economic impact on businesses has been stark. Brick-and-mortar industries such as retail and hospitality, which traditionally were open to hiring PwD have suffered tremendous losses. Many small businesses in the community have shut down either temporarily or permanently. Several firms reported having trouble hiring and retaining staff due to prevailing economic conditions and fear of the virus. Several companies are compelled to revisit and review their policies and procedures to strategically protect high potential employees, customers, and operations. Therefore, to begin with, some new approaches, or reinforcing what worked, becomes relevant for the inclusion of people with disabilities and their talent:

1) *Reducing risk*. As many people with disabilities could be medically fragile or immunocompromised, partnering with civic authorities and local healthcare centres to validate and enable dynamic individual testing and status in relation to the virus can help.
2) *Safety in the workplace and new protocols*. As safety cannot come at the cost of inclusion in the workplace, it's important for organizations to abide by COVID-19

safety protocols. With several businesses reopening and initiating operations, it is important to thoughtfully create guidelines to keep employees and workers with disabilities safe. New protocols may include requiring workers to maintain social distancing as reiterated by the Government of India motto 'Do gaj doori, mask hai zaroori', stressing that it is important to maintain a distance of two-yards and wear face masks and to ensure face/hand hygiene at all times in the fight against COVID-19.

3) *Awareness and understanding disability.* As the term disability can comprise of several varied functional boundaries ranging from physical, neural and mental, congenital or acquired, permanent or transitory, and can vary in degree/severity, awareness of disability, its causes and the rights of the disabled is generally low. Hence, as disability is not an inability, it's important for organizations to develop an operational definition of disability and appreciate the business reasons to hire diverse talent and PwD, besides social responsibility or tax incentives from the government.
4) *Hiring.* Hiring activities have begun to surge among sectors such as e-commerce, logistics, e-services, technology, and banking. Further, several businesses such as departmental stores, drugstores, and warehouses are witnessing the swell in customer demand and are needing to hire employees for several open positions during this time of the pandemic. Employers may need to revisit job profiles/postings, job descriptions/specifications to suit a disability-inclusive format. Nevertheless, building a strong pool of candidates and streamlining the hiring approach by partnering with job placement agencies/services usually involving no costs, can lay the foundation to support and include people with disabilities and their talent deployment. Thus, employers can leverage disability employment services to find the right candidates.

5) *Transportation.* Many individuals with disabilities rely on public transportation to get to work. With few public transportation networks around the country that are fully accessible to people with disabilities, alternative arrangements such as ridesharing, remote working, telepresence, and other technology-enabled measures can be implemented more easily than ever before.
6) *Workplace accessibility.* Employers can ensure the new work environment is accessible not only for new PwD recruits but also for those employees with disabilities who are comfortable and willing to come back to the workplace. Providing a safe environment in terms of handrails on all walking paths and other assistive tools/devices can help deploy new talent. Simple arrangements such as sanitation stations, automatic hand sanitizer dispensers within reach, storing disinfectant wipes on lower shelves/cabinets, communicating expectations in writing and signs, as well as in team meetings can create enabling working conditions.
7) Opting to *redesign workspaces* based on *universal design principles.*
8) *Flexibility.* As workplace needs change significantly depending on the spread of the virus and subsequent requirements of workers with disabilities, it's important to acknowledge that reasonable accommodations are an ongoing duty and not a one-time exercise. This necessitates policies to be flexible and frequently reviewed. It is important to engage in a conversation to better understand what the employees with disabilities need especially when the employer is unclear on those needs. A prescription from their doctors can help provide this clarity. Some people with sensory difficulties may find it difficult to wear masks/gloves at all times or others may have difficulties observing social distancing etiquette. Thus, as no one size fits all, telework/remote working may work for some, while others may be amenable to work where there is little contact with

others. Financial aid/concessions or non-financial aid in terms of delivery of essentials, hygiene kits, and other services including the provision of home-based care or accessible information or smart devices can help deploy PwD resourcefulness.

9) *Education and training.* This helps in skilling and becomes key to upskilling or cross-skilling especially for advanced technical competence/proficiency in newer technologies.
10) *Counselling and support.* Connecting and engaging with families/caretakers to enable smooth integration of people with disabilities into the organization through necessary support and counselling.
11) *Building a positive work culture/environment.* This is important and can be achieved through awareness programmes/forums within the organization for co-workers on diversity, disability and equal opportunities.
12) *Disability sensitization.* With new/alternate modes of working to counter the effects of the COVID pandemic, remote work can potentially exacerbate disability and inclusion-related challenges. To minimize the risks of any potential disability-related discrimination/harassment under the new working norms, contracting with the workforce through education and sensitization on disability types/risks for the effective enablement of policies, to prevent/deal with specific challenges, may be initiated.
13) *Leadership engagement.* Disability inclusion cannot be confined to mere hiring them as progression and development are important human goals. Hence it's important to connect and engage with employees with disabilities within the organization through the right interventions. While several organizations are also making efforts to support employees with disabilities, it is important to move beyond hiring and reasonable accommodations, to more inclusive integration by providing employees with disabilities a

career progression path, coaching, mentorship, targeted training and leadership opportunities.

Towards combating arbitrary obstacles which block people from realizing their ambitions, substantive equality of opportunity is key to address issues regarding PwD recruitment, hiring, training, promotions, responsibility, wages, sick leave, vacation, overtime, insurance, retirement, pensions, and various other issues. Since equal opportunity can be seen as a factor correlating positively with deploying diverse talent and social mobility, it can benefit society in general in maximizing well-being for all.

CONCLUSION

As an invisible microbe proved a deadly adversary wreaking havoc on the lives and livelihoods of a generation, it has also provided an unprecedented opportunity to shatter all disparities stemming from decades of prejudice and discrimination against people with visible disabilities. Hence, the responsibility to craft meaningful and dignified lives for all and those with visible disabilities lies squarely with all of us more than ever before. Sensible collective action is needed now to overcome the short-sightedness in planning for human development. As investments across the social spectrum promise improved human productivity besides creating opportunities for people in disadvantaged positions, a greater realization must dawn upon various stakeholders and policy-makers on the importance of investment in the social sector promoting social mobility and fluidity.

THE EMBERS REMAIN

Kirtika Kain

We've been wearing masks since December 2020. As the Black Summer bushfires were raging with no end in sight, smoke and ash swept through the city and heralded the New Year with a phenomenon I never thought I would see in my lifetime: Delhi air transposed onto a Sydney skyline.

The only silver lining in the dense plumes was a taste of unprecedented disaster. Before the rest of the world, we were being primed with the language of crises and as the blazes dwindled, the changing season brought new versions of 'hotspots' and daily toll counts with COVID-19.

There was, however, no preparing for the micro assailant that was to dismantle, disrupt and defy every structure of our creation. In March, case numbers followed a dreaded trajectory and a temporary lockdown ensued. I packed my materials, transported my canvases and before I knew it, my artist studio and living space were one.

In the immense stillness of lockdown, all that had been sidelined by maintaining a constant busyness could be avoided no longer. Impending exhibitions and projects fell away and my books ushered me into their parallel worlds.

I was well acquainted with the first text on my reading list. I had been carrying *The Prisons We Broke* like a talisman for months, skirting the pages, keeping a safe distance by holding it close. My hesitation was not for its incomprehensibility, but quite the opposite —I was never ready for its searing clarity.

Until April.

Through Babytai Kamble's words, I was transported to Veergaon, into the world of the Mahars of Maharashtra. Kamble's historical account is the first Dalit feminist autobiography written in Marathi. Although it is a short read, it carries the weight of a tome and the monumentality of an epic. Her scope is vast as she follows the transformation of society at the dawn of the Ambedkarite era, and yet attends to each detail in her immediate reality.

Nothing is amiss. Kamble recounts that which only a woman could—the passing of each day in domestic spaces, the festivals, local deities and rituals, the physical toll of violent spiritual possessions and superstitious beliefs.

Kamble's descriptions are vivid and visceral. Through her eyes, we see the lice-infested rags stitched together to cover the women's bodies, we sense the layers of dust and dirt upon our own skin, taste the stew of decaying food and smell the acrid stench of animal carcasses in the waste pits.

Woven in are the most graphic accounts of the lives of the Mahar women. The child brides are battered by floggings, torture and dismemberment at the hands of their in-laws. Kamble details childbirth in abject poverty—the repeated prodding of unlearned midwives, the gnawing hunger in the empty belly of the new mother and the dirty rags used to stop the incessant bleeding. Whilst some women plan a treacherous escape from their marital homes, others are forced into heavy iron stocks that lacerate their feet. Miraculously, the women are not broken by the rage of caste and patriarchy; every morning they sing sweet songs to their children as they grind stones.

Kamble describes these harrowing instances of deprivation without a grain of self-pity or glorification. The emotion she withholds makes the rawness of her writing more palpable and confronting. She speaks as one with her community, in a voice that does not censor the carnage of caste.

The pages that trace Dr Babasaheb Ambedkar's arrival in Jejuri radiate with light. A small gathering is planned on an auspicious day for the family deity Khandoba. As crowds of Mahars gather, there is talk of a man who speaks in the sahib's tongue and has studied beyond the seven seas.

Babasaheb arrives in a vehicle and captivates all. He asks the crowd what Khandoba has ever done for them and urges them to stop worshiping idols and their own ignorance. In an epoch of neglect and disillusionment, he inspires knowledge and education. He is the light that shines through a millennium of darkness. Kamble describes Babasaheb as the essence of truth grown from the soil upon which many lives have been sacrificed. This truth is met with resistance as some Mahars continue to eat the decaying flesh of dead animals. Yet it is the women who safeguard his vision.

For every Dalit, *The Prisons We Broke* stirs that which cannot be described. It unstitches a century-old wound and awakens remnants of memories that are our birth right. There is an unborn and imperishable cord that connects us to each Dalit life and generation. The impressions and sensations held within us are pre-language, yet are evoked powerfully through Babytai Kamble's words.

For myself, the only way I am able to stand firmly upon this sacred ground is through my art. Everything else seems abstract—to ponder, to write, to intellectualize it. Within the studio, I can receive each line and not be swept away by the torrents of this moving text. I am at a knife's edge—held by the ancient history in my cells and abandoned to the spontaneity and newness of creation. Whilst making art, I feel simultaneously closest to the imprint of this historical wound, as well as complete freedom from it.

As I received each word, Babytai Kamble's visual language guided my material expression. I sought to create a work that was as monumental as her writing. When I closed my eyes, in the darkness I saw centuries of accrual compressed like geological strata. Familiar materials presented themselves: cow dung—used by the Mahars to polish the walls and floors, thick tar in all its tonal ranges, wax as smooth and impressionable as skin, the roughened edges of coir rope, laaldhaga from my travels that had now been worn down to a lifeless red, Indian cotton soaked in black charcoal and oil, vats of human hair, coconut husk, broom sticks from a jhadu and radiant gold leaf.

I set about forming the landscape I saw in *The Prisons*. I was led by intuition through a process that was much like drawing from images in my peripheral vision. Upon large wooden panels, I assembled my materials layer by layer and melted wax with charcoal, coating the surface with a thick black pitch. Punctuating each line of material was pure gold leaf. I imagine gold to be a metaphor for the Dalit body. As ancient as the Earth itself, its qualities have been managed by an arbitrary value system, yet gold is so luminous, it remains untainted by it.

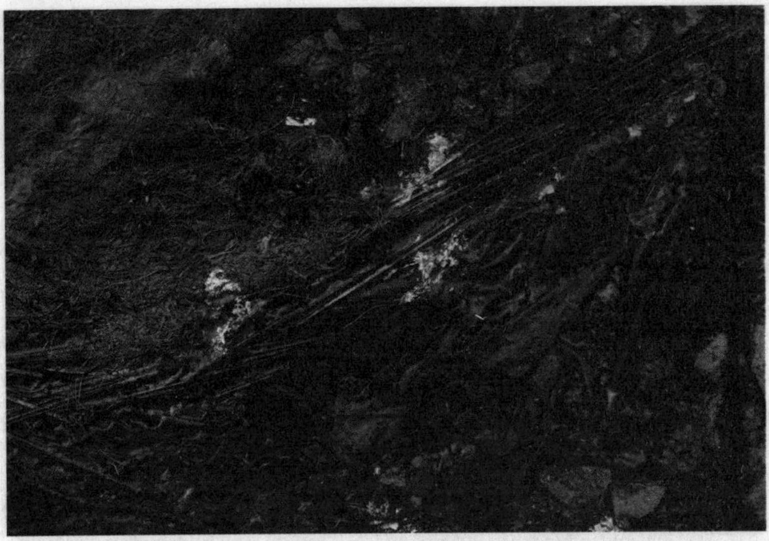

Kirtika Kain, 'Jina Amucha', 2020, beeswax, charcoal, coconut husk, rope, gold leaf, plaster, cow dung, Indian cotton, tar, coconut broom grass, religious thread, human hair, 8 panels, each 110 x 100 cm. Photo by Luis Power. Image courtesy of the artist and Roslyn Oxley9 Gallery, Sydney.

The lockdown stretched from weeks to months as the piece was composed. Each layer and panel responded to the previous one. My materials are my words and they are not dictated, they come from the same embryonic silence from which the art is born. They are potent and charged with the politics of my body. In the cacophony of these heightened times, it is this silence that I return to, that I know to be true.

I shared my time with Urmila Pawar and her extraordinary writings in *The Weave of My Life*. I was moved by the words of young Muktabai in her essay *The Grief of the Mahars and the Mangs*. I returned to Dr Ambedkar's early anthropological and political writings. As I traced the development of his ideas, I could read the real-life implications through the social and domestic lens of Kamble and Pawar. Hindu rituals, wedding songs, and practices were abandoned as there were mass conversions to a new Dalit consciousness.

~

I continue to survey my history to understand myself as the continuation of this thread. As a beneficiary of Reservation, a first-generation migrant and the daughter of this revolution, my freedom is not mine until it can be shared by all.

As I watch the heroes march, my fellow migrants walk hundreds of kilometres, I see the waves of progress ebb away further than ever. As I watch stones being laid for new temples, I see time contract and the structures of ignorance fortified. The light has more layers to penetrate, it will now have to be stronger and brighter than ever.

Kirtika Kain, 'Jina Amucha' (detail), 2020, beeswax, charcoal, coconut husk, rope, gold leaf, plaster, cow dung, Indian cotton, tar, coconut broom grass, religious thread, human hair, 8 panels, each 110 x 100 cm. Photo by Luis Power. Image courtesy of the artist and Roslyn Oxley9 Gallery, Sydney.

A critical epoch has come to the fore again. Our work is cut out for us. Yet we are the children who would rest our heads in our mother's laps and hear their sweet songs. We are the children of a father who guided us not to lamps in shrines, but the flame within us.

We create with this light.

SOUTH ASIANS IN THE UNITED KINGDOM DURING COVID-19: A REALIST VIEW

Dave Sookhoo

INTRODUCTION

The severe acute respiratory syndrome coronavirus 2 (SARS-CoV-2), often referred to as COVID-19, after the contagious disease that it causes, is exacting an unprecedented toll at the personal, social, and economic levels globally, and it is not showing any sign of disappearing from the face of the planet any time soon. Since January 2020, the global community has been desperately trying to find health solutions to prevent the transmission and spread of the virus, containing and averting high mortalities across nations (World Health Organization 2020). In the discourse about the global impact of COVID-19, comparisons have been drawn with pandemics going back centuries, and the recent ones including the Spanish Flu (1918–20), the Asian Flu (1957–58), and the 2009 influenza pandemic (Petersen et al. 2020). Furthermore, among the many stark realities of the impact of the virus on humanity, one that has become a source of grave concern is the disproportionally high fatalities associated with COVID-19 among ethnic groups in European and Western countries. This is an exploration of the factors associated with ethnicity and its concomitants in the UK that have caused this. With daily changes in what is known about the spread of the virus, policies and practices, information and legal measures, the public response to the threats and human cost has been remarkable and courageous. In demographic terms, this paper focuses on the UK South Asian communities, who are often referred to as part of the Black, Asian, and Minority Ethnic (BAME) groups. The purpose is to understand the impact of COVID-19 on these groups against the backdrop of shifting evidence and guidance on minimizing health and social effects on the population.

RESPONSIVENESS

The World Health Organization (WHO) declared a global health emergency on 30 January 2020, followed by a declaration of a global pandemic on 11 March 2020 (Cucinotta and Vanelli 2020). The WHO Director-General expressed his organization's deep concern at 'both the alarming levels of spread and severity and...the alarming levels of inaction', asking countries to take measures to contain the virus and prevent its worldwide spread. The UK government was preparing for the challenges by creating field hospitals and stockpiling medical supplies and equipment. With increasing numbers of cases being reported, hospitalizations and deaths, the UK government imposed a lockdown on 23 March 2020. From containment to the prevention of the spread of the virus, staying at home, advocating hand washing and hand hygiene, self-isolation, there were measures put in place designed to reduce the potential peak that could overwhelm hospitals. A delay phase was observed—containment plus social distancing, social isolation, quarantining; limiting travel and social gatherings; closing businesses and enforcing lockdowns. With the rise in reported COVID-19 cases and mortality, the UK government imposed a lockdown on 23 March 2020. Many questions were being asked about the supplies of personal protective equipment (PPE) for frontline National Health Service (NHS) workers. When the extensive health, economic, and social effects of the pandemic were felt across the UK, at its height between April and May 2020, questions were being asked about the vulnerability of people across their lifespan and the implications of risk assessment for 'segments' of the population. Reassurance was given to the public about the availability and supplies of PPEs and other equipment but public concerns grew with reports from the health and social care sectors about a lack of supplies which was putting staff and patients at increased risk of being infected.

Since early February 2020, the UK government was alert to the threats of the coronavirus, yet not much action was taken. Even the scientific advice was that of being cautious about transmission and the precautions needed to be put in place to protect the population. Much noise was made in several administrative quarters, but was not reflected in the provision of resources and preparedness to deal with the pandemic, leading to a clear and worrying series of kneejerk reactions. Stocking up of essential equipment (gloves, masks, sanitizers, respirators), preparing of field hospitals to receive patients and protect the NHS, discharge of patients from hospitals to care homes without testing, ensuing lockdowns, social distancing, advice about handwashing and hand hygiene, and addressing economic concerns became points of reference for commentators on how proactive or reactive the political and healthcare professionals were on a daily basis. What was becoming clear was the lack of personal protective equipment, and the strategy of attaining herd immunity with apparently little concern or respect for the large numbers of people dying in their homes, hospitals or care homes as reported in the daily briefings and updates in the media. It can be argued that it was governance by neglect. The consequences of indecisiveness and poorly communicated guidance meant that prevarication cost people their lives, including those of healthcare professionals and public sector workers. The vulnerability of South Asians to COVID-19 became abundantly clear when the deaths of BAME doctors working with patients at the beginning of the pandemic were the first mortalities reported (BMA 2020). As the reported deaths were linked to people most vulnerable in society, and the lack of cohesive action and monitoring of what was happening with a lack of compliance, the rallying cry was for us to be 'led by the science', dismissing any dissenting voices. Many have argued that the steps taken by the government have been slow and not communicated clearly over the course of the pandemic.

PSYCHOLOGICAL IMPACT OF COVID-19

Fear is a common response when we are faced with uncertainties and threats. The fear of being infected by the coronavirus was very real for all, with uncertainties about the early symptoms and the excessive fear experienced when triggered by shielding and isolation. With self-isolation being advised, the effects of isolation on mental health and necessary support mechanisms were not made clear. However, local organizations and communities were mobilized with volunteers supporting the vulnerable. Local governments played their part in information sharing and guidance on mental health (LGA 2020). Public Health England (2020a) put out guidance on mental health and well-being with a range of information about what to do and the services available. However, it isn't clear if the public was able to access this guidance and what the impact was on the mental health of individuals with existing mental health conditions and those exposed to COVID-19.

Soon after the lockdown was imposed, commentators observed how the public had shown restraint with a high level of compliance but expressed concerns about the risks of isolation, fears about the old and frail, the psychosocial impact on children missing out on schooling, a possible rise in domestic abuse, and the economy. In time, commentators expressed disappointment at the ambiguities in communication and the continued uncertainties about the implications of the strategies being followed to mitigate the effects of COVID-19 on individuals, families, and businesses.

Measures taken to reduce the risk of infection from the coronavirus such as self-isolation, social distancing and quarantine can trigger psychological distress, and this should be borne in mind when designing psychological interventions. A coordinated and interdisciplinary approach is needed (Hotopf et al. 2020).

ETHNICITY AND COVID-19

The point of reference for population data is commonly the 2011 UK census data for England and Wales. Asian ethnic groups made up 7.5% of the UK population (ONS 2011). Self-ascribed as British Asians, settled here by migration and by birth in the country, are people of Indian (2.5%), Pakistani

(2.0%) and Bangladeshi (0.8%) origin. The ethnic groups most likely to live in urban areas were Pakistani (99.1%) and Bangladeshi (98.7%). In England in 2013, it was estimated that around 262,247 South Asians lived in London, the largest group, followed by 37,202 in Leicester, 27,206 in Birmingham, 15,190 in Sandwell and 14,955 in Wolverhampton. Other cities which have a sizeable South Asian population include Blackburn (34.3%), Bradford (26.83%), and Manchester (15%). The geographical demographics of the South Asian groups and the emerging patterning of COVID-19 cases and mortality can be referenced against this backdrop.

Aldridge et al. (2020) showed that the BAME groups were at higher risk of death than their white counterparts. In the data reported in April 2020 (ONS 2020a), out of the 16,272 deaths, the largest number of deaths in ethnic minority groups were among Indians (492 deaths) and Black Caribbean (460 deaths). The standard mortality rate (SMR) was 3.29 for Pakistanis, 2.41 for Bangladeshis, and 1.70 for Indians. Similarly, among COVID-19 related deaths of critically ill patients, 34% were from minority ethnic groups even though they make up only 14% of the population, highlighting how minority ethnic groups were disproportionally affected (Bhala et al. 2020; Kings Fund 2020). More recent data up to 15 May 2020 (ONS 2020b) showed that COVID-19 related deaths (1,011) were 2.7% of all deaths, of which 551 (1.5%) were Pakistanis and 222 (0.6%) Bangladeshis, with more male deaths than female deaths. By religious group, for people aged 8–64 years, deaths were recorded as follows: 297 Muslim males and 125 Muslim females; 90 Hindu males and 43 Hindu females; and 42 Sikh males and 20 Sikh females. For recorded deaths of adults aged 65 years and above, the numbers were higher: 584 Muslim males and 301 Muslim females; 271 Hindu males and 190 Hindu females; and 119 Sikh men and 77 Sikh women.

With the number of cases and deaths rising during March–May 2020, concerns were raised about the likelihood of people from ethnic minority backgrounds being exposed to the coronavirus and deaths among healthcare professionals working in frontline services. A large percentage of doctors and other healthcare workers are from BAME groups. Reportedly, 21% of all staff are from BAME groups (BMA 2020), of which about 20% are nursing staff and 44% are medical staff. There was an outcry about the lack of action, being directed into examining the factors underpinning this emerging pattern in the deaths of frontline health professionals. Questions were raised about the lack of concern about possible contributing factors such as racial discrimination, bullying and lack of risk assessment and testing. In a response under pressure to act, Public Health England (PHE) subsequently launched a review in May and the report was published in June 2020 (PHE 2020b) but it was disappointing that the report did not make any recommendations on how to reduce disparities (Science Media Centre 2020), even with questions asked in parliament about the failure to make recommendations.

Underlying health conditions make the South Asian communities more susceptible and vulnerable to COVID-19, consequently requiring hospitalization and medical interventions, including life-saving artificial ventilation (Pan et al. 2020). It is known that severe cases of COVID-19 were associated with comorbidities such as cardiovascular disease (CVD), hypertension, and diabetes. Evidence suggests that having non-communicable diseases such as these increases the risk of hospitalization. South Asians have high rates of diabetes (GOV.UK, 2016) and cardiovascular diseases which make them more vulnerable to COVID-19. Moreover, help-seeking behaviour and adherence to treatment have been shown to be associated with patients' beliefs about illness, medicines, stigma, and communication barriers (Kumar et al. 2016). Diversity in beliefs about infections and transmission, lack of understanding of the seriousness of COVID-19, working in confined spaces, language, and communication barriers need further exploration.

HEALTH INEQUALITIES

Health inequalities in the UK are not a recent phenomenon. They've been documented for decades. Marmot (2020) has deplored the policy of the UK government since 2010, when the publication of *Fair Society, Healthy Lives*, the report of an independent review chaired by Marmot, had identified six policy objectives that required action in combating health inequalities (Marmot et al. 2010). About the response of the UK government to the health crisis brought about by the COVID-19 pandemic, Marmot (2020, 1414) has argued that the UK government made a political choice then, and 'one that failed to take seriously a national crisis of a slower, more fundamental and enduring kind: health and health inequalities. The government was prepared to do what it takes to deal with the conflagration of the pandemic but not, a decade ago, with the slow-burning injustice of health inequalities'. Referring to the findings of *Health Equity in England: The Marmot Review 10 Years On* (Marmot et al. 2020), Marmot concluded that life expectancy has stalled, inequalities in health have continued to increase and life expectancy for women living in the poorest areas of England outside London has declined. Given the austerity years following the 2008 financial crisis, it is not surprising that generally health disparities and inequalities have widened.

Long-standing structural inequalities, related socio-economic factors such as deprivation and poverty may account for the disproportionate effects and poor health outcomes among South Asian groups in England. Previous studies have shown that 11% of South Asian households are overcrowded (more people than bedrooms); the highest among this group were Bangladeshi (30%) and Pakistani (26%) households (English Housing Survey 2018). Multigenerational living is not uncommon and given that Bangladeshis and Pakistanis are more likely to live in deprived neighbourhoods, social distancing and isolation could be more difficult, thus possibly increasing the vulnerability of older adults and those with comorbidities to the risk of COVID-19.

MENTAL HEALTH IN THE TIME OF COVID-19

Mental health has in the recent past been under sharp focus nationally. Mental health has been associated with underlying long-term conditions such as diabetes and cardiovascular diseases (Chaddha et al. 2016).

Depression is prevalent among South Asian individuals and is a comorbidity of diabetes. Anxiety and depression have been found in South Asian patients with diabetes to be higher compared to their white European counterparts (Razieh et al. 2019). The complexities of comorbidities and mental health cannot be underestimated, given that existing mental health problems could be accentuated by the lack of support and healthcare interventions during isolation and lockdown. Accessing services and help-seeking behaviours among South Asian individuals have been shown to be predicated by cultural beliefs about mental illness, shame and guilt. Cultural beliefs about the causation of diseases, the effectiveness of treatment, and the use of alternative interventions are well documented issues in the acceptance of mental illness. However, there is a need to address mental health and illness in the South Asian communities for change and to remove the stigma with approaches that reflect cultural congruity and competence. With COVID-19, the complexities around mental health are compounded because of reactions to unexpected deaths, inability to mourn loss and grief, little time for customary rituals and absence of physical and psychological support.

Fear of contagion, psychological distress, and stressors have hardly been given the attention they should generally have and even less has been observed in relation to South Asian communities. As usual, it would not be inaccurate to surmise that amidst the chaos, psychological health and well-being get relegated to the sidelines. In contrast, however, optimism in the resilience of common people, hope, support and compassion for each other invariably confounds those who are quick to judge and apportion blame to others. The South Asian communities have had much to bear, living in deprived inner-city areas, actively supporting themselves and, like many, trying to make sense of the contradictions in messages from administrators during the lockdown.

CULTURAL STIGMA OF MENTAL ILLNESS

It is known that there are underlying factors such as poor housing, cohabiting and large families living in poorer parts of cities. Unemployment with a disability is likely to be higher among Bangladeshis and Pakistanis (13%) (GOV.UK 2020). Mental health and well-being among South Asian adults with comorbidities, physical and mental health disorders related to the social environment, cultural values and practices are also factors. Notwithstanding the enormity of the task in terms of interventions and community actions, challenges posed by social distancing, isolation and social inequalities have implications for how well COVID-19 can be prevented among overcrowded households in densely populated towns and cities.

Stigmatization is a pervasive phenomenon, inflicted more on the already harmed and at risk of further psychological distress. Fear of stigmatization prevents South Asian patients from seeking help and treatment for mental illness. The stigma of mental illness can lead to delay in seeking treatment, breakdown in social relationships, and hinder performance in the workplace (Jorm and Reavley 2013). South Asian individuals do not come forward to access mental health services (Karasz et al. 2019). Stigma as a consequence of having COVID-19, in addition to blame targeted at communities affected by the outbreak, could have long-term detrimental socio-cultural effects and impact on health outcomes. Due care needs to be taken to erase the stigma associated with or caused by disease, racism, religious propaganda, which requires regular discussions with trained and specialist healthcare personnel. For this are needed task forces and execution teams which are directly engaged in healthcare delivery systems without creating any communication gaps between policy-makers and ground-level workers (Bruns et al. 2020). Furthermore, tailored interventions have been suggested to address the psychosocial impact of COVID-19 on different strata of society, including marginalized communities and psychiatric patients (Dubey et al. 2020).

In pursuance of a targeted local lockdown strategy, Leicester became the first city in the UK to remain in lockdown. The reason given was the second spike in COVID-19. A closer look at the 2011 household census shows that Leicester, with 15% overcrowded households, has one of the highest levels of overcrowding outside London (Leicester.gov.uk). According to Nazareth et al. (2020), the new cases in Leicester were concentrated in an area where 72.5% of the population are from BAME backgrounds, mostly South Asian communities. Nazareth et al. (2020) went on to argue that 'the opportunity to escalate interventions locally have been stymied by the inadequacy of information sharing' (ibid., e4). Not unlike Marston, Renedo and Miles (2020) who argued that participation of vulnerable and marginalized communities can help identify solutions with possibilities of greater compliance, Nazareth et al. (2020) have called for 'effective community engagement' as a strategy to enhance adherence to measures, which otherwise seem to be imposed and risk being unpopular or misunderstood.

At the end of July 2020, a similar targeted lockdown was imposed on north-western counties, cities and towns with a high percentage of South Asian people. Implicit in the action taken was the notion that people were not adhering to the strict guidance, mixing socially, and therefore, contributing to the spike in cases. Scapegoating and stigmatization of South Asian communities across the north-western cities and towns could not be dismissed as non-consequential as these communities felt unfairly treated compared to others. It is important that sections of the population are not made to feel ostracized, humiliated, and alienated, compounding concerns about 'othering' in society, which can have detrimental effects on the health and well-being of everyone concerned. Logie and Turan (2020) argued that much has been learned about stigma-reduction through decades of dealing with and researching HIV/AIDS and suggested that applying an intersectional perspective can enhance our understanding of how COVID-19 stigma intersects with race, housing security and health. Taking the prevention of stigmatization forward, Bruns and colleagues (2020) have suggested the implementation of timely and culturally appropriate interventions along with proper screening, treatment and follow-up of affected individuals. It is expected that evidence of the effectiveness of any psychosocial interventions applied in the management of mental health issues associated with COVID-19 will emerge soon.

CONCLUSION

COVID-19 has had devastating effects on South Asian communities in Europe. South Asian communities are just as vulnerable to COVID-19 as others but have a higher rate of infection and related mortality. Underlying comorbidities such as diabetes and cardiovascular diseases contribute to the risk of hospitalization and interventions that include artificial ventilation in intensive care units. Affected South Asian communities live in cities and towns with high levels of deprivation and overcrowding. Strategies adopted and the lack of consistency in communication have placed these communities at further risk from COVID-19 given that comorbidities known to heighten vulnerability are also high among them. Furthermore, the psychosocial impact of COVID-19 could be overwhelming, with growing feelings of stigma and the exacerbation of crippling mental health problems. To address the already deep impact of COVID-19 among South Asian communities there is a profound need to ensure strategies that reflect engagement and support in addition to clear communication of strategies at the local level. As COVID-19 is not showing any signs of being driven down any time soon, the South Asian communities need to play their part in full to mitigate the effects of comorbidities (cardiovascular diseases, diabetes, obesity) and COVID-19 on their physical and psychosocial health outcomes with healthcare and community measures. While social and physical distancing must always be adhered to, messages concerning the prevention of COVID-19 should also be clear and culturally compatible.

PLAGUE IS THE GREAT TRUTH-TELLER: HOW CAN WE TALK BACK?

Alison Scott-Baumann and Hina J. Shahid

In these times of 'fake news', 'cancel culture' and 'viral' posts and videos, it is important—perhaps more than at any other time in our history—that we heed and respond to research. It is also, for the very same reasons, more difficult to do so than it has ever been.

Let us look at specific examples—for the purpose of this essay, the work undertaken by the School of Oriental and African Studies (SOAS), University of London; the Muslim Doctors Association (MDA), a grassroots organization which works with Muslim, minority and marginalized communities in the UK; and the activist website Corridors of Power (COP).

SOAS, through the work of Professor Laura Hammond and others, uses long-term research expertise to urge the European Union to improve migration corridors. MDA works with professional groups and community organizations to lobby government and policy-makers, while COP disseminates urgent and accurate information to both Houses of the British Parliament and helps MPs and peers put informed pressure on government. Each initiative complements the recent surge in the demand to be heard, celebrated in 2019 by policy analyst Claudia Chwalisz as a new wave of deliberative democracy. Chwalisz understands this to mean that political decisions should be the result of reasonable discussion among citizens. Such discourse is vastly enhanced by accepting that we understand ourselves better by seeing ourselves reflected in others and in our relationships with them, as French philosopher Ricoeur explains in his seminal text *Oneself as Another* (1992). This insight is much needed in plague times, such as now, when injustices are multiplied and the sick and the dead cannot talk.

Millions have died of COVID-19 worldwide, with several

nations struggling to manage the crisis as opposed to what they might have us believe. For example, in the UK, the death toll relative to population is one of the highest in the world. The patterns of illness and death in the British population hold a mirror to the shortcomings of liberal democracy. Sickness and death have been disproportionally high among those in Britain who are disadvantaged by compromised health, poverty, colour, ethnicity and type of employment. This tragic situation also reflects an often disregarded characteristic of systemic and institutionalized racism: concerns raised as a poor person or person of colour are simply not considered valid. This form of epistemic injustice can be demonstrably evidenced in university populations, and as a result of COVID-19, it has recently and shockingly become apparent in hospital staff populations and among care workers in other parts of the health sector.

Social distancing is mandatory to reduce infections, yet many simply do not have this privilege, such as those living in cramped conditions, caring for the ill at close quarters, and being part of large families or community groups. Self-isolation during illness is also an impossible privilege for those lacking income protection, the ones who literally have to choose between their lives and livelihoods. In addition, on the international stage, racism, class, and nationalism are being used to argue for the protection of borders and the pandemic is being used as the latest opportunity to restrict people's movements. This, as another form of social distancing, is understandable, but these solutions are being deployed by the privileged to keep themselves safe. Rather, solutions must be societal, not individualistic.

COVID-19 further compromises those already at risk due to health, poverty, skin colour, and type of employment. Excess morbidity and mortality is therefore affecting the most vulnerable: those who least need another negative intersectional force exerted against them. Many of these people have strong religious faith that shapes their identity and way of life and affects their health beliefs and personal, household, and community practices. Such practices offer a range of protective health effects (Hill and Pargament 2003) but may also increase risks and affect outcomes from COVID-19. In the UK, religion is a legally protected characteristic under the Equality Act, 2010, and therefore, by definition, religious minorities are vulnerable. Members of minority religious groups are more likely to be from Black, Asian, and Minority Ethnic (BAME) backgrounds, and they may experience multiple intersecting risk factors simultaneously, thus contributing to increased risks and poorer COVID-19 outcomes. A government report (ONS 2020) has shown that Muslims are at the highest risk of dying from COVID-19 among all religious groups. This should not be unexpected—Muslims in the UK already face some of the highest levels of age-standardized ill health, disability, poverty, and deprivation (Laird 2007a).

Dangerous intersections include socioeconomic factors; structural and societal stigma; disruption to social, cultural, and religious practices; barriers to accessing healthcare; religious discrimination; increased prevalence of underlying disorders; and healthcare worker discrimination, all which have been exacerbated during the pandemic (Shahid 2020a, 2020b). If we consider each of these factors, we can see how two or more of these intersectional factors can increase morbidity in an individual and in their community through increasing exposure, transmission, and risk of serious outcomes and reducing protection through access to health promoting and lifesaving information and resources. We take Muslims as a specific example, as they are consistently 'othered' in Britain—viewed as the source of difference and risk.

Socioeconomic factors are clear: 50 per cent of Muslims live in poverty in Britain, are more likely to live in poor quality overcrowded housing, and work in shut-down industries or in the informal sector and gig economy (Ali 2015). These factors result in high occupational hazards through inadequate income, health or safety protection, worsening health and economic inequalities. Over half of the UK Muslim population is also born outside the UK (ibid.), and immigration policies, therefore, disproportionately target them. This has shown to contribute to delayed access to healthcare out of fear of deportation and/or the financial burden of treatment (MedAct 2019). Muslims are also more likely to work in high-risk roles with increased exposure and no protective equipment due to lack of appropriate worker rights. It is well-documented that Muslims face barriers in accessing healthcare, reporting reduced satisfaction and poorer quality healthcare predating COVID-19 which are grounded in prejudice, discrimination, and Orientalist attitudes (Laird 2007b). Additionally, the background of higher prevalence of underlying cardio-metabolic disorders and nutritional deficiencies are associated with high morbidity and mortality from COVID-19 disorders among Muslims and other South Asian religious minorities (SAHF 2020).

There is also structural, societal stigma—due to a long history of alienation by media and politicians, and policies around austerity, immigration, and security that affect them most directly, Black and minority communities often understandably mistrust the authorities. This contributes to a well-documented phenomenon of mistrust in medical advice, which is even more marked in Black communities since the Black Lives Matter movement gave them some voice. Police brutality and increasing publicity about the deaths of Black people at the hands of police in the US also contribute to the mistrust of government advice, as well as the attraction of conspiracy theories as alternative explanatory models, and fake news—all of which are harmful to public health. A recent report has shown the racial and religious disproportionality of Prevent, the counterterror legislation in the National Health Service (NHS), causing a conflict in doctors' duty of care and exacerbating physical and mental health problems (MedAct 2020). This can result in delays in accessing testing and treatment, resulting in increased community transmission and delayed presentation, as well as more advanced levels of disease.

Among the minor religious communities, disruptions to social, cultural, and religious practices such as congregational prayers, grieving, and burial practices and the inability to visit the sick have increased mental health and post-traumatic stress disorders. We have yet to fully understand the deep trauma this has and will leave on BAME communities. Furthermore, faith institutions that ordinarily open their spaces for comfort and support for distressed individuals and communities have had to close their doors. Many of these institutions also depend on donations and have suffered a loss of income due to the combined effects of the suspension of routine activities and the economic impact of the pandemic on the communities they serve; this while trying to offer exceptionally demanding crisis support virtually. These vital community spaces for healing now face an existential threat.

Religious discrimination, anti-Semitism, Islamophobia, and racism based on skin colour have increased during COVID-19, with racist memes and fake news blaming certain groups as being super spreaders or non-compliant with public health guidance (Anti-Muslim Hatred Working Group 2020). This results in religious minorities being targets of abuse and blame, undermining social cohesion and well-being, and leading to reduced feelings of agency. Social cohesion is vital to overcome a pandemic, which requires solidarity, compassion, and collective action. Issues of trust are crucial here, and we have seen fear and hysteria generated by the scapegoating of minority communities for systematic government failings in handling the crisis intensified recently during local lockdowns. Currently, in the UK, we are witnessing a narrative of 'blame the BAME' as photos of mosques and headscarf wearing women are splashed across media outlets accompanied by warnings of rising cases. This is despite mosques in the UK closing one week ahead of government advice through grassroots community-led efforts.

On the frontline, we have seen institutional discrimination and oppression resulting in loss of lives among keyworkers. Over 90 per cent of doctors who have died have been from a BAME background (BMA 2020). It is known that Muslims are the most discriminated religious group in the NHS (West 2015). A 'triple penalty' exists in the NHS (Abdulkareem and Shahid 2017) which was also highlighted in a recent survey showing that over 80 per cent of Muslims in the NHS have experienced

Islamophobia ('Muslim Medics Taunted', 2020). However, when we look deeper, the penalties compound beyond the triple effect of gender, ethnicity and religion to include other overlapping marginalized identities, worsening discrimination (Shahid 2019). Discrimination against healthcare workers makes it difficult to raise concerns about inadequate access to culturally appropriate personal protective equipment and risk assessments, testing, or unfair redeployment to high-risk areas, which contributes to increased viral exposure, stress, anxiety, burnout, and death. Additionally, local doctors, over-represented by ethnic minorities and Muslims, have reported significant income losses and financial strain. These concerns point towards institutional Islamophobia in the NHS.

Faith is an overlooked determinant of health but an important tool for health promotion. Faith-based organizations have a long history of serving vulnerable communities that are marginalized and medically underserved, and they have been at the forefront of community efforts, providing mental health and spiritual support services such as bereavement counselling. They provide practical support by organizing delivery of food, medicines, and essential supplies to the elderly, vulnerable, and isolated households and have provided guidance for issues such as end of life care, hospital visitation, and safe religious practices. They also help integrate public health and faith-based messages that are relevant and accessible to marginalized communities thus filling a void in mainstream sources.

Faith-based health promotion is effective and saves lives (DeHaven et al. 2004). Failure to consider the important role of faith beliefs, practices, and institutions risks missing important lessons and opportunities to prevent a second wave of infection and inequality. To prevent further loss of lives and unequal impact on Muslim and other minority communities, we recommend a whole system, a multi-sectoral approach supported by local contextualized community-led action with transparent governance and reporting systems and with independent monitoring and accountability. This means recognizing racism as a major driver of the disproportionate impact of COVID-19 among Muslim and Black communities, patients, and frontline workers.

The government needs to, as a matter of urgency, re-establish trust and transparency by engaging with grassroots organizations to co-produce and implement immediate and long-term risk mitigation strategies with adequate funding, resources, and community ownership. There needs to be mandatory data collection and reporting of outcomes and experiences by religion, recognizing this as a protected characteristic and thus essential for health inequalities monitoring. These data must be made freely available for patients and NHS staff at surveillance, prevention, primary and secondary care levels, and death certification to monitor for equality and effectiveness of interventions. Policies that entrench structural inequalities should be eliminated, for example, policies on austerity, immigration, or security, and increased media accountability must be ensured with robust action against reports that misrepresent, blame, and stigmatize vulnerable and marginalized communities and increase individual and public health risks.

In the NHS, personalized risk assessments and occupational health and well-being support must be mandated for all workers. These must be faith and culturally sensitive, with inclusive policies that guarantee health, safety, and income protection as well as citizenship rights to family members of healthcare workers. Diverse, supportive, and inclusive workplaces are essential, enabling leadership development and career progression with resourced and funded faith networks and initiatives, psychological safe routes for raising concerns, and rigorous implementation of zero tolerance policies against Islamophobia and broad-spectrum racism. For Muslim and other minority patients, there needs to be improved access and quality of healthcare for thorough provision of linguistic, cultural, and faith-sensitive public health messaging with awareness, dialogue, and training on anti-Islamophobia among healthcare providers to eliminate healthcare provider-associated discrimination.

Religious minority groups have borne the brunt of excess

deaths and trauma; it is time for the government to repay their sacrifices through authentic allyship built on agency and accountability, thereby ensuring optimal health, well-being, peace, and security for all. Deliberative democracy is necessary to achieve this.

NATIONAL HEALTH SERVICE: RESPONDING TO THE PLAGUE DOMESTICALLY

As a result of COVID-19 and the epistemic injustice that dismisses the opinions of certain groups, great inequities have recently and shockingly been revealed in hospital staff populations and among care workers in other parts of the health sector (Shahid 2020a). So how do we draw attention to these multiple wrongs? Dr Hina Shahid is among those at the forefront of this struggle. She is chair of MDA, a non-profit organization of multi-disciplinary health professionals in the UK. They work both at grassroots and policy levels to reduce health inequalities in Muslim and ethnic minority communities and improve equity and inclusion in the NHS. During COVID-19, the MDA has worked with a range of community, professional, academic, and media organizations to reduce the impact of COVID-19 on Muslim communities and to highlight structural discrimination, racism, and Islamophobia as key drivers of an alarming number of deaths both in the community and on the front line.

They have written policy briefings and reports, including with SOAS-COP and presented evidence to a number of MPs, parliamentary committees, and government advisors on the impact of COVID-19 on the Muslim community along with recommendations to mitigate risks. Many of these were included in Public Health England's review on health disparities.

Their campaigning has also resulted in the publication of data on COVID-19 deaths by religion and raised the profile of religious discrimination including in the NHS where they are now working to develop a formal system of support and accountability for those affected by religious discrimination.

At the grassroots level, they have created toolkits and

guidance for physical and mental well-being. They have also held public webinars and social media campaigns to disseminate evidence-based and culturally sensitive information to the community on public health and safety, mental health, and palliative care. They have also provided community insights on improving the effectiveness and efficiency of the testing programme and culturally sensitive risk communication to the Muslim community in particular as well as to the rest of the population.

RESPONDING TO THE PLAGUE INTERNATIONALLY

In addition, when SOAS scholars look beyond the UK's problems, at the international stage they find more evidence that racism, class, and nationalism are being used to argue for the protection of borders, with COVID-19 becoming the latest opportunity to restrict people's movements. So how do we engage those with the power to address these injustices? The need, first, to investigate injustices and provide solutions is essential in times of crisis. The current global tragedy highlights the urgent need for sustained high-quality research.

SOAS academics work tirelessly to support countries exploited historically and which are still weakened by crises. Louisa Brain explains COVID-19 and morbidity, conflict, and development in the Horn of Africa by stating, 'It overlaps with and exacerbates existing political and social inequalities to generate impacts that are felt unevenly.' Brain is part of Professor Laura Hammond's team. Hammond has been working for years with the European Union, the United Nations, and with national and regional authorities in the Horn of Africa. Displacement is a widespread response to war, famine, drought, and flood and is often local, not international. Hammond's Research and Evidence Facility (REF) has influenced the design and delivery of EU-funded programmes related to migration and displacement in the Horn of Africa and such work improves social cohesion between migrant/displaced populations and their hosts, in addition to creating economic opportunities for mobile populations (Hammond 2019).

Hammond now uses her long-term and effective social science research in the Horn of Africa to guide the analysis of the current COVID-19 pandemic. Mobility has for a long time been known to be an essential survival strategy for the region's refugees and displaced populations, including poorer families who have to diversify their livelihoods to survive. To respond to COVID-19, governments all over the world are imposing border closures, internal movement restrictions, and social distancing orders, and the economic implications of the closures of businesses and workplaces are all having specific and harmful effects in such areas. In these circumstances, mobile populations do become greater targets of suspicion, fear, and hostility. Hammond's research at SOAS focuses on mobile populations in the Horn and helps inform the agencies she already works with about COVID-19 preparedness and response strategies (Brain 2020, 19).

WESTMINSTER AND THE VOICE OF YOUTH AND RESEARCH

These are tragic situations that demonstrate an often invisible characteristic of systemic and institutionalized racism—not being heard when you raise concerns because what you say as a poor person or as a person of colour is quite simply not considered valid. This form of epistemic injustice can be demonstrably evidenced in university populations (Scott-Baumann et al. 2020).

To return our attention to issues closer home, and in the understanding that the international and the local are potent when they come together, we now consider ways in which the voice of the young, such as university students, could be much more effective in Westminster. Students are citizens and, as Chwalisz (2017) points out, 'the public is a resource to be tapped, not a risk to be managed'.

To tackle this, we have developed the Influencing Corridors of Power (ICOP) project, a SOAS initiative that aims to help parliament have an impact in government by mobilizing students, academic staff, and activists to inform parliamentarians. ICOP has been running since November 2020, and we hope to transform its great success as an information disseminator into a training model for rights and justice, bringing the higher education sector and democratic potential of parliament together and bringing the disenfranchised into Westminster to speak truth to power (Scott-Bauman et al. 2020).

ICOP is unique in that it fills the current vacuum at the heart of fact-finding in parliament by communicating directly with the members of both houses to whom we issue regular one-page briefings and offer specialist advice on urgent matters such as the Coronavirus Act and immigration legislation (ibid.). With ICOP, we hope to step up a gear to transform democratic processes into decision-making. It can help develop live connections between academics, students, politicians, and civil servants and create a new space underpinned by the voices of young people, by evidence-based academic authority and research to guide parliament in its commitment to hold government accountable in preserving rights, liberties, and justice. ICOP aims to guide participants in using structures of government effectively, for example, in lobbying select committees and setting up APPGs (all-party parliamentary groups). These procedures are vastly underused and vitally important in the current government with a presidential style that seeks to bypass parliament.

At the heart of ICOP's work is policy advocacy and campaigning to protect and promote the overarching framework of human rights for the most vulnerable. Through our briefings and reports, we hold government and public bodies to account for their implementation of human rights. We look forward to working through ICOP to build a bridge between public intellectuals and academic experts who are often disconnected from the decision-making circles and those with political power and influence. As such, we seek to widen access to the sphere of power by establishing and making the fundamental connections for knowledge exchange between academia and parliament and ensure justice in the decision-making process.

It is more vital now than ever because COVID-19

exacerbates systemic discrimination. We need to promote the political empowerment of the young, of women, and ethnic and religious minorities within the wider society through greater inclusion and representation.

CONCLUSIONS

This plague reveals the cracks and fissures in society and deepens and broadens them to such an extent that the more fortunate may risk falling on top of the less fortunate and crushing them while the poor cushion their fall. Steep rises in billionaire fortunes have been documented in 2020 as a result of COVID-19 and countries such as the US and the UK are being governed by those with more influence than understanding. Those who do not have a voice in these markets of power and money, the young and the minorities, will inherit the mistakes of their elders and those with influence, so they need to seize influence themselves. Deliberative democracy is a viable expression of the ways in which those without a voice can work together to talk and articulate possible solutions. Accurate research is vital for informing such democratic impulses. The activism of a university like SOAS with a truly global reach must also bring together the national and the international and show clearly how we are all interconnected—remittances from Somalian refugees in Europe to their families in Africa, for example, are vital and are under threat due to COVID-19. We live in the same cities and have to accept that we are reflected in each other's destinies—we are the other.

EPILOGUE

COVID and Beyond

CORONAVIRUS: RETROSPECT 2040

Christopher Norris

It's twenty years ago and more
Coronavirus hit.
It hit the sick, it hit the poor,
And shares went crashing through the floor,
But we said, 'Wait a bit, you lot,
Stay calm and wait a bit.'

For we saw how it just might go,
This re-run of old scenes
That pitched the high against the low,
The boss-class guy with loads of dough
Against us might-have-beens, us lot
Of low-class might-have-beens.

We saw it coming, just the same
As when *Titanic* sank,
A life-boat place booked in their name
But nary a space for us to claim:
We've their class-law to thank, you lot,
Their boss-class law to thank.

The virus had a tale to tell,
A most instructive tale.
It said: I'm here on time to spell
It loud and clear, the future hell
You face if they prevail and plot,
Your fate if they prevail!

A virus is a curious beast,
It's neither live nor dead,
A hybrid thing that, once released,
Has death to bring from 'the Far East',
For that's the fear they spread, that's what
The racist papers spread.

But we got wind of how things stood,
Of what they had in mind,
Those swine who thought 'the common good'
Meant 'you go short, as your sort should;
You're just the common kind, you lot,
You're just the common kind'.

Oh yes, we clocked the message then,
We commoners got the gist:
'They're at their tricks and games again,
Their schemes to fix just where and when
To brandish the iron fist they've got,
That thinly gloved iron fist.'

It's capital that ran the show,
That told us, 'Listen up:
You paupers may, with luck, pull through
If you'll just pay and join the queue,'
But we were sold a pup, that's what—
Us lot were sold a pup.

So listening up taught us to trust
Our wits, not boss-class lies.
It told us how the doubters must
Cease doubting now and deem it just,
The rage that bid us rise, you lot,
The rage that bid us rise!

We knew all crises had a close,
However long they took,
And so it went, as anger rose
And all you spent-out paupers chose
To bring their crimes to book, that lot,
To bring their crimes to book.

First it was 'Put all plans on hold
And let the virus run',
Until a graph too plainly told
It might kill half the sick and old:
Who'll hold the smoking gun, big shot,
Who'll hold the smoking gun?

Then they got panicky and tried
To bolt the stable door
With new rules each time someone died,
Though rules whose reach they strove to hide:
They knew the insurance score, that lot,
They knew the pay-off score.

We've kicked them out with all their rules,
We've kicked them good and hard.
We cleared the land of public schools,
And took in hand the flannelled fools,
And flashed them our red card, you lot,
Just flashed them our red card.

Coronavirus showed the way
To cast their idols down.
It showed how crass the part that they,
The governing class, had come to play—
The role of licensed clown and sot,
Of corporate-licensed clown.

For there were viruses out there
Ten times more virulent
Since spread abroad by those who'd dare
Have lies and fraud supplant all care
For those they represent—you lot
They claim to represent.

Let's not thank god the virus struck:
It brought us death and grief.
But let's concede that we were stuck,
In desperate need of devil's luck
To turn a greener leaf, that's what:
To turn a greener leaf!

They'd screw things up for good and all,
Those tools of corporate greed.
They'd foul our nest and have a ball
At power's behest or fortune's call
And pay the rest no heed, that lot,
And pay the rest no heed.

Act now, strike back, don't blow your chance!
That's what the virus taught.
Else who knows when they'll next advance,
Through pathogen or high finance,
And bring your lives to naught, you lot,
And bring your lives to naught.

ACKNOWLEDGEMENTS

This book is the outcome of the authors unconditionally sharing their creative and thought-provoking research, despite conditions of intense turbulence. They readily accepted our invitation to write, notwithstanding their pressing commitments and schedules. Our deep gratitude to the authors in this volume.

The September 2020 issue of the University of Mumbai's online journal *Sambhāṣaṇ* is reprinted in the experiential section (Part II) of this book (with the exception of Ruxandra Anghel's essay, which is an additional piece). Some of these essays have been revised by the authors. We thank the *Sambhāṣaṇ* team of Assistant Editors for their assistance.

We additionally appreciate Meera Mahadevan and Biraj Mehta's valuable inputs and suggestions.

We thank Ravi Singh, Nazeef Mollah and their colleagues at Speaking Tiger Books for their encouragement, feedback, patience, assistance and time with this book.

CONTRIBUTORS

Ruxandra Anghel is developing her second career in Psychology, following a successful career in Communications. She is currently training as an existential psychotherapist, undertaking a doctoral programme in psychotherapy at the New School of Psychotherapy and Counselling in London. Her doctoral research project focuses on Generation Z and explores their experience of 'joy of living' in times of crisis. She is a psychology teaching fellow in academia, and she is the founder of a well-being programme for students. She worked with young people as a senior mentor in personal development programmes. Since 2020 she is a registered BACP psychotherapist in the UK, currently working on developing The Cartesian Experience, a project dedicated to supporting young adults and the mediation between generations. In September 2021, she returned to teaching in higher education as a counselling lecturer, developing training programmes in counselling and psychotherapy.

Brunella Antomarini has a PhD in Aesthetics (Gregoriana University in Rome) and teaches Aesthetics and Contemporary Philosophy at John Cabot University, Rome. She has a pluri-disciplinary formation in contemporary epistemology, aesthetics, anthropology, and post-humanism. Her current research concerns the analysis of the common functions of the organic body and a retroactive machine through an epistemological convergence of different views, such as pragmatism, cybernetics, and systems theory. Some of her publications include *Le machine nubili* (2020); 'Peirce and Cybernetics: Retroduction, Error and Auto-Poiesis in Future Thinking' (*Cognitio*, São Paulo, vol. 18, no. 2, pp. 187–204); *The Maiden Machine: Philosophy in the Age of the Unborn Woman* (2013); *Thinking Through Error: The Moving Target of Knowledge* (2012); as a co-editor with Adam Berg, *Aesthetics in Present Future: The Arts in the Technological Horizon* (2013); *La preistoria acustica* *della poesia* (2013); *L'errore del maestro: Una lettura laica dei Vangeli* (2006); *La percezione della forma: Trascendenza e finitezza in Hans Urs von Balthasar* (2004); and as a co-author with A. Berg, Vladimir D'Amora, Alessandro De Francesco, and Miltos Manetas, *Haephestus Re-Loaded* (2019). She is also a translator from English into Italian and the author of a children's book, *Denizens of the Forest* (1992).

İclal Eskioğlu Aydın is a clinical psychologist and supervisor at Ibn Haldun University Center for Psychotherapy Research and İnsula Psychotherapy Center. She graduated from the Psychology Department and received her Master's Degree in Clinical Psychology. Currently, she is a PhD student of Clinical Psychology at Ibn Haldun University in Istanbul, Turkey. She has been a narrative practitioner for four years. She is working with young people, adults, couples and groups.

Elena Baskina is the co-founder of Reconnect, a global movement and course encouraging authentic connections. She has focused her career on shifting culture through the playful solutions of narrative and other postmodern approaches in education, therapy and community work. She was educated as a lawyer, after which she pursued her post-graduate education at the Dartmouth MALS programme. Later on she obtained a degree in Psychology from Moscow State University. Then she got trained in the narrative approach through a variety of international programmes including those by: Nkazelo Nkube (South Africa), Ana Dumitrascu (Spain), Maggie Carey (US) and Hugh Fox (UK). She also got certified as an EMDR therapist by EMDR Russia and received mindfulness training under the Harvard CE programme. She started the 'You Are Not Alone' programme addressing infertility issues in Russia, challenging societal stereotypes and giving women with fertility difficulties support and choice. She has also launched the 'Future is Now' foundation that trained psychology students in fast and effective approaches in therapy, giving hope to people in difficult situations in life. She is a member of faculty of the non-profit Re-authoring Teaching together with colleagues from all over the world.

Jude Clark is an independent consultant and practitioner within the social justice and development arena, a clinical psychologist with expertise in the area of trauma, gender and group process. She was awarded a PhD from Manchester Metropolitan University (UK) in 2006 and lectured at the University of KwaZulu-Natal, South Africa for 14 years. She has published 12 articles and book chapters and has been a guest editor for special issue editions of three journals. Her previous research focused on Black women's experience of the Truth and Reconciliation Commission in South Africa as well as the representation of trauma in Black women's life narratives. She also has over 20 years of experience in facilitating processes around issues of transformation, diversity, inclusion and healing—for individuals, communities, academic institutions, non-governmental organizations, and corporate entities. Her current focus is on creating spaces and processes that enable Black womxn to overcome the obstacles that stand in the way of our well-being, through an initiative called 'Deep Wellness for Black womxn'.

Sara Dang is Save the Children's Advisor for Early Childhood Development for Asia. She offers technical support to ensure the creation and delivery of quality early childhood education curricula and programmes. She focuses on designing, implementing and advocating for innovative and affordable ECCD programmes that allow the most vulnerable children to reach their full potential in safe and sustainable environments. At the regional level, she chairs the Asia Pacific Regional Network for Early Childhood steering committee, where she provides strategic guidance in the network's vision, actions and strategy. She has over 15 years of professional experience, including eight years of experience with Save the Children, and has worked in Asia, Africa, the Caribbean, and the Pacific.

Basantsingh Deerpaul has completed a Masters' Degree in Psychology from the University of Mumbai and currently works as a psychologist at the Mauritius Institute of Training and Development. Besides his full-time employment, he also lectures part time at the University of Technology, Mauritius, and is an independent researcher in the field of applied spirituality and positive psychology. While being involved with institutions engaged in promoting alternative and complementary therapies, he is an authorized Instructor of Pranic Healing® and runs a wellness centre.

Lata Dyaram is an Associate Professor in the Department of Management Studies, IIT Madras. She studies volitional and discretionary phases at work, spontaneous mental states and goal directed behaviour across contexts, team/group dynamics and related constructs in workplace behaviour. In collaboration with students, she employs mixed research methods, qualitative measures, large-scale organizational surveys and field experiments to study varied phenomena.

Andrew Edgar (DPhil, Sussex) retired from teaching in 2018, and is now Emeritus Reader in Philosophy at Cardiff University, and an honorary member of staff at Swansea University, UK. He continues his research and writing in philosophy. His research interests include twentieth-century German philosophy, having completed his DPhil on Adorno's aesthetics. He is the author of *The Philosophy of Habermas* (2005) and *Habermas: Key Concepts* (2006). He has written and published extensively on the philosophy of medicine, having been a participant in European Commission funded projects on health-related quality of life, chronic illness, and dignity and ageing. He was for some time the editor of the journal *Health Care Analysis*. He currently works on the philosophy of sport. He is the editor of *Sport, Ethics and Philosophy*, and the author of *Sport and Art: An Essay in the Hermeneutics of Sport* (2014). He is also president of the European Association for the Philosophy of Sport.

Maurice Hamington is Professor of Philosophy, and Affiliate. He is a care ethicist interested in both the theory and application of care. Hamington is a Member of the International Consultants for The Melete Center of Philosophy for Care, University of Verona, and a Steering Committee Member of the international

Care Ethics Research Consortium, Utrecht, The Netherlands. He has authored or edited twelve books including *Care Ethics and Poetry* (2019) authored with Ce Rosenow, *Care Ethics and Political Theory*, with Daniel Engster (2015), *Applying Care Ethics to Business*, with Maureen Sander-Staudt (2011), *Socializing Care*, with Dorothy C. Miller (2006) and *Embodied Care* (2004). He is currently working on two collections of original contributions, one addressing care ethics and precarity and the other focusing on care ethics and religion. For more information on his other works, see https://pdx.academia.edu/MauriceHamington

Ernest W.B. Hess-Lüttich was Full Professor, University of Berne (1992–2014; since 2015, Prof Emer), Honorary Professor at the Technical University, Berlin (since 2015), Honorary Professor at University of Stellenbosch (2007–17), Honorary Professor UCT, Cape Town (since 2020). His main areas of research are dialogue analysis and discourse studies in various fields of theory and application (sociology of language, literary studies, theatre studies, intermedial, intercultural, intra-/subcultural, institutional, public, political, technical, and urban communication). He has written and edited some 70 books and published approximately 400 scholarly articles in journals and collective volumes. His monographs include books on the foundations of dialogue linguistics, on communication and aesthetics, on the semiotics of theatre and drama, on Gerhart Hauptmann, on applied sociology of language, on literary theory and media practice, on urban and medical discourse, on German grammar and language use. He is a founding member of the editorial boards of several journals and book series, like *Kodikas International Journal of Semiotics*, *Journal of Intercultural German Studies*, *Cross Cultural Communication* and a member of numerous other academic advisory boards, including one at the Austrian Academy of Sciences (ICLTT, until 2016). He is an Honorary Member of the Hungarian Association of German Studies and was (vice) president of various scholarly associations, among them the German Assocication for Semiotic Studies, Association of Applied Linguistics, International Association of Dialogue Analysis, and the Association of Intercultural German Studies. He has held academic positions at the universities of London, Bonn, Berlin, Bloomington/IN, Berne, and has been invited as a guest professor or visiting scholar to more than 30 renowned universities around the world.

Kirtika Kain is a Delhi-born artist based in Sydney, Australia. She received her Bachelor of Fine Arts in 2016 for which she was awarded the Bird Holcomb MFA Scholarship. Upon completing her Masters of Fine Arts in 2018, she received the University Medal at the National Art School, Sydney. In 2019, Kain completed two consecutive artist's residencies in New Delhi, India and at the prestigious British School at Rome NAS International Residency, Italy followed by her first solo exhibition *Corpus* in Sydney. She is presently a recipient of the Artist-in-Residence (AIR) programme of the Parramatta Artist Studios and a finalist in the 2020 Create NSW Emerging Artist Fellowship, in partnership with Artspace. Kain is represented by the Roslyn Oxley9 Gallery, Sydney.

Ada Kot was born and grew up in Hong Kong. She has demonstrated strong commitment in working with disadvantaged groups since her university life by conducting assessments and supporting students for primary education in rural China. Upon graduation from the University of Hong Kong, she joined different local and international non-governmental organizations, working with the most vulnerable groups, including people suffering from natural disasters in China and ethnic minorities in Hong Kong. She further studied counselling in 2014 and is now a certified counsellor under the Hong Kong Professional Counselling Association, a Level 2 professional member under Australian Counselling Association and a Registered Member of the British Association for Counselling and Psychotherapy. She is a narrative practitioner, her counselling and co-research interest is in areas of intercultural identity, intergeneration relationships, gender and sexuality, as well as people with mental health problems and special education needs. At present, she is conducting research, as well as teaching psychology and counselling courses at universities. She is dedicated to promoting narrative practices among Chinese communities on social media platforms by producing podcasts, videos and writing blogs.

Vinay Lal is Professor of History and Asian American Studies at the University of California, Los Angeles (UCLA). He writes widely on Indian history, historiography, the Indian diaspora, colonialism, the architecture of nonviolence, Gandhi, American politics, contemporary culture, and the global politics of knowledge systems. His 18 books include the two-volume *Oxford Anthology of the Modern Indian City* (2013); *The Future of Knowledge and Culture: A Dictionary for the Twenty-first Century*, co-edited with Ashis Nandy (2005); *Of Cricket, Guinness and Gandhi: Essays on Indian History and Culture* (2005); *The History of History: Politics and Scholarship in Modern India* (2003); *Empire of Knowledge: Culture and Plurality in the Global Economy* (2002); and, most recently, *India and Civilizational Futures: Backwaters Collective on Metaphysics and Politics II* (2019) and (co-edited) *A Passionate Life: Writings by and on Kamaladevi Chattopadhyay* (2017). *The Fury of COVID-19: The Passions, Histories, and Unrequited Love of the Coronavirus* is published by Pan Macmillan in October 2020. He blogs at vinaylal.wordpress.com and maintains an academic YouTube channel at youtube.com/user/dillichalo which has two million views. He also blogs at abplive.in.

Sebastiano Maffettone is an Italian philosopher, currently Full Professor of Political Philosophy at Luiss Guido Carli University in Rome, where he was formerly also the Dean of the Faculty of Political Science. He specialized in Social Philosophy at the London School of Economics, and among other appointments, has been a visiting professor at Harvard, Tufts and New York University. He is a member of many scientific committees supported by Adriano Olivetti, Einaudi and Ernst & Young foundations. Professor Maffettone is also Director of *Filosofia* *e Questioni Pubbliche*, a semi-annual review of political, moral and social philosophy and applied ethics. Professor Maffettone's research concerns the development of an original vision of public ethics within the context of Italy and international themes of contemporary political philosophy. He also takes interest in the philosophy of John Rawls and has produced an Italian translation of *A Theory of Justice*.

Christopher Norris is Emeritus Professor in Philosophy at Cardiff University. In his early career he taught English Literature, then moved to Philosophy *via* literary theory, and has now moved back towards creative writing. He has published widely on the topic of deconstruction and is the author of more than 30 books on aspects of philosophy, literature, politics, the history of ideas, and music. More recently he has turned to writing poetry in various genres, among them—unusually—that of the philosophical verse-essay. His collections include *The Cardinal's Dog* (2014), *The Winnowing Fan* (2015), *For the Tempus-Fugitives* (2017), *The Matter of Rhyme* (2018), *A Partial Truth* (2019), and *Socrates at Verse* (2020). He has also published two collections of political-satirical verse, *The Trouble with Monsters* (2018) and *The Folded Lie* (2019).

Raji Manjari Pokhrel grew up in Kathmandu, Nepal. Her specialization lies in labour and community organizing and mental health and her passion is to integrate the two at the intersection of gender. She has a therapy practice, and she loves to do collaborative work using narrative practices and somatic awareness to envision queer ways of being. She is forever grateful for her education and know-how of the world to the Nepali-speaking domestic and elder care workers' community in Queens, New York, who taught her to see emotional labour otherwise rendered invisible in everyday life. She has a Master's degree in Social Work from the Columbia University School of Social Work, New York (2013).

Prathama Raghavan is from Hyderabad, India. She currently works as a school counsellor and mental health and disability support worker and facilitator in Kathmandu, Nepal. She has been working in child, young person, adult and family well-being through therapeutic conversations using the narrative approaches. She has worked in the humanitarian mental health sector in conflict, refugee crisis and post-disaster environments in South Asia doing mental health coordination work. Her work and life are informed by narrative approaches, principles of disability justice, neurodiversity and transformative justice and poetry. She has recently become interested in working towards building 'imperfect solidarities' through group conversations in a far from perfect world. Prathama has a PhD in Developmental Psychology from Université Paul-Valéry, France (2012).

Aarti Ramaswami is the Deputy Dean of ESSEC Business School, Asia-Pacific, and Professor in the Department of Management. Her specialities are transformational leadership and education. She co-creates and drives strategy implementation for academic/corporate initiatives in line with group strategy. Her research work focuses on systems used to identify, select, and develop managerial and executive talent, with a particular interest in career success, diversity and inclusion, expatriation, and cross-cultural management. Her research has appeared in top international peer-reviewed journals. She teaches various leadership and management topics to MBA, Executive Education, and doctoral programme participants. She graduated with a PhD in Organizational Behaviour and Human Resource Management from the Kelley School of Business at Indiana University, Bloomington. She has a highly international profile, having lived and worked in India, USA, France, UAE, and now in Singapore.

Sanjay G. Reddy is an Associate Professor of Economics at The New School for Social Research. He is an Affiliated Faculty Member of the Politics Department of the New School for Social Research. He teaches development economics, microeconomics, philosophy and economics, and other subjects. He has published widely in academic journals in economics and related subjects and given many prominent academic lectures.

Yvonne Sandoval is a mother, poet, artist, farmer living in the borderlands in New Mexico in the US. She is an executive at the El Valle Women's Collaborative and a therapist in private practice. She is committed to dismantling oppressive systems that keep us separated from land and food. Her experience as a community organizer has helped connect young people to the natural world and see themselves as positive agents for change. Sandoval works in collaboration with neighbours and friends to run the Bueno Para Todos ('Good for all') Farm in northern New Mexico. In recent months they have increased their efforts to create a local food hub to provide aid while inspiring others to rematriate land. As part of the process Ms Sandoval is actively seeking to liberate land and create a land trust so that others may be in reciprocity with the plants and water. She is working on her studies in curanderismo and becoming a permaculture consultant. She graduated with her BSW and a minor in Chicanx Studies; she earned her Master's degree at the University of Denver in 2001.

Peggy Sax is the founder and Executive Director of Re-authoring Teaching—a global learning community of narrative therapy practitioners, teachers and enthusiasts. Having apprenticed herself to narrative therapy since the early 1990s, she also works in independent practice as a licensed psychologist, consultant, international teacher, and trainer. During the last decade, she has visited India several times and is proud of her association with The Ummeed Mental Health Team. She is an author of several publications. Whether online, on-the-road (pre-COVID-19) or within her beautiful home state of Vermont, it gives her great joy to bring together her favourite people, ideas and practices—to learn, engage, play and replenish together.

Alison Scott-Baumann is Associate Director, Research, Impact and Public Engagement and Professor of Society and Belief at the School of Oriental and African Studies (SOAS), London University. She is an internationally respected academic and researcher and applies Continental Philosophy to issues of social justice. From 2015 to 2018, she led an Arts and Humanities

Research Council (AHRC) project about Islam on campus. This research and her work on free speech shows how State-imposed counter-extremism measures have a chilling effect on freedom of expression for all, not only for minorities. She speaks on BBC radio and writes in the Guardian Higher Education journal. Her intellectual pursuits include the philosophy of Paul Ricoeur.

Hina J. Shahid is a family physician with a background in public health and is Chairperson of the Muslim Doctors Association. She is an honorary clinical tutor at the Imperial College Medical School and an honorary faculty member at An-Najah National University, Palestine. She has worked in a number of research and humanitarian settings in Europe, Asia and the Middle East. Her research interests are the impact of Islamophobia on health and healthcare. She is a frequent contributor to the media on health issues affecting Muslims in Britain.

Arundhati Sharma is an international educator with over eight years of teaching experience. She is currently based in Guangzhou, China, and is teaching the Cambridge International AS and A-level Psychology Curriculum at Ulink College, Guangzhou. She has experience teaching the International Baccalaureate Diploma Programme, International Baccalaureate Middle Years Programme, Cambridge IGCSE programme, College Board Advanced Placement programme, and has also taught various humanities subjects such as Psychology, Geography, and Sociology. She has an MA in Psychology from the University of Mumbai, MSc in International Employment Relations, and has studied Human Resource Management from the London School of Economics. She is currently pursuing her Post Graduate Certificate in Education from the University of Sunderland. Her interest lies in developing metacognition skills and the use of questioning to develop critical thinking. She is also an amateur writer and enjoys travelling.

Dave Sookhoo is a nurse educator and researcher with considerable experience in health and social care. He is a peer reviewer for journals and the Joanna Briggs Institute and teaches research methods. He fervently collaborates with colleagues in conducting primary research and systematic reviews across disciplines. His areas of interest span health and cross-cultural psychology, education and long-term conditions, and their impact on health outcomes.

Masha Tiunova is the co-founder of Reconnect, a global movement towards forming authentic connections. While studying Sociology at Dartmouth College through a post-graduate leadership programme, she volunteered at the Women's Resource Center developing campaigns connecting alum female leaders with a newer generations of students. As a Head of People and Culture for the Leo Burnett global ad agency, she was a part of the global team developing HumanKind that was focused on creating safe, enjoyable, and empowering professional environments. Having become fascinated by the playfulness and depth of narrative approach, she founded Communa, helping companies and communities connect through their values. She connects the narrative approach with vocational counselling and critical education to develop leadership, soft skills and relationships courses for the Moscow Institute of Physics and Technology. She has also created courses for the MADS creative school in Moscow and the Teen Power project at World Skills 2019.

Joan C. Tronto is Professor Emerita of Political Science at the University of Minnesota and the City University of New York. A graduate of Oberlin College, she received her PhD from Princeton University. She is the author of *Moral Boundaries: A Political Argument for an Ethic of Care* (1993) and *Caring Democracy: Markets, Equality and Justice* (2013) and nearly 50 articles about care ethics. In 2015, she was awarded an honorary doctorate by the University for Humanistic Studies in the Netherlands. She has served as a Fulbright Fellow in Bologna, Italy.

Slavoj Žižek is a Professor of Philosophy at The European Graduate School, a senior researcher at the Institute for Sociology and Philosophy at the University of Ljubljana, Global Distinguished Professor of German at New York

University, International Director of the Birkbeck Institute for the Humanities, and founder and president of the Society for Theoretical Psychoanalysis, Ljubljana. His works address psychoanalytical, political and cultural issues, while articulating the relevance of Western philosophical texts such as Hegel's to contemporary contexts.

REFERENCES

FOREWORD

'Coronavirus live news EU rollout of Pfizer vaccine may be disrupted'. 2021. *The Guardian*, 2 January (https://www.theguardian.com/world/live/2021/jan/01/coronavirus-live-news-new-covid-variant-b117-in-united-states-since-october?page=with%3Ablock-5fef17518f08d08389ae7f37, accessed on 15 January 2021).

'Missionaries of Charity'. 2021. *Wikipedia* (https://en.wikipedia.org/wiki/Missionaries_of_Charity, accessed on 25 February 2021).

Allen, Woody. 1979. 'My Speech To the Graduates'. *The New York Times*, 10 August (https://www.nytimes.com/1979/08/10/archives/my-speech-to-the-graduates.html, accessed on 20 May 2020).

Davey, Melissa. 2020. 'WHO warns COVID-19 pandemic is "not necessarily the big one"'. *The Guardian*, 29 December (https://www.theguardian.com/world/2020/dec/29/who-warns-covid-19-pandemic-is-not-necessarily-the-big-one, accessed on 23 January 2021).

Hitchens, Christopher. 2013. *The Missionary Position: Mother Theresa in Theory and Practice*. London: Verso Books.

Schwering, Markus. 2020. 'Jürgen Habermas über Corona: So viel Wissen über unser Nichtwissen gab es noch nie'. *Frankfurter Rundschau* (https://www.fr.de/kultur/gesellschaft/juergen-habermas-coronavirus-krise-covid19-interview-13642491.html, accessed on 10 May 2020).

von Rainer Volk. 2020. 'Hölderlin-Trost in der Corona-Krise: "Wo aber Gefahr ist, wächst das Rettende auch"'. *SWR2* (https://www.swr.de/swr2/literatur/hoelderlin-geburtstag-trost-auch-in-der-coronavirus-krise-104.html, accessed on 10 June 2020).

INTRODUCTION

Butler, Judith. 2009. *Frames of War: When is Life Grievable*. London: Verso.

Camus, Albert. 1948. *The Plague*. Translated by Stuart Gilbert. New York: The Modern Library.

Flett, Gordon. 2018. *The Psychology of Mattering: Understanding the Human Need to be Significant*. London, San Diego: Academic Press, Elsevier.

Foucault, Michel. 1979. *Discipline and Punish. The Birth of the Prison*. Translated by Alan Sheridan. New York: Vintage Books.

———. 1988 (1986). *The Care of the Self: The History of Sexuality*, Vol. 3. New York: Vintage Books.

Henry, W.P., T.E. Schacht and H.H. Strup. 1990. 'Patient and therapist introject, interpersonal process, and differential psychotherapy outcome'. *Journal of Consulting and Clinical Psychology* 58(6): 768–774.

Kosambi, Meera, ed. 2016. *Pandita Ramabai: Life and Landmark Writings*. Oxon and New York: Routledge.

Lal, Vinay. 2020. *The Fury of COVID-19: The Politics, Histories and Unrequited Love of the Coronavirus*. New Delhi: Macmillan.

McWhir, Anne. 1998. 'Introduction'. In *The Last Man* by Mary Wollstonecraft Shelley, xiii-xxxvi. Broadview Literary Texts.

———. 2002. 'Mary Shelley's Anti-Contagionism: *The Last Man* as "Fatal Narrative"'. *Mosaic: An Interdisciplinary Critical Journal* 35(2): 23–38.

Melville, Peter. 2007. 'The Problem of Immunity in *The Last Man*'. *Studies in English Literature, 1500-1900* 14(4): 825–846.

Misra, Udit. 2021. 'Explainspeaking: What 2020 taught us about India's internal migration'. *Indian Express*, 18 February (https://indianexpress.com/article/explained/what-2020-taught-us-about-indias-internal-migration-explainspeaking-7189053/, accessed on 18 February 2021).

Neff, Kristen D. 2012. 'The Science of Self-Compassion'. In *Compassion and Wisdom in Psychotherapy*, edited by C. Germer and R. Siegel, 79–92. New York: Guilford Press.

Schwering, Markus. 2020. 'Habermas on the Corona crisis—and what his new book has to add to this. [Translation of an interview, 10 April 2020]', interview with Markus Schwering in *Frankfurter Rundschau*, 10 April. From Federick van Gelder's Research Gate profile (https://www.researchgate.net/publication/340610680_Habermas_on_the_Corona_crisis_-_and_what_his_new_book_has_to_add_to_this_Translation_of_an_interview_-_April_10th_2020, accessed on 5 March 2021).

Sharma, Harikishan. 2021. 'Pandemic sent migrants home, record 11 crore turned to rural job scheme'. *Indian Express*, 2 April (https://indianexpress.com/article/india/coronavirus-pandemic-sent-migrants-home-record-11-crore-turned-to-rural-job-scheme-7255071/, accessed on 3 April 2021).

Shelley, Mary Wollstonecraft. 1998. *The Last Man*. Edited by Anne McWhir. Ontario: Broadview Literary Texts.

PAUSE, PRIVILEGE, SACRIFICE, AND A MORE CARING SOCIETY

Arora, Maneesh. 2020. 'How the Coronavirus Pandemic Helped the Floyd Protests become the Biggest in U.S. History'. *The Washington Post* (https://www.washingtonpost.com/politics/2020/08/05/how-coronavirus-pandemic-helped-floyd-protests-become-biggest-us-history/, accessed 20 August 2020).

Black Lives Matter. n.d. 'About'. Website of Black Lives Matter (https://blacklivesmatter.com/about/, accessed 20 July 2020).

Blanchard, Jeremiah S. 2020. '4 Reasons Why the Great Pause is Exactly What We All Needed'. *Medium* (https://medium.com/@jeruhmaya/4-reasons-why-the-great-pause-is-exactly-what-we-all-needed-6082a8e6bb8e, accessed 17 August 2020).

Branicki, Layla J. 2020. 'COVID-19, Ethics of Care and Feminist Crisis

Management'. *Gender, Work, and Organization* 27(5): 872–883 (https://onlinelibrary.wiley.com/doi/full/10.1111/gwao.12491, accessed 20 August 2020).

Dalmiya, Vrinda. 2016. *Caring to Know: Comparative Ethics, Feminist Epistemology and the Mahābhārata*. New Delhi: Oxford University Press.

Engster, Daniel. 2007. *The Heart of Justice: Care Ethics and Political Theory*. Oxford: Oxford University Press.

Gilligan, Carol. 1982. *In a Different Voice: Psychological Theory and Women's Development*. Cambridge: Harvard University Press.

Gray, John. 2020. 'Why This Crisis is a Turning Point in History'. *The New Statesman* (https://www.newstatesman.com/international/2020/04/why-crisis-turning-point-history, accessed 21 August 2020).

Hamington, Maurice. 2018. 'Care, Competency and Knowledge'. In *Evaluation for A Caring Society*, edited by Merel Visse and Tineke Abma, 27–50. Charlotte, NC: Information Age Publishing.

Held, Virginia. 2006. *The Ethics of Care: Personal, Political, and Global*. New York: Oxford.

Lorey, Isabell. 2015. *State of Insecurity: Government of the Precarious*. London: Verso.

Mohammed, Amina J. 2020. 'COVID-19 Exposing Inequalities, Cost of Weak Health, Social Protection Systems, Deputy Secretary-General Tells New York City Webinar Series'. United Nations Press Release (https://www.un.org/press/en/2020/dsgsm1412.doc.htm, accessed 20 August 2020).

Monbiot, George. 2016. 'Neoliberalism—The Ideology at the Root of all Our Problems'. *The Guardian*, 15 April (https://www.theguardian.com/books/2016/apr/15/neoliberalism-ideology-problem-george-monbiot, accessed 20 August 2020).

Noddings, Nel. 1984. *Caring: A Feminine Approach to Ethics and Moral Education*. Berkeley: University of California Press.

Puig de la Bellacasa, Maria. 2017. *Matters of Care: Speculative Ethics in More Than Human Worlds*. Minneapolis: University of Minnesota Press.

Roberts, Alasdair. 2020. '"Whatever It Takes": Danger, Necessity, and Realism in American Public Policy'. *Administration & Society* 52(7): 1131–1144.

Shiu-Ching, Wu. 2016. 'On the Priority of Relational Ontology: The Complementarity of Heidegger's Being-With and Ethics of Care'. *Kemanusiaan* 23(2): 71–87.

Slote, Michael. 2007. *The Ethics of Care and Empathy*. New York: Routledge.

Tronto, Joan. 1993. *Moral Boundaries: A Political Argument for an Ethic of Care*. New York: Routledge.

United Nations. 2016. 'Racism, Xenophobia Increasing Globally, Experts Tell Third Committee, amid Calls for Laws to Combat Hate Speech, Concerns over Freedom of Expression'. Press Release (https://www.un.org/press/en/2016/gashc4182.doc.htm, accessed 20 August 2020).

van Nistelrooij, Inge. 2015. *Sacrifice: A Care-Ethical Reappraisal of Sacrifice and Self Sacrifice*. Leuven, Belgium: Peeters Publishing.

Westoby, Peter, and Verne Harris. 2020. 'Community development "yet-to-come" during and post the COVID-19 pandemic: From Derrida to Zuboff'. *Community Development Journal* 55(4): 1–17.

Wirth, Mathias, Laurel Rauschenbach, Brian Hurwitz, Heinz-Peter Schmiedebach, and Jennifer A. Herdt. 2020. 'The Meaning of Care and Ethics to Mitigate the Harshness of Triage in Second-Wave Scenario Planning During the COVID-19 Pandemic'. *The American Journal of Bioethics* (https://doi.org/10.1080/15265161.2020.1777355, accessed 20 August 2020).

Zaki, Jamil. 2019. *The War for Kindness: Building Empathy in a Fractured World*. New York: Broadway Books.

CONSPIRACY THEORIES, FAKE NEWS, AND COVID-19

Butter, Michael, and Peter Knight, eds. 2020a. *Routledge Handbook of Conspiracy Theories*. London: Routledge.

———. 2020b. 'General Introduction'. In Michael Butter and Peter Knight, *Routledge Handbook of Conspiracy Theories*, 1-8. London: Routledge.

Camus, Albert. 1975. *The Myth of Sisyphus*. Harmondsworth: Penguin.

Charon, Rita. 2006. *Narrative Medicine: Honoring the Stories of Illness*. Oxford: Oxford University Press.

Descartes, René. 1996. *Meditations on First Philosophy with Selections from the Objections and Replies*. Translated and edited by John Cottingham. Cambridge: Cambridge University Press.

Fenster, Mark. 1999. *Conspiracy Theories: Secrecy and Power in American Culture*. Minneapolis: University of Minnesota Press.

Frank, Arthur W. 1995. *The Wounded Storyteller: Body, Illness and Ethics*. Chicago: Chicago University Press.

Jones, Mary Paumier. 1996. 'The Storytelling Animal'. *The Georgia Review* 50(4): 649–666.

Ricoeur, Paul. 1991. 'Narrative Identity'. *Philosophy Today* 35(1): 73–81.

CONTACT IN ABSENTIA: TOWARDS A CYBERTOUCH

Benjamin, Walter. 2000. 'The Work of Art in the Age of Its Technological Reproducibility'. In *The Work of Art in the Age of Its Technological Reproducibility and Other Writings on Media*, edited by Michael Jennings et al., 19–55. Cambridge, Mass: Harvard University Press.

Brenda, Laurel. 1993. *Computers as Theatre*. Boston: Addison-Wesley.

Guerrero, Juan Christian, ed. 2011. *Antoine-Louis-Claude Destutt de Tracy's Elements of Ideology*, Vols. 1 & 5. American University of Paris.

Hume, David. 2009. *A Treatise of Human Nature*. Ebook: The Floating Press.

Lister, Martin et al. 2009. *New Media. A Critical Introduction*. New York: Routledge.

Noe, Alva. 2012. *Varieties of Presence*. Cambridge, Mass: Harvard University Press.

Stelarc. 2020. '"STELARC: Reclining Stickman" at 2020 Adelaide Biennial of Australian Art: Monster Theatres'. YouTube (https://www.youtube.

com/watch?time_continue=10&v=Vg-oHiKra9Y&feature=emb_logo, accessed on 8 December 2020).

Varela, Francisco. 2001. 'Intimate Distances: Fragments for a Phenomenology of Organ Transplantation'. *Journal of Consciousness Studies* 8(5–72): 259–271.

DISCOURSE, CRISIS AND CORONA: SOME ETHICAL IMPLICATIONS OF THE GERMAN DEBATE ON THE COVID-19 PANDEMIC

Auswärtiges Amt. 2020. 'COVID-19 Informationen für Beschäftigte und Reisende'. Auswärtiges Amt, Gesundheitsdienst, Stand 25.03.2020 (accessed on 1 May 2020).

Bartsch, Matthias, Annette Bruhns, Jürgen Dahlkamp et al. 2020. 'Geisterland'. *Der Spiegel* 12 (14 March): 29.

BfR. 2020. 'Zoonosen'. Bundesinstitut für Risikobewertung (https://www.bfr.bund.de/de/zoonosen.html, accessed on 17 April 2020).

Breuer, Uta, and Dieter Genske, eds. 2020. *Ethik in den Ingenieurwissenschaften: Eine Annäherung*. Wiesbaden: Springer.

Deutscher Bundestag. 2013. 'Bericht zur Risikoanalyse im Bevölkerungsschutz 2012'. Unterrichtung durch die Bundesregierung 17/12051: 88. Berlin: Deutscher Bundestag.

Deutscher Ethikrat. 2020. 'Solidarität und Verantwortung in der Corona-Krise'. [Eine] ad-hoc Empfehlung, 20 March (https://www.aem-online.de/fileadmin/user_upload/DER_ad-hoc-empfehlung-corona-krise.pdf, accessed on 18 April 2020).

di Lorenzo, Giovanni. 2020. 'Die Welt steht still'. *Die Zeit* 13, 19 March: 1.

Gisanddata. 2020. COVID-19 Dashboard by the Center for Systems Science and Engineering (CSSE) at Johns Hopkins University (https://gisanddata.maps.arcgis.com/apps/opsdashboard/index.html#/bda7594740fd40299423467b48e9ecf6, accessed on 27 April 2020).

Grolle, Johann. 2020. 'Das Jahrhundertvirus'. *Der Spiegel* 17, 18 April: 100–104.

Hackenbroch, Veronika, Kerstin Kullmann, Martin Schlak, and Thomas Schulz. 2020. '30 473 rettende Zeichen'. *Der Spiegel* 13, 21 March: 100–103.

Hess-Lüttich, Ernest W.B. 2020. 'Dürfen wir (immer, alles), was wir können? Für eine Diskursethik der Ingenieurwissenschaften'. In Breuer and Genske, *Ethik in den Ingenieurwissenschaften*, 51–77.

———, Uta Breuer, and Dieter D. Genske. 2020. 'Ethik in Zeiten globaler Krisen: die Corona-Pandemie'. In Breuer and Genske, *Ethik in den Ingenieurwissenschaften*, 419–468.

Johns Hopkins. 2020. COVID-19 Dashboard by the Center for Systems Science and Engineering (CSSE) at Johns Hopkins University (https://coronavirus.jhu.edu/map.html, accessed on 15 April 2020).

Klafki, Wolfgang. 1996. *Neue Studien zur Bildungstheorie und Didaktik: Zeitgemäße Allgemeinbildung und kritisch-konstruktive Didaktik*, 4. Aufl., Weinheim: Beltz.

Kohlenberg, Kerstin. 2020. 'Wenn es nicht für alle reicht'. *Die Zeit* 18, 23 April: 29.

Minkmar, Nils. 2020. 'Endlich ist nichts mehr so, wie es war'. *Der Spiegel* 12, 14 March: 78.

OECD. 2020. 'Flattening the COVID-19 peak: Containment and mitigation policies'. Organization for Economic Cooperation and Development OECD, 24 March.

Rengeling, David. 2017. *Vom geduldigen Ausharren zur allumfassenden Prävention: Grippe-Pandemien im Spiegel von Wissenschaft, Politik und Öffentlichkeit*. Baden-Baden: Nomos.

RKI. 2020. 'SARS-CoV-2 Steckbrief zur Coronavirus-Krankheit-2019 (COVID-19)'. Robert Koch Institut website (https://www.rki.de/DE/Content/InfAZ/N/Neuartiges_Coronavirus/Steckbrief.html, accessed on 31 March 2020).

Schäuble, Wolfgang. 2020. 'Schäuble will dem Schutz des Lebens nicht alles unterordnen'. *Der Tagesspiegel*, 26 April (https://www.tagesspiegel.de/politik/bundestagspraesident-zur-corona-krise-schaeuble-will-dem-schutz-des-lebens-nicht-alles-unterordnen/25770466.html, accessed on 30 April 2020).

Snowden, Frank. 2020. 'Wie blind kann man eigentlich sein?'. *Der Spiegel* 18, 25 April: 104–106.

Spinney, Laura. 2018. *1918—Die Welt im Fieber: Wie die Spanische Grippe die Gesellschaft veränderte*. München: Hanser.

Vogt, Paul Robert. 2020. 'COVID-19—Eine Zwischenbilanz'. *Die Mittelländische Zeitung*, 8 April (https://www.mittellaendische.ch/2020/04/08/covid-19-eine-zwischenbilanz-oder-eine-analyse-der-moral-der-medizinischen-fakten-sowie-der-aktuellen-und-zukünftigen-politischen-entscheidungen/, accessed on 17 April 2020).

WHO. 2005. 'WHO global influenza preparedness plan: The role of WHO and recommendations for national measures before and during pandemics'. World Health Organization website (https://apps.who.int/iris/handle/10665/68998, accessed on 25 March 2020).

———. 2020a. 'Coronavirus disease (COVID-2019) situation report 65: 25 March 2020'. World Health Organization website (https://www.who.int/emergencies/diseases/novel-coronavirus-2019/situation-reports, accessed on 25 March 2020).

———. 2020b. WHO COVID-19 Dashboard (https://who.sprinklr.com/, accessed on 27 April 2020).

———. 2020c. 'Coronavirus disease (COVID-2019) situation report 81: 10 April 2020'. World Health Organization website (https://www.who.int/emergencies/diseases/novel-coronavirus-2019/situation-reports, accessed on 10 April 2020).

Worldometers. 2020. 'COVID-19 Coronavirus Pandemic' (https://www.worldometers.info/coronavirus/, accessed on 1 May 2020).

WWF. 2020a. 'Hintergrundpapier Umweltzerstörung und Gesundheit Naturschutz und Pandemie-Gefahr'. World Wide Fund website (https://www.wwf.de/fileadmin/fm-wwf/Publikationen-PDF/WWF-Hintergrundpapier_Umweltzerstoerung_und_Gesundheit.pdf, accessed on 4 April 2020).

———. 2020b. 'Opinion survey on COVID-19 and wildlife trade in 5 Asian Market'. World Wide Fund website (https://www.wwf.de/fileadmin/fm-wwf/Publikationen-PDF/WWF-Survey_on_Covid-19_and_Wildlife_Trade.pdf, accessed on 4 April 2020).

Zhu, Tuofu, Bette T. Korber, Andre J. Nahmias, Edward Hooper, Paul M. Sharp, and David D. Ho. 1998. 'An African HIV-1 sequence from 1959 and implications for the origin of the epidemic'. *Nature* 39: 594–597.

THE LIMITS OF RESPONSIBLE CARING IN THE COVID-19 PANDEMIC

Allen, Danielle. 2004. *Talking to Strangers: Anxieties of Citizenship Since Brown v. Board of Education*. Chicago: University of Chicago Press.

Brown, W.O. 1933. 'Rationalization of Race Prejudice'. *International Journal of Ethics* 43(3): 294–306.

Engster, Daniel. 2015. 'Care in the State of Nature: The Biological and Evolutionary Roots of the Disposition to Care in Human Beings'. In *Care Ethics and Political Theory*, edited by Daniel Engster and Maurice Hamington, 227–251. New York: Oxford.

Gilens, Martin. 1999. *Why Americans Hate Welfare: Race, Media, and the Politics of Antipoverty Policy, Studies in Communication, Media, and Public Opinion*. Chicago: University of Chicago Press.

Harris, Cheryl I. 1995. 'Whiteness as Property'. In *Critical Race Theory: The Key Writings That Formed the Movement*, edited by Kimberle Crenshaw, Neil Gotanda, Garry Peller and Kendall Thomas, 276–292. New York: The New Press.

Hochschild, Adam. 2011. *To End All Wars: A Story of Loyalty and Rebellion, 1914–1918*. New York: HMH Books.

Hochschild, Arlie. 2016. *Strangers in Their Own Land: Anger and Mourning on the American Right*. Brooklyn, NY: The New Press.

Jones, Janelle, and Valerie Wilson. 2017. 'Low-wage African American workers have increased annual work hours most since 1979'. Economic Policy Institute website (https://www.epi.org/blog/low-wage-african-american-workers-have-increased-annual-work-hours-most-since-1979/, last modified 27 March 2017, accessed on 20 August 2017).

Jones, Kimberly Latrice. 2020. 'Kimberly Latrice Jones BLM Video Speech Transcript'. Transcript available on Rev (website) (https://www.rev.com/blog/transcripts/kimberly-latrice-jones-blm-video-speech-transcript, last modified 8 June 2020).

Katznelson, Ira. 2005. *When Affirmative Action Was White: An Untold History of Racial Inequality in Twentieth-Century America*. New York: WW Norton.

Lipsitz, George. 2006. *The Possessive Investment in Whiteness: How White People Profit from Identity Politics*. Philadelphia: Temple University Press.

Merritt, Keri Leigh. 2017. *Masterless Men: Poor Whites and Slavery in the Antebellum South*. New York: Cambridge University Press.

Putnam, Robert D. 1993. *Making Democracy Work: Civic Traditions in Modern Italy*. Princeton, NJ: Princeton University Press.

Tronto, Joan. 2017. 'There is an alternative: Homines curans and the limits of neoliberalism'. *International Journal of Care and Caring* 1(1): 27–43.

———. 2013. *Caring Democracy: Markets, Equality and Justice*. New York: New York University Press.

Walker, Margaret Urban. 2007. *Moral Understandings: A Feminist Study in Ethics*. 2nd ed. New York: Oxford University Press.

White, Julie Anne. 2020. 'Time for Caring Democracy: Resisting the Temporal Regimes of Neoliberalism'. In *Care Ethics, Democratic Citizenship and the State*, edited by Petr Urban and Lizzie Ward, 161–177. London: Palgrave MacMillan.

Young, Iris Marion. 2003. 'The Logic of Masculinist Protection: Reflections on the Current Security State'. *Signs: Journal of Women in Culture & Society* 29(1): 1–24.

PANDEMIC: PHILOSOPHY AND PUBLIC POLICY

'Call to Action to the Tech Community on New Machine Readable COVID-19 Dataset'. 2020. White House press release, 16 March (https://web.archive.org/web/20210120122215/https://www.whitehouse.gov/briefings-statements/call-action-tech-community-new-machine-readable-covid-19-dataset/).

Casaglia, Anna, Raffaella Coletti, Christopher Lizotte, John Agnew, Virgine Mamadouh, and Claudio Minca. 2020. 'Interventions on European Nationalist Populism and Bordering in Time of Emergencies'. *Political Geography* 82 (https://doi.org/10.1016/j.polgeo.2020.102238).

Diamond, Larry, and Marc F. Plattner, ed. 2015. *Democracy in Decline?*. Baltimore, MD: John Hopkins University Press.

Flinders, Matthew. 2020. 'Democracy and the Politics of Coronavirus: Trust, Blame and Understanding'. *Parliamentary Affairs* (https://doi.org/10.1093/pa/gsaa013, accessed on 1 December 2020).

Fukuyama, Francis. 2020. 'The Thing that determines a country's resistance to corona virus'. *The Atlantic Monthly*, 30 March (https://www.theatlantic.com/ideas/archive/2020/03/thing-determines-how-well-countries-respond-coronavirus/609025/, accessed on 23 April 2020).

———. 2020. 'The Pandemic and Political Order'. *Foreign Affairs*, July/August.

Han Byung Chul. 2020. 'The Viral Emergency and the World of Tomorrow'. *El País*, 22 March.

Honig, Bonnie. 2009. *Emergency Politics: Paradox, Law, Democracy*. Princeton: Princeton University Press.

Landman, Todd, and Luca Di Gennaro Splendore. 2020. 'Pandemic Democracy: Elections and COVID-19'. *Journal of Risk Research* (https://doi.org/10.1080/13669877.2020.1765003, accessed on 12 December 2020).

Nussbaum, Martha. 2018. *The Monarchy of Fear: A Philosopher Looks at Our Political Crisis*. New York: Simon and Schuster.

———. 2019. *The Cosmopolitan Tradition: A Noble but Flawed Ideal*. Cambridge, MA: Harvard University Press.

COVID-19 AND THE 'RETURN OF THE NORMATIVE' IN ECONOMIC POLICY

'Spend as Much as You Can, IMF Head Urges Governments Worldwide'. 2021. *Reuters*, 15 January (https://www.reuters.com/article/us-russia-imf/spend-as-much-as-you-can-imf-head-urges-governments-worldwide-idUSKBN29K1XJ).

Acharya, A., and S.G. Reddy. 2020. 'The Economic Case for a People's Vaccine'. *Boston Review*, 15 September.

Babones, S. 2018. *The New Authoritarianism: Trump, Populism, and the Tyranny of Experts*. Polity Press.

Barry, C., and S.G. Reddy. 2008. *International Trade and Labor Standards: A Proposal for Linkage*. New York: Columbia University Press.

Berlin, I. 1958. *Two Concepts of Liberty*. Oxford: Clarendon Press.

Bhagwati, J., V. Ramaswami, and T. Srinivasan. 1969. 'Domestic Distortions, Tariffs, and the Theory of Optimum Subsidy: Some Further Results'. *Journal of Political Economy* 77(6): 1005–1010.

Collier, P. 2020. 'The problem of modelling: Public policy and the coronavirus'. *Times Literary Supplement*, 24 April.

Friedman, M., and F. Friedman. 1980. *Free to Choose: A Personal Statement*. Harcourt.

Godelier, M. 1972. *Rationality and Irrationality in Economics*. London: New Left Books.

Polanyi, K. 1944. *The Great Transformation*. New York: Farrar & Rinehart.

Ramakrishnan, V. 2020. 'Following the science'. *The Royal Society Blog* (https://royalsociety.org/blog/2020/05/following-the-science/, accessed on 28 February 2021).

Reddy, S. 2005. 'The Role of Apparent Constraints in Normative Reasoning: A Methodological Statement and Application to Global Justice'. *Journal of Ethics* 9: 119–125.

———. 2020a. 'Coronavirus and the Limits of Economics'. *Foreign Policy*, 31 March.

———. 2020b. 'Population health, economics and ethics in the age of COVID-19'. *BMJ Global Health* 5.

Robbins, L. 1932. *An Essay on the Nature and Significance of Economic Science*. London: Macmillan.

Scitovsky, T. 1941. 'A Note on Welfare Propositions in Economics'. *Review of Economic Studies* 9(1): 77–88.

Sen, A. 1982. 'Rights and Agency'. *Philosophy & Public Affairs* 11(1).

———. 1995. *Inequality Reexamined*. Oxford: Clarendon Press.

———. 1999. *Development as Freedom*. New York: Knopf.

———. 2020. 'Overcoming a pandemic may look like fighting a war, but the real need is far from that'. *Indian Express*, 8 April.

Spivak, G.C. 2021. Interview with *Raisons Politiques*, forthcoming.

Stiglitz, Joseph E., Amartya Sen, Jean-Paul Fitoussi. 2009. *Report by the Commission on the Measurement of Economic Performance and Social Progress*. Paris.

Tribe, K. 1978. *Land, Labour and Economic Discourse*. Routledge and Kegan Paul.

United Nations Development Programme. 1990. *Human Development Report*. Oxford: Oxford University Press.

WHO, UNICEF, and UNESCO. 2020. 'Considerations for school-related public health measures in the context of COVID-19: Annex to Considerations in adjusting public health and social measures in the context of COVID-19'. WHO website, 14 September (https://www.who.int/publications/i/item/considerations-for-school-related-public-health-measures-in-the-context-of-covid-19, accessed on 28 February 2020).

THE 'GREAT RESET'? YES, PLEASE—BUT A REAL ONE!

'Hungarian cultural commissioner lights powder keg of controversy after describing Europe as "George Soros' gas chamber"'. 2020. *RT World*, 29 November (https://www.rt.com/news/508146-soros-hungary-nazi-hitler-comparison, accessed on 6 December 2020).

Adorno, T.W. 2008. *Philosophische Elemente einer Theorie der Gesellschaft*. Frankfurt: Suhrkamp.

Baer, Jason. 2020. 'Leading into the Unknown: Coronavirus and the Great Reset'. SYPartners (https://www.sypartners.com/insights/leading-unknown-coronavirus-great-reset/, accessed on 18 December 2020).

Dean, Jodi. 2020. 'Neofeudalism: The End of Capitalism?'. *Los Angeles Review of Books*, 12 May (https://lareviewofbooks.org/article/neofeudalism-the-end-of-capitalism/, accessed on 1 December 2020).

Galloway, Scott. 2020. *Post Corona. From Crisis to Opportunity*. New York: Portfolio.

Schwering, Markus. 2020. Jürgen Habermas über Corona: "So viel Wissen über unser Nichtwissen gab es noch nie". *Frankfurter Rundschau* (https://www.fr.de/kultur/gesellschaft/juergen-habermas-coronavirus-krise-covid19-interview-13642491.html, accessed on 10 May 2020).

Shapiro, Adam. 2020. 'Capitalism "will collapse on itself" without more empathy and love: Scott Galloway'. *yahoo/finance*, 1 December (https://in.finance.yahoo.com/news/capitalism-will-collapse-on-itself-without-empathy-love-scott-galloway-120642769.html, accessed on 29 December 2020).

Thunberg, Greta. 2020. 'We now need to do the impossible: Greta Thunberg on Fighting Climate Change During COVID-19'. *Time*, 8 December (https://time.com/5918448/greta-thunberg-coronavirus-climate-change/, accessed on 15 December 2020).

Žižek, Slavoj, 2017. *Defense of Lost Causes*. London: Verso Books.

A NARRATIVE GROUP PROJECT FROM TURKEY: EXPLORING DIVERSE RESPONSES TO COVID-19

Denborough, David. 2008. *Collective Narrative Practice: Responding to Individuals, Groups, and Communities Who Have Experienced Trauma*. Adelaide: Dulwich Centre Publications.

———. 2014. *Retelling the Stories of Our Lives: Everyday Narrative Therapy to Draw Inspiration and Transform Experience*. WW Norton & Company.

Russell, Shona, and Maggie Carey. 2004. *Narrative Therapy: Responding to Your Questions*. Adelaide: Dulwich Centre Publications.

White, Michael, and David Epston. 1990. *Narrative Means to Therapeutic Ends*. New York: WW Norton & Company.

———. 2006. 'Working with people who are suffering the consequences of multiple trauma: A narrative perspective'. In *Trauma: Narrative Responses to Traumatic Experience*, edited by David Denborough, 25–85. Adelaide: Dulwich Centre Publications.

———. 2007. *Maps of Narrative Practice*. New York: WW Norton & Company.

———. 2011. *Narrative Practice: Continuing the Conversations*. New York: WW Norton & Company.

———. 2020. 'Challenging the Culture of Consumption: Rites of Passage and Communities of Acknowledgement'. Dulwich Centre (https://dulwichcentre.com.au/articles-about-narrative-therapy/deconstructing-addiction/challenging-the-culture-of-consumption/, accessed on 14 December 2020).

SOCIALIZED HEALTHCARE AND MEDICAL INTERNATIONALISM: CUBA AND THE CORONAVIRUS

'Coronavirus worsens Cuba's economic woes'. 2020. *Deutsche Welle*, 29 June (https://www.dw.com/en/coronavirus-worsens-cubas-economic-woes/a-53981899, accessed on 10 July 2020).

Augustin, Ed. 2020. 'Cuba sets example with successful programme to contain coronavirus'. *The Guardian*, 7 June (https://www.theguardian.com/world/2020/jun/07/cuba-coronavirus-success-contact-tracing-isolation, accessed on 1 July 2020).

Dantés, Octavio Gómez. 2018. 'The Dark Side of Cuba's Health System: Free Speech, Rights of Patients and Labor Rights of Physicians'. *Health Systems & Reform* 4(3): 175–182.

Fritz, Don. 2020. 'How Che Guevara Taught Cuba to Confront COVID-19'. *Monthly Review*, 1 June (https://monthlyreview.org/2020/06/01/how-che-guevara-taught-cuba-to-confront-covid-19/, accessed on 6 July 2020).

Gorry, Conner. 2019. 'Six Decades of Cuban Global Health Cooperation'. *MEDICC Review* [*International Journal of Cuban Health and Medicine*] 21(4): 83–92 (https://scielosp.org/article/medicc/2019.v21n4/83-92/en/, accessed on April 2020).

Graham, Bill. 2020. 'Cuba—The Country That Dares to be Wise'. *Magic Pills*, 7 May 7 (https://magicpillsmovie.com/cuba-the-country-that-dares-to-be-wise/, accessed on 5 June 2020).

Hackel, Joyce. 2020. 'As Cuba battles coronavirus, activists see an opening to protest police brutality'. *The World*, 28 July (https://www.pri.org/

stories/2020-07-28/cuba-battles-coronavirus-activists-see-opening-protest-police-brutality, accessed on 1 August 2020).

Hoffman, Sarah Z. 2004. 'HIV/AIDS in Cuba: A model for care or an ethical dilemma?'. *African Health Services* 4(3): 208–209 (https://www.ncbi.nlm.nih.gov/pmc/articles/PMC2688320/, accessed on 3 March 2020).

Kirk, John M. 2015. *Healthcare without Borders: Understanding Cuban Medical Internationalism*. Gainesville: University Press of Florida.

Kornbluh, Peter. 2020 'Cuba's Welcome to a Covid-19-Stricken Cruise Ship Reflects a Long Pattern of Global Humanitarian Commitment'. *The Nation*, 21 March (https://www.thenation.com/article/world/coronavirus-cuba-cruise-ship/, accessed on 3 May 2020).

Lowenberg, Sam. 2016. 'Cuba's focus on preventive medicine pays off'. *The Lancet* 387, 23 January (https://www.thelancet.com/journals/lancet/article/PIIS0140-6736%2816%2900155-0/fulltext?rss=yes, accessed on 6 March 2020).

Morris, Emily, and Ilan Kelman. 2020. 'Coronavirus response: Why Cuba is such an interesting case'. *The Conversation*, 15 April (https://theconversation.com/coronavirus-response-why-cuba-is-such-an-interesting-case-135749, accessed on 5 May 2020).

Sananes, Rebecca. 2016. 'Love, Loss and Beauty Pageants: Inside a Cuban HIV Sanitarium'. *National Public Radio*, 26 March (https://www.npr.org/sections/goatsandsoda/2016/03/26/471765424/love-loss-and-beauty-pageants-inside-a-cuban-hiv-sanitarium, accessed on 5 March 2020).

Schell, Patience A. 2010. 'Beauty and Bounty in Che's Chile'. In *Che's Travels: The Making of a Revolutionary in 1950s Latin America*, edited by Paul Drinot, 53–87. Durham: Duke University Press.

Starr, Paul. 1992. *The Social Transformation of American Medicine*. New York: Basic Books.

Torres, Nora Gámez. 2020 'Cuba promotes homeopathy as effective "weapon" against the coronavirus'. *Miami Herald*, 7 April (https://www.miamiherald.com/news/nation-world/world/americas/cuba/article241803371.html, accessed on 5 May 2020).

UN News. 2020. 'Lift Cuba embargo or risk many lives lost to COVID-19, UN rights experts warn US'. UN website, 30 April (https://news.un.org/en/story/2020/04/1062982, accessed on 15 May 2020).

US Central Intelligence Agency. 1968. *The Life of Che Guevara: A Series of Failures*. CIA website (https://www.cia.gov/library/readingroom/docs/CIA-RDP78-03061A000400030027-7.pdf, accessed on 7 May 2020).

———. 1986. *The Cuban-Soviet Connection: Costs, Benefits, and Directions: An Intelligence Assessment*. CIA website (https://www.cia.gov/library/readingroom/docs/CIA-RDP04T00794R000100080001-0.pdf, accessed on 7 May 2020).

Warner, Rich. 2016. 'Is the Cuban healthcare system really as great as people claim?'. *The Conversation*, 30 November (https://theconversation.com/is-the-cuban-healthcare-system-really-as-great-as-people-claim-69526, accessed on 10 March 2020).

WHO. 2018. 'Medical doctors (per 10,000 population)'. WHO website (https://www.who.int/data/gho/data/indicators/indicator-details/GHO/medical-doctors-(per-10-000-population), accessed on 7 May 2020).

Yaffe, Helen. 2020. 'The world rediscovers Cuban medical internationalism'. *Le Monde Diplomatique*, 30 March.

COVID-19: COLLECTIVE RESPONSES TO CHALLENGES IN HONG KONG

Cheung, Elizabeth. 2020. 'Hong Kong activates "serious response level" for infectious diseases as Wuhan pneumonia outbreak escalates'. *South China Morning Post*, 4 January. Archived from the original on 10 April 2020, accessed on 26 July 2020.

Dulwich Centre. 2020. 'Documents & Audiences'. Dulwich Centre website (https://dulwichcentre.com.au/lessons/documents-audiences/, accessed 30 July 2020).

HKU. 2020. 'Flaws in the system behind Hong Kong's third wave'. Fight COVID-19 (Hong Kong university website). Archived from the original on 31 July 2020, accessed on 13 August 2020.

Hung, Lee Shiu. 2003. 'The SARS epidemic in Hong Kong: What lessons have we learned?'. *Journal of the Royal Society of Medicine* 96(8): 374–378.

Newman, David. 2008. '"Rescuing the Said from the Saying of It": Living Documentation in Narrative Therapy'. *International Journal of Narrative Therapy & Community Work* 3: 24.

Ting, Victor. 2020. 'To mask or not to mask: WHO makes U-turn while US, Singapore abandon pandemic advice and tell citizens to start wearing masks'. *South China Morning Post*, 4 April. Archived from the original on 18 May 2020, accessed on 26 July 2020.

DISCOVERING THE JOY OF LIVING IN TIMES OF CRISIS, INSPIRATION FOR GROWTH

Camus, A. 2002 (1947). *The Plague*. London: Penguin Books.

Frankl, V. 2004 (1949). *Man's Search for Meaning: The classic tribute to hope from the Holocaust*. London: Penguin Random House.

Nietzsche, F. 2006 (1910). *The Gay Science*. New York: Dover Publications.

van Deurzen, E. 2015. *Paradox and Passion in Psychotherapy: An Existential Approach*. 2nd ed. New York: Willey-Blackwell.

———. 2021. *Rising from Existential Crisis*. Monmouth: PCCS Books.

Vos, J. 2018. *Meaning in Life: An Evidenced-Based Handbook for Practitioners*. London: Palgrave Macmillan.

———. 2021. *The Psychology of Covid-19: Building Resilience for Future Pandemics*. London: Sage Publications.

Yalom, I.D. 2011. *When Nietzsche Wept: A novel of obsession*. New York: Harper Collins.

———. 2017. *Becoming Myself: A Psychiatrist's Memoir*. New York: Basic Books.

EARLY LEARNING ROADMAP IN RESPONSE TO COVID-19: KEEPING YOUNG CHILDREN SAFE, LOVED AND LEARNING

Almond, D. 2006. 'Is the 1918 influenza pandemic over? Long-term effects of in utero influenza exposure in the post-1940 US population'. *Journal Political Economy* 114: 672–712.

Black, Maureen M. et al. 2017. 'Early Childhood Development Coming of Age: Science Through the Course of Life'. *Lancet*, January (https://www.thelancet.com/pdfs/journals/lancet/PIIS0140-6736(16)31389-7.pdf, accessed on 5 May 2020).

Edwards, Jess. 2020. 'Protect a Generation: The Impact of COVID-19 on Children's Lives'. Save the Children website (https://www.savethechildren.org/us/about-us/media-and-news/2020-press-releases/during-covid-19-children-in-poverty-experience-greatest-financial-education-loss-highest-risk-of-violence, accessed on 2 August 2020).

King, S., and D.P. Laplante. 2015. 'Using natural disasters to study prenatal maternal stress in humans'. *Advances in Neurobiology* 10: 285–313 (https://pubmed.ncbi.nlm.nih.gov/25287546/, accessed on 15 March 2020).

Lumey, L.H., A.D. Stein, H.S. Kahn, K.M. van der Pal-de Bruin, G.J. Blauw, and P.A. Zybert. 2007. 'Cohort profile: The Dutch Hunger Winter families study'. *International Journal of Epidemiology* 36(6): 1196–1204 (https://pubmed.ncbi.nlm.nih.gov/17591638/, accessed on 15 March 2020).

National Scientific Council on the Developing Child. 2014. 'Excessive Stress Disrupts the Architecture of the Developing Brain: Working Paper 3' (https://developingchild.harvard.edu/wp-content/uploads/2005/05/Stress_Disrupts_Architecture_Developing_Brain-1.pdf, accessed on 5 May 2020).

Save the Children. n.d. 'Save our Education'. Save the Children website (https://www.savethechildren.net/save-our-education, accessed on 15 August 2020).

Shonkoff, J.P., A.S. Garner. 2012. 'Committee on Psychosocial Aspects of Child and Family Health; Committee on Early Childhood, Adoption, and Dependent Care; Section on Developmental and Behavioral Pediatrics. The lifelong effects of early childhood adversity and toxic stress'. *Pediatrics* 129: e232–e246.

World Bank. 2018. 'World Bank warns of "learning crisis" in global education'. World Bank website (https://www.worldbank.org/en/news/press-release/2017/09/26/world-bank-warns-of-learning-crisis-in-global-education, accessed on 15 May 2020).

Yoshikawa, H., A.J. Wuermli, P. Britto, B. Dreyer, J. Leckman, S.J. Lye, A. Ponguta, L. Richter, and A. Stein. 2020. 'Effects of the Global Coronavirus Disease-2019 Pandemic on Early Childhood Development: Short- and Long-Term Risks and Mitigating Programme and Policy Actions'. *Journal of Pediatrics* 223: 188–193 (https://doi.org/https://doi.org/10.1016/j.jpeds.2020.05.020, accessed on 15 August 2020).

RE-AUTHORING CONFINEMENT: ENDURING COVID-19 AND CREATING A COLLABORATORY

Blanc-Sahnoun, Pierre. 2020. 'On Behalf of the Galactic Federation of Narrative Planets 2020—Together Enduring COVID-19: Events and Resources'. Re-authoring Teaching website (https://reauthoringteaching.com/resources/together-enduring-covid-19-events-and-resources/ accessed on 1 September 2020).

Carey, M., and Russell, S. 2004. 'Re-Authoring: Some answers to commonly asked questions'. In *Narrative Therapy: Responding to your Questions*, compiled by Shona Russell and Maggie Carey, 19–62. Dulwich Centre.

Combs, G., and J. Freeman. 2012. 'Narrative, Poststructuralism, and Social Justice: Current Practices in Narrative Therapy'. *The Counselling Psychologist* 40(7): 1033–1060.

Dickerson, V.C. 2020. [In process.] 'The "Flip"—Sustaining Complexity and Multiplicity Post Quarantine'. *Family Process* (doi:10.1111/famp.12583, accessed on 1 September 2020).

Epston, D. (with Peggy Sax). 2011. 'Re-authoring Teaching: New developments in creating a collaborator'. *Journal of Systemic Therapies* 30(2): 98–104.

———. 1999. 'Co-research: The Making of Alternative Knowledge'. In *Narrative Therapy and Community Work: A Conference Collection*, 137–157. Adelaide: Dulwich Centre Publications.

———, and M. White. 1990. *Narrative Means to Therapeutic Ends*. New York: WW Norton.

Freire, P. 1970. *Pedagogy of the Oppressed*. New York: Herder and Herder.

Gremillion, H. 2013. 'Special Section: Community Approaches to Problems: Beyond Individual and Family Solutions'. *Journal of Systemic Therapies* 31(1): 27–29.

Hancock, F., and D. Epston, D. 2005. Personal communication.

Hoffman, L. 2007. 'The art of "withness"'. In *Collaborative Therapies: Relationships and Conversations That Make a Difference*, edited by H. Anderson and D. Gehart, 63–79. New York: Taylor & Francis Group (Routledge).

———. 2009. 'Notes for a Starfish Federation'. *Scribd* (https://www.scribd.com/document/22377210/Notes-for-a-Starfish-Federation, accessed on 11 April 2020).

Ingamells, K. 2016. 'Learning how to counter-story in narrative therapy with David Epston & Wilbur the Warrior'. *Journal of Systemic Therapies* 35(4): 58–71.

Lewis, D., and A. Cheshire. 2007. 'TeWhakaakona: Teaching and Learning as One'. *Journal of Systemic Therapies* 26: 43–56.

McNamee, Sheila. 2009. 'Postmodern Ethics'. *Human Systems* 20(1): 57–71.

Sax, P. 2013. 'Reclaiming Community Out of Personal Catastrophe: Communal Practices That Build on Naturally Sustaining Webs'. *Journal of Systemic Therapies* 32(1): 30–42.

Solnit, R. 2009. *A Paradise Built in Hell: The Extraordinary Communities That Arise in Disaster*. New York: Viking.

White, M. 1997. *Narratives of Therapists' Lives*. Adelaide, South Australia: Dulwich Centre Publications.

———. 1997. 'The ethic of collaboration & decentered practice'. In M. White, *Narratives of Therapists' Lives*, 193–216.

———. 2004. 'Folk psychology and narrative practice'. In *Narrative Practice and Exotic Lives: Resurrecting Diversity in Everyday Life*, edited by M. White, 59–118. Adelaide, Australia: Dulwich Centre Publications.

———, and D. Epston. 1990. *Narrative Means to Therapeutic Ends*. New York: WW Norton.

INTERNATIONAL EDUCATION AS A RESPONSE TO COVID-19: AN INDIAN PERSPECTIVE

'Timeline of WHO's response to COVID-19'. 2020. World Health Organization website (https://www.who.int/news-room/detail/29-06-2020-covidtimeline, accessed on 20 August 2020).

Atack, Patrick. 2019. 'ISC report notes increase in Chinese private international schools'. *The Pie News*, 23 April (https://thepienews.com/news/isc-report-notes-increase-in-chinese-private-schools/, accessed on 4 August 2020).

Cadell, Cate. 2019. 'Class dismissed: Surge in arrests of foreign teachers in China'. *Reuters*, 13 August (https://www.reuters.com/article/us-china-education/class-dismissed-surge-in-arrests-of-foreign-teachers in-china-idUSKCN1V2233, accessed on 8 August 2020).

Carless, David. 2011. 'From Testing to Productive Student Learning: Implementing Formative Assessment in Confucian-Heritage Settings'. *Journal of Second Language Teaching and Research* 1(2): 55–158.

Daskal, Lolly. 2015. 'The 100 Best Leadership Quotes of All Time: Sometimes the most powerful and meaningful things come from words that touch our heart and lead us forward to our potential'. *Inc.*, 3 April (https://www.inc.com/lolly-daskal/the-100-best-leadership-quotes-of-all-time.html, accessed on 17 August 2020).

Huang, Futao. 2003. 'Policy and Practice of Internationalization of Higher Education in China'. *Journal of Studies in International Education* 7(3): 225–240.

Kennedy, Peter. 2002. 'Learning cultures and learning styles: Myth-understandings about adult (Hong Kong) Chinese learners'. *International Journal of Lifelong Education* 21(5): 430–445.

Nyomi, Nunana. 2020. 'International education perpetuates structural racism and anti-racism is the solution'. Council of International Schools website, 10 June (https://www.cois.org/about-cis/news/post/~board/perspectives-blog/post/international-education-perpetuates-structural-racism-and-anti-racism-is-the-solution, accessed on 21 August 2020).

The Search Associates Team. 2020. 'Black lives Matter'. Search Associates website, 5 June (https://www.searchassociates.com/news-events/black-lives-matter/, accessed on 8 August 2020).

RECONNECTING IN A POST-PANDEMIC WORLD

'Pandating: Coronavirus and the language of love'. 2020. *The Economist* (https://www.economist.com/1843/2020/07/15/pandating-coronavirus-and-the-language-of-love, accessed on 31 August 2020).

Mikado, Mikita. 2020. Facebook post (https://www.facebook.com/mikita.mikado/posts/10158685311839592, accessed on 13 August 2020).

Orenstein, Peggy. 2020. *Boys & Sex: Young Men on Hookups, Love, Porn, Consent, and Navigating the New Masculinity*. New York: Harper.

GLIMPSES OF SERVANT LEADERSHIP IN MAURITIUS: A BOLD AND EFFECTIVE RESPONSE TO COVID-19

'Due to extreme urgency to procure our needs, recourse to emergency procurement was the only alternative, underlines PM'. 2020. Government of Mauritius website, 21 July (http://www.govmu.org/English/News/Pages/Due-to-extreme-urgency-to-procure-our-needs,-recourse-to-emergency-procurement-was-the-only-alternative,-underlines-PM.aspx).

Allison, Simon, and Abdul Brima. 2020. 'How Mauritius beat the pandemic'. *Mail & Guardian* (https://mg.co.za/coronavirus-essentials/2020-05-21-how-mauritius-beat-the-pandemic/, accessed on 30 May 2020).

Barbuto, John E., and Daniel W. Wheeler. 2006. 'Scale Development and Construct Clarification of Servant Leadership'. *Group & Organization Management* 31(3): 300–326 (https://digitalcommons.unl.edu/aglecfacpub/51, accessed on 6 May 2020).

Bechler, Curt, and Scott D. Johnson. 1995. 'Leadership and listening: A study of member perceptions'. *Small Group Research* 26(1): 77–85 (https://doi.org/10.1177%2F1046496495261004, accessed on 3 May 2020).

Chan Sun, Marie, and Claud Bernard Lan Cheong Wah. 2020. 'Lessons to be learnt from the COVID-19 public health response in Mauritius'. *Public Health in Practice* 1 (https://doi.org/10.1016/j.puhip.2020.100023, accessed on 21 June 2020).

COVID-19 in Mauritius STUDY YouTube. 2020. Official Statements from the Government of Mauritius (COVID-19) [Playlist]. YouTube (https://www.youtube.com/playlist?list=PLbzHFuDxBTGSpOyFenxXRAGEcCh9nt2I3, accessed on 12 May 2020).

de Melo, Jaime, Verena Tandrayen-Ragoobur, and Boopen Satanah. 2020. 'COVID-19 in Mauritius and other tourist paradises: A progress report'. *VoxEU.org*, 28 May (https://voxeu.org/article/covid-19-mauritius-and-other-tourist-paradises, accessed on 30 June 2020).

De Pree, Max. 1992. *Leadership Jazz*. New York, NY: Dell.

Fisher, Dale, and Annelies Wilder-Smith. 2020. 'The global community needs to swiftly ramp up the response to contain COVID-19'. *The Lancet* 395(10230) (https://doi.org/10.1016/S0140-6736(20)30679-6, accessed on 2 September 2020).

Focht, Adam, and Michael Ponton. 2015. 'Identifying primary characteristics of

Servant Leadership: Delphi Study'. *International Journal of Leadership Studies* 9(1): 44–61.

Graham, Jill W. 1991. 'Servant-leadership in organizations: Inspirational and moral'. *Leadership Quarterly* 2(2): 105–119 (https://doi.org/10.1016/1048-9843(91)90025-W, accessed on 6 May 2020).

Greenleaf, Robert. 1977. *The Servant as Leader*. Indianapolis, IN: Greenleaf Center.

Heymann, David L., and Nahoko Shindo. 2020. 'COVID-19: What is next for public health?'. *The Lancet* 395(10224): 542–545 (https://doi.org/10.1016/S0140-6736(20)30374-3).

Jeeneea, Ramanand, and Kaviraj Sharma Sukon. 2020. 'The Mauritian response to COVID-19: Rapid bold actions in the right direction'. *VoxEU.org*, 9 May (https://voxeu.org/article/mauritian-response-covid-19, accessed on 25 May 2020).

Jit, Ravinder, C.S. Sharma, and Mona Kawatra. 2017. 'Healing a Broken Spirit: Role of Servant Leadership'. *Vikalpa* 42(2): 80–94 (https://doi.org/10.1177/0256090917703754, accessed on 5 May 2020).

Johnson, Scott. D., and Curt Bechler. 1998. 'Examining the relationship between listening effectiveness and leadership emergence: Perceptions, behaviours, and recall'. *Small Group Research* 29(4): 452–471 (https://doi.org/10.1177%2F1046496498294003, accessed on 4 May 2020).

Liden, Robert C., Alexandra Panaccio, Jeremy D. Meuser, Jia Hu, and Sandy J. Wayne. 2014. 'Servant leadership: Antecedents, consequences, and contextual moderators'. In *The Oxford Handbook of Leadership and Organizations*, edited by David V. Day, 357–379. Oxford, UK: Oxford University Press.

Mauritius National Assembly. 2020. Parliamentary Question B/297, 21 July (https://mauritiusassembly.govmu.org/Documents/PQ/PQ2020/pq21july2020.pdf).

Reinke, Saundra, J. 2004. 'Service before self: Towards a theory of servant-leadership'. *Global Virtue Ethics Review* 5(3): 30–57.

Slaughter, Richard A. 1995. *The Foresight Principle: Cultural Recovery in the 21st Century*. London: Adamantine.

Song, JiYing. 2018. 'Leading through awareness and healing: A servant leadership model'. *The International Journal of Servant-Leadership* 12(1): 245–284 (https://digitalcommons.georgefox.edu/dps_fac/14).

Spears, Larry C. 1995. 'Tracing the growing impact of servant leadership'. In *Insights on Servant Leadership: Service, Stewardship, Spirit, and Servant-Leadership*, edited by Larry C. Spears, 1–12. New York, NY: John Wiley and Sons.

WHO. 2020. Virtual Press Conference on COVID-19, 11 March. WHO website (https://www.who.int/docs/default-source/coronaviruse/transcripts/who-audio-emergencies-coronavirus-press-conference-full-and-final-11mar2020.pdf, accessed on 16 March 2020).

Wong, Enoch. 2014. 'Not just simply looking forward: An Exploration of Greenleaf's Servant-Leadership Characteristic of Foresight'. *The International Journal of Servant-Leadership* 10(1): 89–118.

World Bank. 2020. 'COVID-19 (coronavirus) drives Sub-Saharan Africa toward first recession in 25 years'. Press Release No. 2020/099/AFR, 9 April (https://www.worldbank.org/en/news/press-release/2020/04/09/covid-19-coronavirus-drives-sub-saharan-africa-toward-first-recession-in-25-years, 9 accessed on 10 June 2020).

COLLECTIVE DOCUMENTATION OF LIVES DURING COVID-19 IN KATHMANDU

Bista, U. 2020. uma.bista. Instagram profile (https://www.instagram.com/uma.bista/, accessed on 8 September 2020).

Narrative Practices Adelaide. 2015. 'What is Narrative Practice?'. Re-authoring Teaching website (https://reauthoringteaching.com/what-is-narrative-practice/2015/, accessed on 1 September 2020).

Denborough, David. 2008. *Collective Narrative Practice: Responding to Individuals, Groups, and Communities Who Have Experienced Trauma*. Adelaide: Dulwich Centre Publications.

Myerhoff, B. 2007. *Stories as Equipment for Living: Last talks and tales of Barbara Myerhoff*. Edited by M. Kaminsky and M. Weiss. Ann Arbor, Michigan: University of Michigan Press.

White, M. 2003. 'Narrative Practice and community assignments'. *International Journal of Narrative Therapy and Community Work* 2: 17–56.

Koyu, P. 2020. '(अ)साहसी उफान'. *Setopati*, 4 June (https://www.setopati.com/literature/207345, accessed on 10 September 2020).

'TAKING CURRENT STRAIN AND FEELING PAST PAIN, AGAIN': A REFLECTION ON BLACK SOUTH AFRICAN WOMXN'S EXPERIENCE WITHIN THE CONTEXT OF COVID-19

Clark, Jude, Shula Mafokoane, and Ntombi Nyathi. 2019. '"Rocking the rock": A conversation on the slogan "Wathinta abafazi, wathint' imbokodo!", intergenerational feminisms and the implications for womxn's leadership'. *Agenda* 33(1): 67–73 (https://doi.org/10.1080/10130950.2019.1598775, accessed on 23 May 2020).

Crenshaw, Kimberle. 2017. *On Intersectionality: Essential Writings*. New York, NY: The New Press.

Herman, Judith. 2015. *Trauma & Recovery: The Aftermath of Violence from Domestic Abuse to Political Terror*. Philadelphia: Basic Books.

Lewis, Desiree. 2003 'Editorial'. *Feminist Africa: Changing Cultures* 2: 1–5.

Mair, Miller. 1989. *Between Psychology and Psychotherapy: A Poetics of Experience*. London: Routledge.

TIME FOR A PARADIGM SHIFT: ENGAGING WITH DISABILITY IN THE AFTERMATH OF COVID-19

'The Persons with Disabilities (Equal Opportunities, Protection of Rights and Full Participation) Act, 1995' (https://legislative.gov.in/actsofparliamentfromtheyear/persons-disabilities-equal-opportunities-protection-rights-and-full).

Government of India, Ministry of Social Justice & Empowerment, Department of Empowerment of Persons with Disabilities (Divyangjan) website (http://disabilityaffairs.gov.in, accessed on 16 October 2020).

Ministry of Law and Justice, Government of India. 2016. 'The Rights of Persons with Disabilities Act, 2016'. Gazette of India (Extraordinary), 28 December (http://www.tezu.ernet.in/PwD/RPWD-ACT-2016.pdf, accessed on 5 October 2020).

Ministry of Statistics and Programme Implementation. 2016. 'Disabled Persons in India—A Statistical Profile, 2016'. MOSPI (http://mospi.nic.in/sites/default/files/publication_reports/Disabled_persons_in_India_2016.pdf, accessed on 5 October 2020).

National Centre for Promotion of Employment for Disabled People (NCPEDP). 2020. *Locked Down and Left Behind: A Report on the Status of Persons with Disabilities in India During the COVID-19 Crisis*. New Delhi: NCPEDP (https://ncpedp.org/reports/Report-locked_down_left_behind.pdf).

Raman, Srinivas. 2017. 'The Disabilities Act in India: What Employers Need to Know'. *India Briefing*, 12 December (https://www.india-briefing.com/news/the-disabilities-act-india-what-employers-need-to-know-15755.html/, accessed on 6 December 2020).

THE EMBERS REMAIN

Kāmbale, Baby, and Maya Pandit. 2009. *The Prisons We Broke*. Hyderabad: Orient BlackSwan.

Muktabai. 1991. 'Mang Maharachya Dukhvisayi' [About the Grief of the Mangs and Mahars]. In *Women Writing in India: 600 BC to the Present*, Vol. 1, edited by Susie Tharu and K. Lalitha, 215–216. City University of New York: The Feminist Press.

Pawar, Urmila. 2008. *The Weave of My Life*. Colombia University Press.

SOUTH ASIANS IN THE UNITED KINGDOM DURING COVID-19: A REALIST VIEW

Aldridge, R.W., D. Lewer, S.V. Katikireddi, R. Mathur, N. Pathak, R. Burns, E.B. Fragaszy, A.M. Johnson, D. Devakumar, I. Abubakar, and A. Hayward. 2020. 'Black, Asian and Minority Ethnic groups in England are at increased risk of death from COVID-19: Indirect standardisation of NHS mortality data'. *Wellcome Open Research* 5: 88 (https://doi.org/10.12688/wellcomepenres.15922.1, accessed on 6 June 2020).

Bhala, N., G. Curry, A.R. Martineau, C. Agyemang, and R. Bhopal. 2020. 'Sharpening the global focus on ethnicity and race in the time of COVID-19'. *The Lancet* 395: 1673–1675.

British Medical Association (BMA). 2020. 'COVID-19: The risk to BAME doctors'. BMA website (https://www.bma.org.uk/advice-and-support/COVID-19/your-health/COVID-19-the-risk-to-bame-doctors, accessed on 2 July 2020).

Bruns, D.P., N.V. Kraguljac, and T.R. Bruns. 2020. 'COVID-19: Facts, Cultural

Considerations, and Risk of Stigmatisation'. *Journal of Transcultural Nursing* 31(4): 326–332.

Chaddha, A., E.A. Robinson, E. Kline-Rogers, T. Alexandris-Souphis, and M. Rubenfire. 2016. 'Mental health and cardiovascular disease'. *American Journal of Medicine* 129(11): 1145–1148.

Cucinotta, D., and M. Vanelli. 2020. 'WHO Declares COVID-19 a Pandemic'. *Acta Biomed* 91(1): 157–160 (doi: 10.23750/abm. v91i1.9397, accessed on 28 December 2020).

Department of Health, UK. 2020. 'Number of coronavirus (COVID-19) cases and risk in the UK'. Government of UK website.

Dubey, S., P. Biswas, T. Ghosh, S. Chatterjee, A.J. Dubey, S. Chatterjee, D. Lahiri, and C.J. Lavie. 2020. 'Psychosocial impact of COVID-19'. *Diabetes & Metabolic Syndrome: Clinical Research & Reviews*, 14: 779–788.

English Housing Survey. 2018. 'Overcrowded households'. Government of UK website (https://www.ethnicity-facts-figures.service.gov.uk/housing/housing-conditions/overcrowded-households/latest, accessed on 14 July 2020).

GOV.UK .2016. 'Chapter 3: Trends in morbidity and risk factors'. In *Health profile for England: 2018* (https://www.gov.uk/government/publications/health-profile-for-england-2018/chapter-3-trends-in-morbidity-and-risk-factors, accessed on 25 June 2020).

———. 2020. 'People living in deprived neighbourhoods'. Government of UK website, 16 June (https://www.ethnicity-facts-figures.service.gov.uk/uk-population-by-ethnicity/demographics/people-living-in-deprived-neighbourhoods/latest, accessed on 28 July 2020).

Hotopf, M., E. Bullmore, R.C. O'Connor, and E.A. Holmes. 2020. 'The scope of mental health research during COVID-19 pandemic and its aftermath'. *The British Journal of Psychiatry* 1–3 (doi: 10.1192/bjp.2020.125, accessed on 5 January 2021).

Jorm, A.F., and N.J. Reavley. 2013. 'Depression and stigma: From attitudes to discrimination'. *The Lancet* 381(10-11) (http://dx.doi.org/10.1016/, accessed on 3 March 2020).

Karasz, A., F. Gany, J. Escobar, C. Flores, L. Prasad, A. Inman, V. Kalasapudi, R. Kosi, M. Murthy, J. Leng, and S. Diwan. 2019. 'Mental Health and Stress Among South Asians'. *J Immigrant Minority Health* 21(7–14) (https://doi.org/10.1007/s10903-016-0501-4, accessed on 15 March 2020).

King's Fund. 2020. 'Ethnic minority deaths and COVID-19: What are we to do?'. The King's Fund website (https://www.kingsfund.org.uk/blog/2020/04/ethnic-minority-deaths-covid-19, accessed on 26 June 2020).

Kumar, K., S. Greenfield, K. Raza, P. Gill, and R. Stack. 2016. 'Understanding adherence-related beliefs about medicine amongst patients of South Asian origin with diabetes and cardiovascular disease patient: A qualitative synthesis'. *BMC Endocrine Disorder* 16: 24 (https://bmcendocrdisord.biomedcentral.com/articles/10.1186/s12902-016-0103-0, accessed on 12 February 2020).

Leicester.GOV.UK. 2011. 'Population comparison between England and Leicester Census 2011' (https://www.leicester.gov.uk/media/177362/comparison-of-2011-census-findings.pdf, accessed 4 July 2020).

Local Government Association (LGA). 2020. 'Loneliness, social isolation and COVID-19'. Government of UK website (https://www.local.gov.uk/publications/loneliness-social-isolation-and-covid-19, accessed on 27 June 2020).

Logie, C.H., and J.M. Turan. 2020. 'How do we balance tensions between COVID-19 public health responses and stigma mitigation? Learning from HIV research'. *AIDS Behav* 7: 1–4 (doi: 10.1007/s10461-020-02856-8, accessed on 5 January 2021).

Marmot, M. 2020. 'Society and the slow burn of inequality'. *The Lancet* 395(2 May): 1413–1414.

———, J. Allan, T. Boyce, P. Goldblatt, and J. Morrison. 2020. *Health Equity in England: The Marmot Review 10 Years On*. London: Institute of Health Equity.

———, J. Allen, P. Goldblatt, T. Boyce, D. McNeish, M. Grady, and I. Geddes. 2010. *Fair Society, Healthy Lives. The Marmot Review*. Strategic Review of Health Inequalities in England Post-2010 (http://www.instituteofhealthequity.org/resources-reports/fair-society-healthy-lives-the-marmot-review/fair-society-healthy-lives-full-report-pdf.pdf, accessed on 24 June 2020).

Marston, C., A. Renedo, and S. Miles. 2020. 'Community participation is crucial in a pandemic'. *The Lancet* 395: 1676–1678.

National Health Service (NHS). 2018. 'Health Profile for England'. Government of UK website (https://www.gov.uk/government/publications/health-profile-for-england-2018/, accessed on 14 July 2020).

Nazareth, J., J.S. Minhas, D.R. Jenkins, A. Sahota, K. Khunti, P. Haldar, and M. Pareek. 2020. 'Early lessons from a second COVID-19 lockdown in Leicester, UK'. *The Lancet* 396: e4.

Office of National Statistics (ONS). 2011. 'Census analysis: Ethnicity and religion of the non-UK born population in England and Wales: 2011'. Government of UK website (https://www.ons.gov.uk/peoplepopulationandcommunity/culturalidentity/ethnicity/articles/2011censusanalysisethnicityandreligionofthenonukbornpopulationinenglandandwales/2015-06-18, accessed on 20 June 2020).

———. 2020a. 'Coronavirus (COVID-19) related deaths by ethnic group'. Government of UK website (https://www.ons.gov.uk/peoplepopulationandcommunity/birthsdeathsandmarriages/deaths/articles/coronaviruscovid19relateddeathsbyethnicgroupenglandandwales/2march2020to15may2020#ethnic-group-differences-in-deaths-involving-covid-19-adjusted-for-socio-demographic-factors, accessed on 14 June 2020).

———. 2020b. 'Coronavirus (COVID-19) related deaths by ethnic group, England and Wales: 2 March 2020 to 15 May 2020'. Government of UK website (https://www.ons.gov.uk/peoplepopulationandcommunity/birthsdeathsandmarriages/deaths/articles/coronaviruscovid19 relateddeathsbyethnicgroupenglandandwales/2march2020to15may2020, accessed 28 July 2020).

———. 2020c. 'Coronavirus (COVID-19) related deaths by religious group, England and Wales: 2 March to 15 May 2020'. Government of UK website (https://www.ons.gov.uk/peoplepopulationandcommunity/birthsdeathsandmarriages/deaths/articles/coronaviruscovid19relateddeathsbyreligiousgroupenglandandwales/2marchto15may2020, accessed on 7 August 2020).

Pan, D., S. Sze, J.S. Minhas, M.N. Bangash, N. Pareek, P. Divall, C.M.L. Williams, M.R. Oggioni, I.B. Squire, L.B. Nellums, W. Hanif, K. Khunti, and M. Pareek. 2020. 'The impact of ethnicity on clinical outcomes in COVID-19: A systematic review'. *EClinicalMedicine* 23(100404) (https://doi.org/10.1016/j.eclinm.2020.100404, accessed on 20 July 2020).

Petersen, E., M. Koopmans, U. Go, D.H. Hamer, N. Petrosillo, F. Castelli, M. Stogaard, and S. Al Khalili. 2020. 'Comparing SARS-CoV-2 with SARS-CoV and influenza pandemics'. *The Lancet* 20(9): E238-E244 (https://www.thelancet.com/journals/laninf/article/PIIS1473-3099(20)30484-9/fulltext, accessed on 3 January 2021).

Public Health England (PHE). 2020a. 'Guidance for the public on the mental health and wellbeing aspects of coronavirus (COVID-19)'. Government of UK website (https://www.gov.uk/government/publications/COVID-19-guidance-for-the-public-on-mental-health-and-wellbeing/guidance-for-the-public-on-the-mental-health-and-wellbeing-aspects-of-coronavirus-COVID-19, accessed on 2 July 2020).

———. 2020b. 'Disparities in the risks and outcomes of COVID-19'. Government of UK website (https://assets.publishing.service.gov.uk/government/uploads/system/uploads/attachment_data/file/892085/disparities_review.pdf, Accessed on 5 September 2020).

Razieh, C., K. Khunti, M.J. Davies, C.L. Edwardson, J. Henson, N. Darko, A. Comber, A. Jones, and T. Yates. 2019. 'Research: Educational and psychological aspects of association of depression and anxiety with clinical, sociodemographic, lifestyle and environmental factors in South Asian and white European individuals at high risk of diabetes'. *Diabet Med* 36: 1158–1167 (doi: 10.1111/dme.13986, accessed on 7 March 2020).

Science Media Centre. 2020. 'Expert reactions to PHE review of disparities in risks and outcomes in COVID-19'. Science Media Centre website, 2 June (https://www.sciencemediacentre.org/expert-reaction-to-phe-review-of-disparities-in-risks-and-outcomes-in-covid-19/, accessed 20 June 2020).

PLAGUE IS THE GREAT TRUTH-TELLER: HOW CAN WE TALK BACK?

'Muslim Medics Taunted About Bacon and Alcohol—By Their Own NHS Colleagues'. 2020. *Huffington Post* (https://www.huffingtonpost.co.uk/amp/entry/islamophobia-nhs-muslim-doctors-institutionalised_uk_5f562e80c5b62b3add43cccb/?__twitter_impression=true&guccounter=1, accessed on 15 November 2020).

Abdulkareem, B., and Hina J. Shahid. 2018. *The Triple Penalty: Muslim Doctors in the NHS*. London: Muslim Doctors Association.

Ali, S. 2015. *British Muslims in Numbers*. London: Muslim Council of Britain.

Anti-Muslim Hatred Working Group. 2020. 'Coronavirus, fear and how Islamophobia spreads on social media'. Blog entry on official website (https://anti-muslim-hatred-working-group.home.blog/2020/04/20/coronavirus-fear-and-how-islamophobia-spreads-on-social-media/, accessed on 15 June 2021).

Brain, Louisa. 2020. 'Covid-19 and morbidity, conflict and development in the Horn of Africa REF'. SOAS website (blog) (https://blogs.soas.ac.uk/ref-hornresearch/files/2020/06/COVID-19-and-mobility-conflict-and-development-in-the-Horn-of-Africa-220620.pdf, accessed on 12 October 2020).

British Medical Association. 2020. 'Tackling COVID-19's effect on BAME doctors'. BMA website (https://www.bma.org.uk/news-and-opinion/tackling-covid-19-s-effect-on-bame-doctors, accessed on 15 October 2020).

Chwalisz, C. 2017. 'The people's verdict: Adding informed citizen voices to public decision-making'. *Policy Network*, 20 June.

———. 2019. 'A New Wave of Deliberative Democracy'. *Carnegie Europe*, 26 November.

DeHaven, Mark J., Irby B. Hunter, Laura Wilder, James W. Walton, and Jarett Berry. 2004. 'Health Programs in Faith-Based Organizations: Are They Effective?'. *American Journal of Public Health*, 94(6): 1030–1036 (doi: 10.2105/ajph.94.6.1030).

Hammond, Laura. 2019. 'Livelihoods and Mobility in the Border Regions of Ethiopia'. In *The Oxford Handbook of the Ethiopian Economy*, edited by Fantu Cheru, Christopher Cramer and Arkebe Oqubay, 269–287. Oxford: Oxford University Press.

Hill, P.C., and K.I. Pargament. 2003. 'Advances in the conceptualization and measurement of religion and spirituality: Implications for physical and mental health research'. *American psychologist* 58(1): 64.

Laird, L.D., Mona M. Amer, Elizabeth D. Barnett, Linda L. Barnes. 2007a. 'Muslim patients and health disparities in the UK and the US'. *Archives of Disease in Childhood* 92(10): 922–926.

———, Justine de Marrais, Linda L. Barnes. 2007b. 'Portraying Islam and Muslims in MEDLINE: A content analysis'. *Social Science & Medicine* 65(12): 2425–2439.

MedAct. 2020. 'False Positives, the Prevent counter-extremism policy in healthcare'. MedAct website (https://www.medact.org/wp-content/uploads/2020/07/MEDACT-False-Positives-WEB.pdf, accessed on 12 December 2020).

Office for National Statistics. 2020. 'Coronavirus (COVID-19) related deaths by religious group, England and Wales: 2 March to 15

May 2020'. Official website (https://www.ons.gov.uk/peoplepopulationandcommunity/birthsdeathsandmarriages/deaths/articles/coronaviruscovid19relateddeathsbyreligiousgroupenglandandwales/2marchto15may2020).

Ricoeur, Paul. 1992. *Oneself as Another*. Chicago: University of Chicago Press.

Scott-Baumann Alison et al. 2020. 'Lobbying and Activism'. SOAS (blog) (https://blogs.soas.ac.uk/cop/wp-content/uploads/2020/05/Lobbying-and-Activism.pdf, accessed on 15 December 2020).

———, Mathew Guest, Shuruq Naguib, Sariya Cheruvallil-Contractor, and Aisha Phoenix. 2020. I*slam on Campus: Contested Identities and the Cultures of Higher Education in Britain*. Oxford: Oxford University Press.

Shahid, Hina J. 2019. 'Faith discrimination in the NHS: Multiple penalties facing Muslim doctors'. *Journal of Holistic Health* 16(2): 48–52.

———. 2020a. 'The Pandemic of Islamophobia'. *Journal of the British Islamic Medical Association* 6(2): 1–4.

———. 2020b. 'Impact of COVID-19 on the Muslim Community'. Muslim Doctors Association (https://muslimdoctors.org/wp-content/uploads/2021/02/Impact-of-COVID-19-on-the-Muslim-Community.pdf, accessed on 20 December 2020).

South Asian Heart Foundation. 2020. 'COVID-19 in Black, Asian and Minority Ethnic populations: An evidence review and recommendations from the South Asian Health Foundation'. SAHF website (https://www.sahf.org.uk/s/Covid19_SAHF_Final-for-Release.pdf, accessed on 20 December 2020).

West, M. et al. 2015. 'Making the difference: Diversity and inclusion in the NHS'. The King's Fund website (https://www.kingsfund.org.uk/sites/default/files/field/field_publication_file/Making-the-difference-summary-Kings-Fund- Dec-2015.pdf, accessed on 15 September 2020).